13

DATE DUE

FEB 27 2014	
JUN 0 6 2018	

PRINTED IN U.S.A.

ALCOHOL AND ILLICIT DRUG USE IN THE WORKFORCE AND WORKPLACE

ALCOHOL AND ILLICIT DRUG USE IN THE WORKFORCE AND WORKPLACE

Michael R. Frone

AMERICAN PSYCHOLOGICAL ASSOCIATION
WASHINGTON, DC

Published by
American Psychological Association
750 First Street, NE
Washington, DC 20002
www.apa.org

To order
APA Order Department
P.O. Box 92984
Washington, DC 20090-2984
Tel: (800) 374-2721; Direct: (202) 336-5510
Fax: (202) 336-5502; TDD/TTY: (202) 336-6123
Online: www.apa.org/pubs/books
E-mail: order@apa.org

In the U.K., Europe, Africa, and the Middle East, copies may be ordered from
American Psychological Association
3 Henrietta Street
Covent Garden, London
WC2E 8LU England

Typeset in Goudy by Circle Graphics, Inc., Columbia, MD

Printer: Maple Press, York, PA
Cover Designer: Berg Design, Albany, NY

The opinions and statements published are the responsibility of the authors, and such opinions and statements do not necessarily represent the policies of the American Psychological Association.

Library of Congress Cataloging-in-Publication Data

Frone, Michael Robert.
  Alcohol and illicit drug use in the workforce and workplace / Michael R. Frone.
    p. cm.
  Includes bibliographical references and index.
    ISBN 978-1-4338-1244-6 (alk. paper) — ISBN 1-4338-1244-4 (alk. paper) 1. Alcoholism and employment—United States. 2. Drugs and employment—United States. 3. Employee assistance programs—United States. 4. Drug testing—United States. I. Title.
    HF5549.5.A4F76 2013
    362.29'12—dc23

                                          2012018252

British Library Cataloguing-in-Publication Data
A CIP record is available from the British Library.

Printed in the United States of America
First Edition

DOI: 10.1037/13944-000

CONTENTS

ACKNOWLEDGMENTS

I express my appreciation to my parents—Mary Ann and the late Henry—for their support over many years and for ensuring that their children had the opportunity they did not have to obtain a college education. I also thank my wife, Joan, for her support and patience over a career that often required long hours and weekend work.

I express gratitude to two former colleagues at the Research Institute on Addictions (RIA)—Marcia Russell (Prevention Research Center, Berkeley, California) and M. Lynne Cooper (University of Missouri–Columbia)—for taking a chance and hiring a graduate student in organizational psychology who had much interest in learning the ropes of research but had no training in the study of substance use. Their support and tutelage are forever appreciated.

I also thank several current colleagues, Julian Barling (Queen's University) and Kathleen Parks (RIA), for reading the manuscript as it unfolded. Each provided valuable comments that forced me to clarify issues and keep the material on task. Any and all errors or omissions that remain are mine. I also extend my gratitude to Ann Sawusch, head librarian at RIA, for immeasurable help in tracking down numerous reports, articles, chapters, and books.

Finally, financial support is essential for research and career development. My research during the past 20 years has been supported by grants from the National Institute on Alcohol Abuse and Alcoholism (NIAAA), including a 6-year mentored scientist development award (1994–2000). In this book, I present data and summarize published findings resulting from a national survey I conducted in 2002–2003 with funding from NIAAA Grant R01-AA12412. I also rely on publicly available data sets from several other studies. These studies were conducted and made available to other researchers with federal and private research funding.

ALCOHOL AND ILLICIT DRUG USE IN THE WORKFORCE AND WORKPLACE

INTRODUCTION

Psychoactive substances have been a universal part of human history for millennia. People have used a wide spectrum of psychoactive substances for ceremony, medicine, social facilitation, and the regulation of affect and performance. Historical accounts of such use can be found for many psychoactive substances, including alcohol, marijuana, opiates, hallucinogens, and cocaine (e.g., Carlson-Berne, 2007; N. Harris, 2005; Maisto, Galizio, & Connors, 2008; Manheimer, 2007; McMullen, 2005; Westermeyer, 1988; M. E. Williams, 2007). Less attention, however, has been paid to the historical nexus between substance use and work. Although the available information is primarily related to the use of alcohol, evidence exists that other psychoactive substances have been closely intertwined with work. For example, prior to 1500 A.D., stimulant use from chewing betel-areca (areca nut wrapped in betel leaf) was associated with heavy, repetitive work from taro farming in Oceania to paddy rice farming in Asia, whereas chewing coca leaf was associated with

DOI: 10.1037/13944-001
Alcohol and Illicit Drug Use in the Workforce and Workplace, by M. R. Frone

long hours and heavy work in the precious metal mines of South America (Meyer & Quenzer, 2005; Westermeyer, 1988).

In preindustrial Europe and America, alcohol was an accepted substitute for water and was used to fight fatigue and relieve aches and pains. Alcohol was given to workers by employers as a reward and as partial payment for work rendered. In effect, the consumption of alcohol during the workday in pre-industrial society was viewed as normative and even necessary for the recruitment of workers and the promotion of health and vigorous work (Ames, 1989; K. M. Fillmore, 1984; Warner, 1995; Westermeyer, 1988). Some employers provided alcohol to workers, and the cost was taken from wages whether or not the alcohol was consumed (Trice & Schonbrunn, 1981). Employers, however, did not condone drunkenness that disrupted the work process. This acceptance of alcohol use at work began to change with industrialization. Employer support began to wane during the late 19th and early 20th centuries with technological innovations that could lead to considerable harm to others, increasing concern over worker efficiency that developed with the beginning of scientific management (F. W. Taylor, 1915), and the emergence of workers' compensation laws holding employers financially responsible for employees injured at work (Trice & Schonbrunn, 1981). Also during this time, the temperance movement exerted pressure to eliminate the provision of alcohol at work and to promote complete abstinence of alcohol during and away from work (Trice & Schonbrunn, 1981). The turn of the 20th century, therefore, began to see some questioning and concern about workers' alcohol use that has continued until today (see Roman & Blum, 1999, for additional details). In contrast, Roman and Blum (1995) suggested that there is virtually no literature from 1900 until the 1970s that described any general pattern or concern regarding nonalcohol drug use in the workplace. They argued that this is suggestive that problem drug use during this period tended to be concentrated among marginal (least likely to be productive and employed) members of society.

At the beginning of the 21st century, in postindustrial societies, interest in employee alcohol use continues, though it has become overshadowed by concern over illicit drug use. For several reasons, interest in employee substance use, especially illicit drugs, has continued to capture the attention of employers, unions, policymakers, researchers, and the media. First, as alluded to previously, the use of alcohol and illicit drugs off and on the job is believed to undermine employee health, productivity, and safety, which can lead to costs being incurred by employers. Second, in the United States, Executive Order No. 12564 (1986)—Drug-Free Federal Workplace—issued by President Ronald Reagan made testing for illicit drug use mandatory for many federal employees. This order also stated that federal employees are required to refrain from the use of illegal drugs, whether on duty or off duty, and those who use them are not suitable for federal employment. Further, the subsequent Drug-Free Workplace Act (1988) mandated that certain employers provide a "drug-free workplace," which required having several components of a work-place drug use program in place. Although this act did not require illicit drug use testing, it implicitly authorized testing as a means of maintaining a drug-free workplace. Also, many U.S. federal agencies do mandate alcohol and illicit drug use testing for specific groups of federal and nonfederal employees. Workplace substance use policies and workforce drug testing also occur in other countries, but the available information suggests that there is little specific legislation mandating them (see Chapter 5). Third, a large industry has developed worldwide to promote the testing of employees for the use of illicit drugs. Finally, the media have played a role in employer concern over illicit drug use and, to some extent, workplace alcohol use by providing wide coverage of memorable, yet rare, events and by creating what some consider an atmosphere of moral panic.

NEED FOR BETTER INFORMATION AND DISSEMINATION

Despite what appears to be a long-standing interest in employee substance use, this issue has not been the subject of much rigorous, systematic research (Roman & Blum, 1995). Although scientific research on employee alcohol use can be traced back at least to the turn of the 20th century (e.g., Sullivan, 1905), systematic empirical research on employee alcohol and illicit drug use is relatively recent. Roman and Blum (1995) noted that this surprising lack of research is the result of several factors in the United States: (a) Federal drug use policy is developed and implemented without the perceived need for a base of research evidence or guidance; (b) research funding for such research is relatively scarce; (c) the study of employee substance use, especially in the workplace, presents a number of difficult obstacles and challenges; and (d) statements by high-level federal policymakers, especially the opinions of former President Reagan, present a perspective that the connection between illicit drug use and poor employee productivity is self-evident and that this connection must be broken. The second and third factors make it difficult to do the required research, whereas the first and fourth factors basically suggest that such research is not even required.

Yet, a lack of systematic research and failure to review adequately the research that does exist allow misinformation about employee substance use to flourish. In the mid-1990s, as I started to explore issues regarding alcohol and illicit drug use in the workplace, I was struck by the fact that many comments on the rate of substance use at work and claims about the organizational outcomes and employer costs of employee substance use were often inconsistent with findings in the scientific literature. Rarely was any concrete evidence cited to support the claims. These inconsistent claims occurred in published articles and on Internet web pages. The latter is particularly important because the Internet has become a pervasive tool for the presentation and acquisition of information. Despite its enormous benefits for learning, the Internet provides naive individuals easy access to information that may be contrived, purposefully misleading, or simply inaccurate. A search of the Internet will produce many web pages from government agencies, drug free or antidrug advocacy groups, antiprohibition advocacy groups, and drug testing companies that provide a myriad of estimates and claims regarding employee substance use. Many of these estimates and claims do not agree with the preponderance of empirical research and cannot be traced back to an actual empirical study. A common strategy is to cite (a) other websites that fail to document their claims, (b) unpublished reports that are unobtainable and may not exist, or (c) nonscientific trade magazine articles that may not provide data or cite credible sources. All of this can lead to questionable information being made available about employee substance use to key stakeholders, such as employers, unions, policymakers, researchers, and the media.

Even when statements about employee substance use are based on documented events and published research, several practices lead to the potential mischaracterization of this issue. I briefly review six such practices because they help set the stage for the remaining chapters and highlight the need to bring more rigor both to future studies and to the interpretation of prior research. The first practice that may lead to mischaracterization of employee substance use is drawing attention to large events that are sensational yet rare. For example, after more than 20 years, many will remember the oil spill disaster caused when the *Exxon Valdez* supertanker ran aground on Bligh Reef, spilling 10.8 million gallons of crude oil into the pristine waters of Prince William Sound. Many will also recall that the ship's captain had consumed alcoholic beverages onshore while the ship was loaded and was not on the bridge when the accident occurred. However, despite the media's narrow attention to Captain Hazelwood's drinking and the use of this accident as an exemplar of the disastrous effect of employee alcohol consumption, the report of the Alaska Oil Spill Commission (1990) pointed out that a disaster of this magnitude has multiple causes. Although the captain's drinking was viewed as a contributory cause, the primary causes were various inadequate technologies and poor management practices, which were fueled by flaws in corporate management and regulatory policies. For example, the Alaska Oil Spill Commission stated,

> Hazelwood's activities in town that day and on the ship that night would become a key focus of accident inquiries, the cause of a state criminal prosecution, and the basis of widespread media sensation. Without

intending to minimize the impact of Hazelwood's actions, however, one basic conclusion of this report is that the grounding at Bligh Reef represents much more than the error of a possibly drunken skipper: It was the result of the gradual degradation of oversight and safety practices that had been intended, 12 years before, to safeguard and backstop the inevitable mistakes of human beings. (p. 7)

A second practice that may lead to mischaracterization of employee substance use is relying on speculation or misapplication of valid information. For example, in the absence of information on the proportion of employees who use illicit drugs at work, it remains common to see presented the employment rate of illicit drug users. The implicit argument is that because most individuals who use illicit drugs are employed, there must be a lot of people using illicit drugs at work. In Chapter 1, I discuss the problems with using the employment rate of illicit drug users or heavy drinkers as an index of substance use in the workforce and workplace. Nonetheless, as discussed in Chapter 6, the employment rate among illicit drug users and heavy drinkers is informative regarding the potential utility of the workplace for intervention efforts.

A third practice that can result in the potential mischaracterization of employee substance use is confusing the correlates of employee substance use with the causes and outcomes of such use. For example, the commonly used cross-sectional study design, where data on substance use and its putative antecedents or outcomes are collected at one point in time, might find a statistically significant positive association between heavy use of alcohol and the frequency of being absent from work. A statistically significant association means that the size of the relation differs from zero and this is not likely due to chance. Subsequently, this association might be cited as evidence that heavy drinking *causes* absenteeism. Although heavy drinking may be a cause of absenteeism, it is just an association in the described research. To infer that heavy drinking is a cause of absenteeism, a study must minimally meet three conditions. The first condition is association, which was just described—it must be shown that more frequent heavy drinking is statistically significantly associated with higher rates or levels of absenteeism. The second condition is temporal precedence of the cause to the outcome—heavy drinking must be shown to precede the occurrence of absenteeism rather than the reverse. The third condition is isolation—all relevant causes of both heavy drinking and absenteeism must be controlled through the design of the study or statistical analysis. Although a cross-sectional study showing that heavy drinking has a statistically significant positive association with absenteeism meets the first condition, it fails to meet the second condition and may fail to meet the third condition. From such a study, we cannot determine whether the heavy drinking occurred before, concurrently with, or after the occurrence of absenteeism. Also, it is often not possible to rule out all relevant common causes of heavy drinking and absenteeism. It might be that individuals with a rebellious personality disposition are more likely to drink heavily and be absent from work. If so, heavy drinking and absenteeism would be associated, but the relation would not be causal. Both heavy drinking and absenteeism would be caused by a rebellious personality, making their relation spurious or noncausal. More complex experimental designs or longitudinal research designs, which obtain multiple assessments over time, are required to provide strong evidence of a causal relation.

A fourth practice that might lead to mischaracterization of employee substance use is related to the reporting of effects. One issue is failing to consider the magnitude of an effect or its practical importance. For example, consider a study that can meet all of the conditions to infer causality noted previously. This study might have found that a statistically significant association exists between heavy drinking and absenteeism, that heavy drinking precedes absenteeism, and that all relevant common causes of heavy drinking and absenteeism have been controlled. In other words, heavy drinking causes absenteeism. However, a statistically significant causal effect merely means that the size of the causal effect is greater than zero and that this is not likely due to chance. More important, statistically significant causal effects vary in size from being weak and of trivial clinical or practical importance to being strong and of crucial clinical or practical importance. Although an important goal of science is to determine the size of causal effects, it is also important to determine the practical importance of the effect. In other words, one needs to ask if the causal effect is large enough to motivate action aimed at (a) modifying the causes of substance use in an effort to reduce use or (b) directly managing employee substance use in an effort to reduce a potential dysfunctional outcome. Even though it is relatively easy to test an association for statistical significance, it is much more difficult to show that the association represents a causal effect. And even if it can be shown that the association is causal, it is often even more difficult to assess the practical importance of a causal effect. Despite this difficulty, focusing on statistically significant effects that are not large enough to be practically important may lead to recommendations for prevention interventions and policies that are unlikely to have notable outcomes. Unfortunately, in many circumstances, researchers use small, statistically significant associations and causal effects to make recommendations regarding interventions and policy rather than concluding that the effect warrants no action.

A second issue is reporting effects in inaccurate and nontransparent ways, which makes it difficult to judge the practical importance of an effect. For example, Halkitis (2009) cited research stating that Quest Diagnostics Incorporated found that methamphetamine use increased by 68% among employees and applicants from 2002 to 2003, which seems like a very large increase. However, Quest Diagnostics actually reported the change in positivity rates from workforce drug testing (see Chapter 5) conducted in the 2 years, not the change in the prevalence of workforce methamphetamine use. Also, because the change was expressed in relative terms, reporting that the positivity rate increased by 68% is uninformative without knowing the base rate (i.e., the positivity rate in 2002). In a detailed report on statistical literacy among physicians, patients (i.e., general population), and journalists, Gigerenzer, Gaissmaier, Kurz-Milke, Schwartz, and Woloshin (2008) pointed out that reporting relative changes without specifying the base rate is bad practice because it can lead the reader to overestimate the extent of the change. They recommended reporting absolute change to avoid this problem. To highlight the issue, consider that the positivity rate for methamphetamine use was 0.19% in 2002 and increased to 0.32% in 2003 (Quest Diagnostics Incorporated, 2004). Although the change represents a seemingly large 68% relative increase, the absolute positivity rates in each year are very low, and the absolute increase in the positivity rate from 2002 to 2003 is only 0.13 of a percentage point.

A fifth practice that may lead to mischaracterization of employee substance use is the selective reporting of research findings. For example, a single supportive study might be cited to make the case that an alcohol hangover is related to or perhaps causes poor work performance. What might go unstated is the fact that many more studies of alcohol hangover and work performance failed to uncover a statistically significant relation. On the other hand, a single study failing to support the relation might be cited to make the case that alcohol use is not associated with work injuries. Again, what might go unstated is the fact that many more studies support the relation. The practice of selective reporting fails to provide appropriate conclusions based on the preponderance of evidence.

A final practice that may lead to an inappropriate portrayal of employee substance use is the overgeneralization of findings. One form of overgeneralization was mentioned previously—relying on a single sensational event to suggest that a broad relation exists between two variables, such as employee alcohol use and workplace accidents. However, other forms occur with respect to aspects of a research study's design, such as sampling and measurement. Much research exploring employee substance use is based on convenience samples (i.e., self-selected volunteers). For example, although a researcher's actual interest might be in generalizing the results of a study to a broad population, such as all employees in the United States or all registered nurses in Finland, data often are collected from employees of a single organization that allowed the researcher access to its employees or from volunteers who have responded to an advertisement. Because a random sample was not drawn from the actual population of interest, the results apply only to the convenience sample of employees used in a specific study. This inability to generalize results beyond the sample studied sometimes is not made clear in research reports, and it is rarely mentioned in press releases and newspaper articles describing a study's results.

Overgeneralization may also occur in regard to the way researchers measure the variables under study. Although there are often several ways to assess a variable, a study may use or report only one of them. For example, several dimensions of alcohol use can be assessed—whether or not alcohol is used during some time period, the frequency of using alcohol, the number of drinks (amount) consumed on a drinking day, the frequency of drinking heavily (five or more drinks per day or occasion), the frequency of drinking to intoxication, the frequency of experiencing a hangover, or whether or not one has a diagnosis of alcohol abuse or dependence. Sometimes a research study uses only one or two measures of alcohol use, which opens the possibility that its results might be overgeneralized. Consider a study showing that alcohol users are more likely than nonusers to be absent from work. This might be taken as evidence that any alcohol use leads to absenteeism. However, if the quantity of alcohol consumed and the frequency of heavy drinking were also assessed, it might be found that only frequent heavy drinkers and not light or moderate drinkers and abstainers are absent. Inadequate measurement can also lead to the failure to find relations. For example, a study might find that frequent exposure to adverse working conditions may not predict whether or not a person uses alcohol. However, because many individuals begin using alcohol before they enter the workforce, frequent exposure to adverse working conditions might more likely be related to frequent heavy drinking among alcohol users. If only drinking status was assessed, it might be concluded erroneously that adverse working conditions have no relation to employee alcohol use. Although these examples focus on the measurement of alcohol use, the same problem extends to inadequate measurement of the potential causes and outcomes of employee alcohol use.

Given the problematic practices just summarized, coupled with the fact that the issue of employee substance use is often a morally, politically, and financially charged topic, it should come as no surprise that there is the potential for (a) the dissemination of misleading and partial information and (b) the development of policies that fail to consider adequately the preponderance of empirical evidence. A number of researchers have pointed out that policy, in particular drug-related policy, has a long history of being devised in the absence of scientific evidence and that policymakers may selectively utilize evidence when it suits their policy platforms (e.g., K. M. Fillmore, 1984; Hughes, 2007; Roman & Blum, 1995). This suggests that all relevant stakeholders (e.g., managers, unions, policymakers, researchers, and the media) should be made aware of what is known and what is not known about employee substance use.

GOALS, AUDIENCE, AND STRUCTURE OF THE BOOK

One way to address the dilemma of potential mischaracterization of employee substance use is to explore a broad set of research studies, identifying their strengths and limitations and determining what the data can and cannot tell us. My goal in writing this book was to take a broad and balanced look at what we know and do not know about key areas of alcohol and illicit drug use in the workforce and in the workplace. This motivation is consistent with recent interests in developing evidenced-based medicine, evidence-based management, and evidence-based policy (e.g., Axelsson, 1998; Brownson, Chriqui, & Stamatakis, 2009; Evidence-Based Medicine Working Group, 1992; Hughes, 2007; Kovner, Elton, & Billings, 2000; Pfeffer & Sutton, 2006; Rousseau & McCarthy, 2007). In each of these instances, the general notion is that practices, decisions, and policies should be informed by a systematic review of available scientific evidence. Thus, any workplace practice or policy should be based on facts, not on managers' own beliefs, what competitors or peers are or are not doing, or the recommendations of consultants who are financially motivated to overpromote their own products and services (e.g., Axelsson, 1998; Kovner et al., 2000; Pfeffer & Sutton, 2006). Thus, this book summarizes the scientific evidence on workforce and workplace substance use in such a way as to be of interest and use to a number of audiences. With regard to employers, unions, and policymakers, this review of what we know and do not know about employee substance use—prevalence, etiology, productivity outcomes, and various types of workplace interventions—will inform workplace policies. With regard to organizational, substance use, and public health researchers,[1] this review will help highlight substantive issues that should be addressed and subgroups of employees that require more attention, as well as set the stage for broader models and stronger research designs. A brief overview of each chapter follows.

Chapter 1 summarizes several issues regarding definitions involving psychoactive substances and employee substance use. A detailed look at the prevalence of workforce and workplace substance use and impairment in the United States is taken, and international data on the prevalence of workforce and workplace substance use are presented. Finally, the prevalence of workforce and workplace substance use and impairment across high- and low-risk

---

[1]I should note that a similarly motivated review of the employee substance use literature was presented in a report produced by the Institute of Medicine entitled *Under the Influence? Drugs and the American Work Force* (Normand, Lempert, & O'Brien, 1994). That review covered literature published before 1994. Nonetheless, it is time to take another in-depth look after nearly 2 decades because data exist for issues that were not addressed in the past and additional, sometimes higher quality, data exist for issues that were addressed in the past. Moreover, an understanding of the current empirical record is eminently useful for guiding future research that can address existing gaps in our knowledge.

groups—defined by gender, age, and occupation—is summarized. Chapter 2 reviews the etiology of employee substance use in terms of major classes of person characteristics and workplace environmental characteristics. The main person characteristics considered are genetic makeup, personality, and substance use expectancies. The workplace environmental factors are substance availability, social control, and work stress.

Chapters 3 and 4 review the outcomes of employee substance use. In particular, Chapter 3 addresses psychopharmacological and workplace simulation research on substance use in relation to basic cognitive and psychomotor performance. Chapter 4 focuses on organizational field research exploring the relation of substance use to three broad classes of productivity outcomes: poor attendance, poor work performance and other dysfunctional work behaviors, and job injuries. In this chapter, I discuss what is known about the cost of employee alcohol and illicit drug use to employers and present a detailed model of employee substance use and productivity that highlights the complexity of these relations.

Chapters 5 and 6 explore workplace intervention efforts. In particular, Chapter 5 reviews major issues involving illicit drug and alcohol use testing including a brief history in the United States and elsewhere, characteristics of organizations that use workforce substance use testing, dimensions of substance use testing, and the major motivations underlying and the effectiveness of workforce substance use testing. Chapter 6 describes broad workplace health promotion programs that have been developed to address employee substance use problems and improve productivity, as well as relevant findings regarding their effectiveness at reducing employee substance use. These programs include employee assistance programs and workplace wellness programs. Finally, Chapter 7 provides some general implications for workplace substance use policy and outlines general issues involving future research.

1

EMPLOYEE SUBSTANCE INVOLVEMENT: DEFINITIONS AND PREVALENCE

What proportion of employees use psychoactive substances? How often do employees use psychoactive substances? Which psychoactive substances are being used by employees? Which employees are using psychoactive substances? When are psychoactive substances being used by employees? What proportion of employees report being impaired by, abuse, or are dependent on psychoactive drugs? Is psychoactive drug use and impairment a problem for all employers? If we want to understand the nature of employee substance use, these are the first questions we need to ask. In other words, we need to begin with an understanding of the scope or landscape of employee substance use. In this chapter, I begin by defining key terms and exploring some important issues that have received little attention in past research. I then take a detailed look at the prevalence of employee substance use and impairment in the United States and the more limited available data on employee substance use and impairment outside the United States.

DOI: 10.1037/13944-002
Alcohol and Illicit Drug Use in the Workforce and Workplace, by M. R. Frone

WHAT IS A PSYCHOACTIVE DRUG?

Broadly defined, a *drug* is any chemical substance that alters biological function or structure. Examples of drugs are insulin, heparin (anticoagulant), Lipitor (atorvastatin calcium used as a lipid-lowering agent), Prevacid (lansoprazole used to suppress gastric acid secretion), marijuana, Prozac (fluoxetine hydrochloride used to treat depressive, obsessive–compulsive, and bulimic disorders), and alcohol. More narrowly, a *psychoactive* (or *psychotropic* or *psychotherapeutic*) *drug* is a chemical substance that acts primarily on the central nervous system, resulting in changes in consciousness, perception, emotion, cognition, or behavior. Among the previous examples of drugs, psychoactive drugs include marijuana, Prozac, and alcohol.

TYPES OF PSYCHOACTIVE DRUGS

Psychoactive drugs can be further classified according to their pharmacological effects. Such classification can be complex because a specific psychoactive substance may have more than one type of pharmacological effect, and individuals may use the substance for one or more of these effects. With one exception, the major classes of psychoactive drugs are presented in Table 1.1 based on their *primary* pharmacological effects on the central nervous system (for more details on specific substances, see Faupel, Horowitz, & Weaver, 2004; Lacy & Ditzler, 2007; Maisto et al., 2008; J. F. Williams & Storck, 2007). The exception is inhalants, which represent a broad class of substances. Although inhalants have effects similar to those of depressants and in some cases hallucinogens, they are the only psychoactive substances grouped by their route of administration.

Narcotic analgesics are substances whose primary effect is to reduce pain, though they also reduce tension and increase euphoria. They include (a) opium, (b) natural derivatives of opium, also called *opiates* (e.g., morphine, codeine), (c) semisynthetic opioids (e.g., heroin, oxycodone, hydrocodone), and (d) synthetic opioids (e.g., methadone). *Depressants* act to slow the central nervous system and produce a drowsy or calm feeling. They include alcohol, barbiturates, benzodiazepines, other sedatives, and antipsychotics. *Stimulants* act to increase central nervous system activity and produce a sense of euphoria. They include amphetamine, methamphetamine, ephedrine, pseudoephedrine, cocaine, caffeine, and nicotine. *Hallucinogens* can alter consciousness in strong and unpredictable ways. There are three categories of hallucinogens—serotonergic hallucinogens (e.g., LSD, mescaline, psilocybin), methylated amphetamines (e.g., MDMA or ecstasy, MDA), and dissociative anesthetics (e.g., PCP, ketamine). *Cannabis* includes marijuana

TABLE 1.1
Pharmacological Classification of Psychoactive Drugs

Type	Pharmacological effects
Narcotic analgesics (opiates and opioids) • Opium • Opiates (codeine, morphine) • Semisynthetic opioids (e.g., heroin, oxycodone, hydrocodone) • Synthetic opioids (e.g., methadone, fentanyl)	Pain relief; reduced tension; increased euphoria; decreased central nervous system activity, especially lowered respiration and body temperature.
Depressants • Alcohol • Barbiturates (e.g., amobarbital, pentobarbital) • Benzodiazepines (e.g., alprazolam, diazepam) • Other sedatives (e.g., methaqualone or quaaludes) • Antipsychotics (e.g., chlorpromazine/Thorazine, haloperidol/Haldol)	Decreased central nervous system activity, producing a drowsy or calm feeling.
Stimulants • Amphetamine, methamphetamine • Ephedrine, pseudoephedrine • Cathinone (khat) • Cocaine, crack cocaine • Caffeine and other xanthines • Nicotine	Increased central nervous system activity, producing a sense of euphoria, heightened mental alertness, and increased energy.
Hallucinogens • Serotonergic hallucinogens (e.g., LSD, mescaline, psilocybin) • Methylated amphetamines (e.g., MDMA or ecstasy, MDA) • Dissociative anesthetics (e.g., PCP or angel dust, ketamine)	Strong and unpredictable effects on consciousness, including altered states of perception and cognition and intensification of extant emotion.
Cannabis • Marijuana • Hashish	Effects include those of several other substances, such as hallucinogens, analgesics, and sedatives.
Inhalants • Volatile solvents (e.g., gasoline, lighter fluids, paint thinners, toluene) • Aerosols (e.g., spray paints, hair sprays, vegetable oil sprays for cooking, and fabric protector sprays) • Gases, including medical anesthetics (e.g., nitrous oxide, ether, chloroform, butane, propane, refrigerants) • Nitrites (cyclohexyl nitrite, isoamyl [amyl] nitrite, and isobutyl [butyl] nitrite, video head cleaner, room odorizer, leather cleaner, or liquid aroma)	Volatile solvents, aerosols, and gases act on the central nervous system to produce effects similar to depressants, especially the effects of alcohol. With high dosage, they may also have effects similar to hallucinogens. In contrast, nitrites do not have psychoactive properties. They cause vasodilation and smooth muscle relaxation and are used primarily as sexual enhancers.

(continues)

TABLE 1.1

Pharmacological Classification of Psychoactive Drugs *(Continued)*

Type	Pharmacological effects
Other psychoactive drugs: Antidepressants • Monoamine oxidase inhibitors (e.g., isocarboxazid/Marplan, tranylcypromine/Parnate, phenelzine/Nardil) • Tricyclic antidepressants (e.g., amitriptyline/Elavil, clomipramine/Anafranil, doxepin/Adapin) • Selective serotonin reuptake inhibitors (e.g., citalopram/Celexa, fluoxetine/Prozac, sertraline/Zoloft, paroxetine/Paxil)	Used to moderate negative mood and other symptoms associated with depression.

and hashish and has many of the same effects reported for hallucinogens, analgesics, and depressants. *Inhalants* produce psychoactive effects similar to those of depressants and, in some circumstances, hallucinogens. They include a variety of volatile solvents (e.g., gasoline, lighter fluids, paint thinners, toluene); aerosols (e.g., spray paints, hair sprays, vegetable oil sprays, fabric sprays); and gases, including medical anesthetics (nitrous oxide, ether, chloroform, butane, propane, refrigerants). Finally, there are other types of psychoactive drugs, such as *antidepressants* that moderate extreme negative mood and other symptoms associated with depression.

DEFINING ILLICIT AND LICIT SUBSTANCE USE

In addition to their pharmacological effects, psychoactive substances can be classified according to their legal availability and the extent of governmental regulation, which are based on their presumed medical value, potential for dependence, and harmfulness. This classification scheme is called *drug scheduling* and is used in a number of countries, though the exact scheduling scheme differs across countries. The classification of any specific drug is often a source of controversy, as are the overall purpose and effectiveness of the entire scheduling scheme (e.g., Caulkins, Reuter, & Coulson, 2011; Kalant, 2010; Nutt, King, Saulsbury, & Blakemore, 2007). Nonetheless, drug schedules underlie the definition of illicit and licit drug use. Table 1.2 presents the five schedules created in the U.S. Controlled Substances Act of 1970, along with a residual category for nonscheduled substances. Consistent with most population studies of substance use, *illicit substance use* refers to (a) the use of psychoactive substances that are illegal and unavailable by medical prescription (Schedule I drugs) or (b) the illicit use of any psychoactive substances that require a

TABLE 1.2
U.S. Drug Schedules

Schedule	Example substances
Schedule I • High potential for abuse • No currently accepted medical use in treatment in the United States • Lack of accepted safety for use under medical supervision • Not available by prescription	• Heroin • Marijuana[a]/hashish • LSD • Mescaline • Ecstasy (MDMA) • Methaqualone
Schedule II • High potential for abuse • Currently accepted medical use in treatment in the United States or a currently accepted medical use with severe restrictions • Risk of severe physical or psychological dependence • Available by prescription but with no refills without seeing health practitioner again	• Opium • Codeine • Morphine • Oxycodone • Cocaine • Amphetamine • Methamphetamine • Short-acting barbiturates (e.g., pentobarbital) • PCP • Methadone
Schedule III • Potential for abuse less than substances in Schedules I and II • Currently accepted medical use in treatment in the United States • Risk of low to moderate physical dependence or high psychological dependence • Available by prescription; may be refilled up to five times in 6 months	• Intermediate-acting barbiturates (e.g., *talbutal, butalbital*) • Ketamine • Codeine combinations (e.g., Tylenol with codeine)
Schedule IV • Low potential for abuse relative to substances in Schedule III • Currently accepted medical use in treatment in the United States • Abuse may lead to limited physical dependence or psychological dependence relative to the drugs or other substances in Schedule III • Available by prescription; may be refilled up to five times in 6 months	• Benzodiazepines (e.g., alprazolam/ Xanax, chlordiazepoxide/Librium, clonazepam/Klonopin, diazepam/ Valium) • Weak opioids (e.g., Darvon)

(*continues*)

TABLE 1.2
U.S. Drug Schedules *(Continued)*

Schedule	Example substances
Schedule V	
• Low potential for abuse relative to substances in Schedule IV	• Cough medications with codeine
• Currently accepted medical use in treatment in the United States	
• Abuse may lead to limited physical dependence or psychological dependence relative to the drugs or other substances in Schedule IV	
• Prescription not required but available only through a licensed pharmacist to persons 18 and older; sale must be recorded	
Unscheduled	
• Not regulated under the Controlled Substances Act	• Alcohol
• Legal for many purposes	• Tobacco
• May be regulated by other laws and regulations (e.g., age restrictions on purchase)	• Caffeine
	• Inhalants

aThere are some exceptions for marijuana. Although the U.S. federal government continues to list marijuana as a Schedule I drug with no accepted medical use and no safe usage even under medical supervision, 14 states (Alaska, California, Colorado, Hawaii, Maine, Michigan, Montana, Nevada, New Jersey, New Mexico, Oregon, Rhode Island, Vermont, and Washington) and the District of Columbia allow the licit use of marijuana for specific medical purposes. The licit use of marijuana for medical purposes is allowed in several countries other than the United States, such as Belgium, Canada, Israel, and the Netherlands.

medical prescription (Schedule II, III, and IV drugs). Illicit use of a prescription psychoactive drug occurs when it is used without a prescription or is used with a prescription but taken more frequently or in higher dosage than prescribed. In contrast, with a few exceptions, *licit drug use* refers to (a) the use of prescription drugs (Schedule II, III, and IV drugs) with a medical prescription and as prescribed, (b) the use of scheduled substances that can be obtained over the counter without a medical prescription (Schedule V drugs), and (c) the use of unscheduled substances (e.g., alcohol, nicotine, caffeine). Thus, alcohol is a licit psychoactive substance for most employed adults.[1]

Inhalants are unscheduled and are not regulated under the Controlled Substances Act in the United States because they constitute products that are universally available and have legitimate uses. Nonetheless, many states

---

[1]There are some exceptions to this. In many countries, alcohol use may be illegal for some or all employed adults. For example, alcohol use is illegal for all individuals 18 to 20 years old in the United States, for individuals 18 years old in some Canadian provinces, and for individuals 18 or 19 years old in Japan. In other countries, such as Afghanistan, Bangladesh, Brunei, Iran, Kuwait, Pakistan, Saudi Arabia, and Yemen, alcohol is illegal more generally.

have introduced fines, incarceration, and/or mandatory treatment for the sale, use, or possession of inhalants for the purpose of intoxication. These legislative efforts are aimed at eliminating inhalant use by children, adolescents, and the impoverished and at reminding society that the use of inhalants for intoxication is not acceptable (J. F. Williams & Storck, 2007). Therefore, past discussion of illicit drugs and assessment of illicit drug use often included inhalants. In this book, when the prevalence of overall illicit drug use is explored, inhalants are included as illicit drugs to maintain consistency with past reports.

WHICH PSYCHOACTIVE DRUGS ARE EXPLORED?

The focus of this book is on the use of alcohol and inhalants and the illicit use of several classes of controlled substances (cannabis, cocaine, hallucinogens, heroin, narcotic analgesics, depressants, tranquilizers, and stimulants). I do not explore employee use of caffeine or nicotine, the licit use of prescription drugs (though this issue is touched on in Chapter 3), or the use of over-the-counter medications. There are several reasons for this focus. First, the use of alcohol and the illicit use of many psychoactive substances are presumed to have the largest potential to impact employee safety and productivity and organizational profitability. Second, alcohol use and the illicit use of the other psychoactive substances have received the most research attention in the population of employed adults. Third, both caffeine and nicotine are classified as minor stimulants, and the typical dose used of either substance does not engender concern for workplace safety or impaired productivity (e.g., Heishman, Kleykamp, & Singleton, 2010; Koelega, 1993; Rees, Allen, & Lader, 1999). Also, the use of over-the-counter medications and the licit use of prescription drugs under the supervision of a licensed medical practitioner are generally expected to have a negligible impact on the workplace. Although tobacco use is associated with long-term health problems, this is the primary outcome of the mode of administration (e.g., inhalation of tobacco smoke and chewing tobacco) and not the result of nicotine use per se. Fourth, little information exists on employee use of caffeine or nicotine and the licit use of prescription drugs or over-the-counter medications.

DEFINING *SUBSTANCE USE*, *IMPAIRMENT*, *SUBSTANCE ABUSE*, AND *SUBSTANCE DEPENDENCE*

The meaning of these four terms may seem self-evident. However, they are used differently within and across various groups—researchers, law enforcement, policymakers, and health professionals. For example, the meaning of *substance abuse* often depends on the legality of the substance under consideration. It is common to see the mere use of illicit drugs referred to as *drug abuse*. In contrast, the mere use of alcohol is not referred to as *alcohol abuse*. *Alcohol abuse* typically refers to alcohol consumption at levels and in contexts that impede role performance and endanger health. Such differences in definitions pose a problem when summarizing research. As a result of this confound between use and abuse for illicit drugs that does not exist for alcohol, comparisons of alcohol abuse with drug abuse are sometimes difficult because fundamentally different things are being compared. As another example of the differential meaning of a specific term, alcohol intoxication has been defined (a) by observable effects on psychomotor performance, such as having slurred speech or being unsteady on one's feet, or (b) by crossing some legally proscribed level of alcohol concentration in blood (i.e., blood alcohol content [BAC] ≥ .08), whether or not there is evidence of cognitive or psychomotor impairment. Therefore, to help structure the presentation of data in this chapter, I define the terms *substance use, substance impairment, substance abuse,* and *substance dependence*. Throughout this book, however, the general term *substance involvement* is used when referring collectively to use, impairment, abuse, and dependence.

Substance Use

Substance use, as a behavior, has several dimensions. *User status* refers to the mere use of a substance. Users are individuals who have used a substance at least once over some fixed period of time (e.g., lifetime user, past year user, past month user). *Frequency* of use refers to the number of days or times that a substance is used over some fixed period of time. *Quantity* of use refers to the dose or number of units (e.g., drinks) consumed on a typical occasion of use. In this chapter, quantity of use is discussed for alcohol but not for other substances. In contrast to alcohol, where standard drinks that contain approximately the same level of absolute alcohol can be defined for individuals, standard dosages or quantity consumed for illicit drugs can be difficult to assess because of differing chemical properties, routes of administration, and levels of purity. Measures of alcohol use can combine the frequency of use and quantity used. For example, *heavy drinking* is often defined as consuming 5 or more drinks in a day. Therefore, it is common for researchers to assess the frequency of consuming 5 or more drinks in a day (i.e., frequency of heavy drinking).

Substance Impairment

Substance impairment has two dimensions: intoxication and withdrawal. *Substance intoxication* refers to acute and reversible central nervous system impairment due to the direct pharmacological action of a substance, resulting in various behavioral, cognitive, and affective changes (e.g., American Psychiatric Association, 2000; Maisto et al., 2008; Rinaldi, Steindler, Wilford, & Goodwin, 1988). *Substance withdrawal* refers to central nervous system impairment due to cessation of or reduction in substance use that has been heavy and prolonged, resulting in various behavioral, cognitive, and affective changes (e.g., American Psychiatric Association, 2000; Rinaldi et al., 1988; Saitz, 1998). Also included in the definition of withdrawal is the "hangover" syndrome typically associated with the use of alcohol. An alcohol hangover represents a general feeling of malaise resulting from a bout of heavy alcohol use after BAC returns to zero, and it is believed to represent, at least in part, a mild form of acute alcohol withdrawal (e.g., R. S. Moore, 1998; Swift & Davidson, 1998; Wiese, Shlipak, & Browner, 2000). The precise signs and symptoms of substance intoxication and withdrawal may differ across types of psychoactive substances (e.g., American Psychiatric Association, 2000; Miller, Gold, & Smith, 1997).

Substance Abuse and Dependence

To identify individuals engaged in harmful levels of substance use, the American Psychiatric Association has developed a diagnostic system to assess substance dependence and substance abuse. The criteria for these two substance use disorders are part of the *Diagnostic and Statistical Manual of Mental Disorders* (4th ed., text revision; *DSM–IV–TR*; American Psychiatric Association, 2000). The same criteria for abuse and dependence apply to all substances. For a given substance (e.g., alcohol), a person cannot be diagnosed with both dependence and abuse; a diagnosis of abuse is made only after a diagnosis of dependence has been ruled out. Nonetheless, a person may meet the criteria for abuse for one substance (e.g., cannabis abuse) and the criteria for dependence for another substance (e.g., alcohol dependence; Maisto et al., 2008).

Substance dependence is defined as "a cluster of cognitive, behavioral, and physiological symptoms indicating that the individual continues use of the substance despite significant substance-related problems. There is a pattern of repeated self-administration that can result in tolerance, withdrawal, and compulsive drug-taking behavior" (American Psychiatric Association, 2000, p. 192). The seven criteria for a diagnosis of substance dependence are presented in Exhibit 1.1. The first criterion is tolerance, which represents a diminished response that occurs after repeated exposure to a fixed dose of a psychoactive substance (see Chapters 3 and 4 for more details). The second criterion is withdrawal, which has been discussed. The third through seventh criteria refer to compulsive drug use. The *DSM–IV–TR* provides an overall diagnosis of current dependence if a person manifests three or more of the

EXHIBIT 1.1
DSM–IV–TR Criteria for Substance Dependence

A maladaptive pattern of substance use leading to clinically significant impairment or distress as manifested by three (or more) of the following, occurring at any time in the same 12-month period:

1. Tolerance, as defined by either of the following:
   (a) A need for markedly increased amounts of the substance to achieve intoxication or the desired effect
   (b) Markedly diminished effect with continued use of the same amount of the substance.
2. Withdrawal, as manifested by either of the following:
   (a) The characteristic withdrawal syndrome for the substance
   (b) The same (or closely related) substance is taken to relieve or avoid withdrawal symptoms.
3. The substance is often taken in larger amounts or over a longer period than intended.
4. There is a persistent desire or unsuccessful efforts to cut down or control substance use.
5. A great deal of time is spent in activities necessary to obtain the substance, use the substance, or recover from its effects.
6. Important social, occupational, or recreational activities are given up or reduced because of substance use.
7. The substance use is continued despite knowledge of having a persistent physical or psychological problem that is likely to have been caused or exacerbated by the substance (for example, current cocaine use despite recognition of cocaine-induced depression or continued drinking despite recognition that an ulcer was made worse by alcohol consumption).

Specify if:
With physiological dependence: evidence of tolerance or withdrawal (i.e., either Item 1 or 2 is present).
Without physiological dependence: no evidence of tolerance or withdrawal (i.e., neither Item 1 nor 2 are present).

Note. From the *Diagnostic and Statistical Manual of Mental Disorders* (4th ed., text revision [*DSM–IV–TR*], pp. 197–198), by the American Psychiatric Association, 2000, Washington, DC: Author. Copyright 2000 by the American Psychiatric Association. Reprinted with permission.

seven criteria during a 12-month period. The first two criteria primarily define physical dependence, whereas the remaining five criteria primarily define psychological dependence. As shown at the bottom of Exhibit 1.1, substance dependence can be diagnosed either with or without physical dependence.

Substance abuse is defined as "a maladaptive pattern of substance use manifested by recurrent and significant adverse consequences related to the repeated use of substances" (American Psychiatric Association, 2000, p. 198). The criteria for substance abuse are presented in Exhibit 1.2. Note that Condition B indicates that to be diagnosed with substance abuse for a specific substance, an individual must not meet the diagnostic criteria for substance dependence for that substance. If the person does not meet the

EXHIBIT 1.2
DSM–IV–TR Criteria for Substance Abuse

Condition A:
A maladaptive pattern of substance use leading to clinically significant impairment or distress as manifested by one (or more) of the following, occurring at any time in the same 12-month period:

1. Recurrent substance use resulting in a failure to fulfill major role obligations at work, school, or home (such as repeated absences or poor work performance related to substance use; substance-related absences, suspensions, or expulsions from school; or neglect of children or household).
2. Recurrent substance use in situations in which it is physically hazardous (such as driving an automobile or operating a machine when impaired by substance use).
3. Recurrent substance-related legal problems (such as arrests for substance-related disorderly conduct).
4. Continued substance use despite having persistent or recurrent social or inter-personal problems caused or exacerbated by the effects of the substance (for example, arguments with spouse about consequences of intoxication and physical fights).

Condition B:
Does not meet the criteria for substance dependence.

Note. From the *Diagnostic and Statistical Manual of Mental Disorders* (4th ed., text revision [*DSM–IV–TR*], p. 199), by the American Psychiatric Association, 2000, Washington, DC: Author. Copyright 2000 by the American Psychiatric Association. Reprinted with permission.

criteria for substance dependence, a diagnosis of substance abuse may be rendered if the person manifests one or more criteria under Condition A during a 12-month period. These criteria focus on impairment in several domains of life resulting from recurrent use of a substance.

IMPORTANCE OF CONTEXT

In terms of substance use and impairment, past research has typically assessed only employees' overall use of or impairment from psychoactive substances. Overall substance use represents the use of a substance across all contexts. Overall substance impairment represents the experience of intoxication or withdrawal due to the use of a substance across all contexts. Thus, past research has primarily explored *workforce substance use and impairment*, which primarily reflects use and impairment away from work and outside an employed individual's normal work hours. In contrast, relatively little research has focused on the temporal context of employee substance use relative to the workday. *Workplace substance use* represents the consumption of a psychoactive substance just before coming to work or during the workday (Ames, Grube, & Moore, 1997; Frone, 2004, 2006a, 2006b; Mangione et al., 1999).

In particular, workplace substance use refers to the consumption of alcohol or illicit drugs (a) within 2 hours of starting one's work shift, (b) during a lunch break, (c) during other work breaks, or (d) while performing one's job. *Workplace substance impairment* represents the experience of intoxication or withdrawal due to alcohol or illicit drug use during work hours. *After work substance use* represents the initiation of substance use within 2 hours of leaving work. *After work substance impairment* represents intoxication experienced as a result of initiating substance use after work. The distinction between overall use and impairment in the workforce, on the one hand, and use and impairment before, during, or after work, on the other hand, may be important for research examining the workplace causes (see Chapter 2) and the productivity outcomes (see Chapter 4) associated with employee substance involvement.

PREVALENCE OF SUBSTANCE USE, IMPAIRMENT, ABUSE, AND DEPENDENCE IN THE WORKFORCE

Before the prevalence data are presented, it should be noted that the employment rate among illicit drug users or heavy drinkers is widely cited. Although there are many examples, consider a recent statement by Marlatt and Witkiewitz (2010): "More than 70% of current illicit drug users and heavy drinkers are employed full time. Thus, the large majority of substance abusers in the United States are in the workplace" (p. 600). The apparent reason for using the employment rate of illicit drug users and heavy drinkers is an indirect attempt to provide information about the proportion of illicit drug users and heavy alcohol users in the workforce and in the workplace. However, as discussed in the Introduction in this volume, this is an example of the misapplication of valid information that can mischaracterize employee substance use. At best, the employment rate among substance users is of little value for employers or policymakers in terms of evaluating the prevalence of heavy drinking and illicit drug use in the workforce and workplace; at worst, this information might be very misleading. From the employment rate of substance users, it is impossible to determine the number or proportion of workers who are heavy drinkers or illicit drug users. Even with a high employment rate, heavy alcohol users or illicit drug users may not represent a large proportion of the workforce. Information on employment rates also fails to provide information about patterns and context of employee substance involvement.

The most direct source of data on workforce substance involvement is epidemiological surveys. However, such surveys rely on self-reports of behavior. This means that some individuals may not be willing to admit to behaviors that are illegal or socially undesirable. Further, even if individuals admit to engaging in heavy drinking or illicit drug use, they may underreport the frequency and quantity of use and may not accurately report the contexts in which their use occurs (e.g., at work). Although some of this underreporting or misreporting may be purposeful, some of it may be due to forgetting as well. Despite their potential limitations, self-reports often may be the best source of data we have on employee alcohol and illicit drug involvement (Baldwin, 2000; Turkkan, 2000). To the extent that a person's substance involvement is hidden from others, the reports of collaterals may not be a useful substitute for self-reports from the target individual (Connors & Maisto, 2003). Also, collaterals may purposefully underreport the undesirable behaviors of someone close to them and suffer from the same cognitive limitations that lead to forgetting and inaccurate reports by the target respondent (Connors & Maisto, 2003). Even biologic tests are limited. Only hair testing will allow estimates of the overall prevalence of illicit drug use and heavy alcohol use over long periods of time (see Chapter 5). However, one might expect that individuals who would not self-report substance use would also be less likely to submit to biologic tests. Moreover, biologic tests cannot provide information on the frequency of use, quantity of use, frequency of impairment, and the context in which substances are used (e.g., away from work or at work). Therefore, to obtain detailed data on the pattern and context of employee substance involvement, one needs to rely on self-reports of individuals participating in epidemiological surveys. These studies expend great effort and expense recruiting random samples of individuals; do not contact individuals through their employers or at their workplace; and try to allay any apprehension regarding the reporting of substance involvement, sometimes with legal protections against the subpoena of data. Detailed prevalence data for workforce substance involvement in the United States are summarized next on the basis of several national surveys. This is followed by a review of available data on workforce substance involvement outside the United States and information on the distribution of substance involvement across the workforce.

U.S. Workforce

In the United States, a number of prior reports have presented data on the prevalence of substance use, abuse, and dependence among employed adults using data from the annual National Survey on Drug Use and Health (NSDUH; formerly called the National Household Survey on Drug Abuse; Hoffmann, Brittingham, & Larison, 1996; Larson, Eyerman, Foster, & Gfroerer, 2007; Normand et al., 1994; U.S. Department of Health and Human Services, 1999). However, these reports provide little or no information on (a) the use of various classes of substances other than alcohol and marijuana, (b) the prevalence of substance impairment, (c) the frequency of substance use or impairment, and (d) the number of alcoholic drinks typically consumed on drinking days. Also, there has been no effort to compare estimates of workforce substance use across multiple national surveys. Therefore, I provide workforce prevalence data for substance use, impairment, abuse, and dependence using data from the NSDUH (conducted in 2002–2003; for more details on this annual survey, see https://nsduhweb.rti.org/ and http://oas.samhsa.gov/nsduh/ reports.htm), the National Survey of Workplace Health and Safety (NSWHS; conducted in 2002–2003; for more details, see Frone, 2006a, 2006b, and the appendix in Schat, Frone, & Kelloway, 2006), the National Epidemiologic Survey on Alcohol and Related Conditions (NESARC; conducted in 2001–2002; for more details, see B. F. Grant & Dawson, 2006), and the National Comorbidity Survey Replication (NCS-R; conducted in 2001–2003; for more details, see Kessler & Walters, 2002; http://www.hcp.med.harvard.edu/ ncs). Data were extracted from each of these studies for employed adults, 18 to 65 years old, in the U.S. workforce.[2] Tables 1.3 to 1.9 provide prevalence estimates for the preceding 12 months from each of the four studies that assessed a specific dimension of alcohol or illicit drug use, impairment, abuse, or dependence. To simplify discussion of the data, these tables also provide (a) the weighted average prevalence estimates across the multiple studies and (b) estimated population totals based on these average prevalence rates.

Workforce Alcohol Use

Table 1.3 reveals that over a 12-month period roughly 75.1% of the workforce (96.7 million workers) used alcohol, with 37.8% (48.7 million workers) doing so infrequently (less than weekly) and 37.2% (47.9 million) doing so frequently (at least once per week). Table 1.4 shows that workers who drank at least 1 day per month consumed an average of 3 drinks on days that they drank. In addition, 17.1% of the workforce (12.5 million workers) who drank alcohol at least monthly and 9.7% of the overall U.S. workforce reported consuming 5 or more drinks on typical drinking days. Table 1.3 shows overall prevalence rates for the frequency of heavy drinking (i.e., 5 or more drinks per day). Over a 12-month period, 26.1% of the workforce (33.6 million workers) reported drinking 5 or more drinks in a day, with 17.0% (21.9 million workers) drinking heavily infrequently and 9.2% (11.8 million workers) drinking heavily frequently.

Table 1.3 does not show the prevalence of heavy drinking for the NCS-R because it was not assessed. The prevalence of heavy drinking is

---

[2]The studies just described provide an opportunity to compare estimates of workforce substance involvement across several national surveys. To determine if the reported prevalence rates reflect current rates of workforce substance involvement, I compared the prevalence rates from the 2010 NSDUH to those from the combined 2002–2003 NSDUH rates reported in Chapters 1 and 3. The 2010 rates are very close to the 2002–2003 rates, suggesting that there has been little if any change in workforce substance involvement. More recent estimates of workplace substance involvement do not exist.

TABLE 1.3
Prevalence of Alcohol Use, Heavy Alcohol Use, and Alcohol Impairment in the Workforce During the Past 12 Months: Overall and by Frequency of Use

Dimension of alcohol use and study	Never	Frequency of alcohol use				Overall prevalence
		Less than monthly	1–3 days per month	1–2 days per week	3 or more days per week	
Alcohol use						
NSWHS	26.6%	21.4%	19.5%	19.0%	13.4%	73.4%
NESARC	26.8%	21.8%	18.1%	18.5%	14.8%	73.1%
NSDUH	23.4%	15.8%	20.6%	21.8%	18.3%	76.6%
NCS-R	29.9%	23.0%	15.7%	15.6%	15.8%	70.1%
Average prevalence[a]	24.9%	18.3%	19.5%	20.3%	16.9%	75.1%
Estimated population[b]	32,060,972	23,562,883	25,107,990	26,138,061	21,760,258	96,697,950
Heavy alcohol use[c]						
NSWHS	70.7%	16.4%	6.1%	4.4%	2.5%	29.3%
NESARC	74.2%	10.6%	5.8%	5.8%	3.6%	25.8%
Average prevalence[a]	73.8%	11.2%	5.8%	5.7%	3.5%	26.1%
Estimated population[b]	95,024,084	14,420,999	7,468,017	7,339,259	4,506,562	33,606,079
Alcohol intoxication[d]						
NSWHS	69.3%	21.1%	6.3%	2.1%	1.2%	30.7%
NESARC	70.6%	21.6%	4.3%	2.4%	1.2%	29.4%
Average prevalence[a]	70.5%	21.5%	4.5%	2.4%	1.2%	29.5%
Estimated population[b]	90,775,040	27,683,168	5,794,151	3,090,214	1,545,107	37,983,882
Alcohol hangover[e]						
NSWHS	77.3%	17.7%	3.6%	1.3%	0.1%	22.7%
Average prevalence[a]	77.3%	17.7%	3.6%	1.3%	0.1%	22.7%
Estimated population[b]	99,530,647	22,790,329	4,635,321	1,673,866	128,759	29,228,275

Note. The National Survey of Workplace Health and Safety (NSWHS; *N* = 2,783) was conducted during 2002–2003. The National Epidemiologic Survey on Alcohol and Related Conditions (NESARC; *N* = 25,026) was conducted during 2001–2002. The National Survey on Drug Use and Health (NSDUH; *N* = 46,271) was conducted during 2002–2003. The National Comorbidity Survey Replication (NCS-R; *N* = 3,590) was conducted during 2001–2003. All prevalence estimates are weighted using the appropriate sampling weights for each study.

[a]The average prevalence represents the weighted average across studies providing information for a given dimension of alcohol use or impairment. [b]The estimated population sizes were based on an overall estimate of 128,758,922 workers in the U.S. workforce during 2001–2003. This overall estimate is the average population based on estimates from the NSDUH (130,049,648), NESARC (129,479, 153), and NSWHS (126,747,965). The NCS-R weights were not scaled to reflect the population size. [c]*Heavy alcohol use* refers to drinking 5 or more drinks in a single day. [d]*Alcohol intoxication* refers to drinking enough to feel intoxicated or drunk. Effects include slurred speech, being unsteady on one's feet, or blurred vision. [e]*Alcohol hangover* refers to drinking enough to feel a hangover after stopping drinking or the next day.

TABLE 1.4

Amount of Alcohol Consumed per Average Drinking Day During
the Past 12 Months Among Those Who Drink at Least 1 Day per Month

Alcohol quantity: No. drinks per drinking day	Prevalence (% or M)					Estimated population total[b]
	NSWHS	NESARC	NSDUH	NCS-R	Average[a]	
1	27.9%	22.2%	28.7%	24.0%	26.7%	19,492,685
2	31.9%	33.5%	29.8%	30.4%	30.9%	22,558,949
3	17.2%	17.8%	16.3%	17.4%	16.8%	12,265,060
4	7.6%	8.7%	8.2%	8.4%	8.4%	6,132,530
5	6.6%	4.6%	4.7%	5.1%	4.7%	3,431,296
6	5.0%	6.9%	5.5%	8.9%	6.0%	4,383,378
7+	3.8%	6.3%	6.7%	5.7%	6.4%	4,672,403
M	2.8	3.2	3.0	3.3	3.0	

Note. The National Survey of Workplace Health and Safety (NSWHS; $N = 2,783$) was conducted during 2002–2003. The National Epidemiologic Survey on Alcohol and Related Conditions (NESARC; $N = 25,026$) was conducted during 2001–2002. The National Survey on Drug Use and Health (NSDUH; $N = 46,271$) was conducted during 2002–2003. The National Comorbidity Survey Replication (NCS-R; $N = 3,590$) was conducted during 2001–2003. All prevalence estimates are weighted using the appropriate sampling weights for each study.
[a]The average percentage or mean is the weighted mean across studies. [b]The estimated population sizes for employees drinking at least 1 day per month were based on an overall estimate of 73,006,309 workers in the U.S. workforce during 2001–2003. This overall estimate was derived from the population totals reported in Table 1.3 for employees who drink at least 1 day per month.

not shown for the NSDUH because this survey used a different set of definitions. Nonetheless, the NSDUH data must be addressed because they are widely cited among substance use researchers and used by policymakers. In the NSDUH, binge drinking is defined as drinking 5 or more drinks on the same occasion at least 1 day in the past 30 days. An occasion means at the same time or within a few hours of one another. The prevalence rate for binge drinking in the prior month was 27.7% in the NSDUH. In contrast, when data averaged across the NSWHS and NESARC are used (see Table 1.3), the prevalence of drinking 5 or more drinks in a day at least monthly is 15.0%. The NSDUH estimate may be 12.7 percentage points higher because the survey focused on alcohol use for just the prior month. That is, some individuals who drink 5 or more drinks per occasion less than monthly may be captured in a given month during data collection in the NSDUH. These individuals are then labeled as binge drinkers even though there may be no consistent pattern of binging over a longer time frame. Finally, the NSDUH defines heavy drinking as 5 or more days of binge drinking during the past 30 days. Using data averaged across the NSWHS and NESARC surveys on heavy alcohol use (i.e., consuming 5 or more drinks per day) during the past 12 months, one can obtain an estimate of NSDUH monthly heavy drinking by looking at the prevalence of workers reporting heavy alcohol use 1 or more days per week during the prior 12 months. The prevalence of monthly heavy drinking was 8.5% in the NSDUH and 9.3% from the combined NSWHS and NESARC studies. The greater consistency between the NSDUH estimate for heavy drinking and the NSWHS and NESARC averaged estimate might be due to the fact that individuals drinking at these levels are likely to do so chronically. Therefore, an estimate of the prevalence of heavy drinking (as defined in the NSDUH) for the past month may reasonably reflect the estimated prevalence over a longer 12-month time span.

Workforce Alcohol Impairment

The overall 12-month prevalence rates for drinking to intoxication and experiencing a hangover are shown in Table 1.3. Drinking to intoxication was reported by 29.5% of the workforce (38.0 million workers), with 26.0% (33.5 million workers) drinking to intoxication infrequently and 3.6% (4.6 million workers) drinking to intoxication frequently. Experiencing a hangover was reported by 22.7% of the workforce (29.2 million workers), with 21.3% (27.4 million workers) experiencing a hangover infrequently and 1.4% (1.8 million workers) experiencing a hangover frequently.

Workforce Alcohol Abuse and Dependence

Table 1.5 presents 12-month prevalence rates for alcohol abuse or alcohol dependence based on DSM–IV–TR criteria (see Exhibits 1.1 and 1.2). As shown in this table, during a 12-month period, 5.4% of the workforce (6.9 million workers) may have an alcohol abuse disorder and 3.9% (5.0 million workers) may have an alcohol dependence disorder. Overall, 9.3% of

TABLE 1.5
Prevalence Estimates for *DSM–IV–TR* Alcohol Use Disorders
in the Workforce During the Past 12 Months

Study	No disorder	Alcohol abuse	Alcohol dependence	Either disorder
NESARC	89.7%	6.0%	4.3%	10.3%
NSDUH	90.8%	5.4%	3.9%	9.2%
NCS-R	96.3%	2.1%	1.5%	3.7%
Average prevalence[a]	90.7%	5.4%	3.9%	9.3%
Estimated population[b]	116,784,342	6,952,982	5,021,598	11,975,580

Note. The National Epidemiologic Survey on Alcohol and Related Conditions (NESARC; *N* = 25,026) was conducted during 2001–2002. The National Survey on Drug Use and Health (NSDUH; *N* = 46,271) was conducted during 2002–2003. The National Comorbidity Survey Replication (NCS-R; *N* = 3,590) was conducted during 2001–2003. All prevalence estimates are weighted using the appropriate sampling weights for each study. *DSM–IV–TR* = *Diagnostic and Statistical Manual of Mental Disorders* (4th ed., text revision). [a]The average prevalence is the weighted average of estimates across relevant studies. [b]The estimated population sizes were based on an overall estimate of 128,758,922 workers in the U.S. workforce during 2001–2003. See note in Table 1.3 for more details.

the workforce (12.0 million workers) may have either an alcohol abuse or an alcohol dependence disorder.

Workforce Illicit Drug Use

Table 1.6 shows the 12-month prevalence of illicit drug use by specific type of drugs. As shown in this table, marijuana is by far the most prevalent drug used by U.S. employees. With the exception of the estimated prevalence of 5.2% for narcotic analgesic use in the NSDUH, the overall prevalence of use of the other classes of drugs is low among employed adults.

TABLE 1.6

Prevalence of Illicit Drug Use by Type of Drug in the Workforce During the Past 12 Months

Illicit drug use and study	Prevalence
Marijuana	
NSWHS	11.1%
NSDUH	12.1%
NCS-R	11.0%
Cocaine	
NSWHS	1.0%
NSDUH	2.8%
NCS-R	1.8%
Inhalants	
NSDUH	0.5%
Hallucinogens	
NSDUH	1.9%
Heroin	
NSDUH	0.1%
Sedatives	
NSWHS	1.1%
NSDUH	0.4%
Tranquilizers	
NSWHS	1.4%
NSDUH	2.3%
Stimulants	
NSWHS	2.1%
NSDUH	1.2%
Narcotic analgesics	
NSWHS	2.3%
NSDUH	5.2%

Note. The National Survey of Workplace Health and Safety (NSWHS; $N = 2,783$) was conducted during 2002–2003. The National Survey on Drug Use and Health (NSDUH; $N = 46,271$) was conducted during 2002–2003. The National Comorbidity Survey Replication (NCS-R; $N = 3,590$) was conducted during 2001–2003. All prevalence estimates are weighted using the appropriate sampling weights for each study. Data from the National Epidemiologic Survey on Alcohol and Related Conditions (NESARC) are not reported because there is evidence that it substantially underestimated the 12-month use of marijuana, the most frequently used illicit drug. The marijuana prevalence estimate from the NESARC is 4.5%, which is less than half the size of the estimates from the other three studies. Including the NESARC estimate would lead to underestimates of the use of marijuana, illicit drugs, and any illicit drug use. The principal investigator of the NESARC recognizes this issue and does not know why the estimate is so low (B. G. Grant, personal communication, August 3, 2007).

Table 1.7 shows the overall 12-month prevalence rates for the use of illegal drugs, illicit use of prescription drugs, and any illicit use of drugs. Using an illegal drug was reported by 12.9% of the workforce (16.6 million workers), with 7.2% (9.3 million workers) reporting infrequent use and 5.6% (7.2 million workers) reporting frequent use. Illicitly using a prescription drug was reported by 6.5% of the workforce (8.4 million workers), with 4.8% (6.2 million workers) reporting infrequent use and 1.7% (2.1 million workers) reporting frequent use. Any illicit use of drugs was reported by 15.9% of the workforce (20.5 million workers), with 9.3% (12.0 million workers) reporting infrequent use and 6.3% (8.1 million workers) reporting frequent use. Finally, the data in Table 1.7 show that the use of illegal drugs, which largely represents marijuana use (see Table 1.6), is more prevalent than the illicit use of prescription drugs.

Workforce Illicit Drug Impairment

Prevalence rates for reported intoxication (i.e., getting high) from the use of illegal drugs, illicit use of prescription drugs, and any illicit use of drugs are shown in Table 1.8. As shown in this table, only one study asked directly about using drugs to the point of being intoxicated. Being intoxicated by an illegal drug was reported by 10.4% of the workforce (13.4 million workers), with 7.2% (9.3 million workers) reporting infrequent intoxication and 3.2% (4.1 million workers) reporting frequent intoxication. Being intoxicated by an illicitly used prescription drug was reported by 2.2% of the workforce (2.8 million workers), with 1.6% (2.1 million workers) reporting infrequent intoxication and 0.6% (0.8 million workers) reporting frequent intoxication. Being intoxicated by any illicit use of drugs was reported by 11.0% of the workforce (14.2 million workers), with 7.5% (9.7 million workers) reporting infrequent intoxication and 3.5% (4.5 million workers) reporting frequent intoxication. Finally, the data in Table 1.8 show that intoxication from the use of illegal drugs is more prevalent than intoxication from the illicit use of prescription drugs.

Workforce Illicit Drug Abuse and Dependence

Table 1.9 presents 12-month prevalence rates for drug abuse or drug dependence based on *DSM–IV–TR* criteria (also see Chapter 3 for overall prevalence rates of substance use disorders for specific substances). For the use of illegal drugs, 0.9% of the workforce (1.2 million workers) may have a drug abuse disorder, 1.0% (1.3 million workers) may have a drug dependence disorder, and 2.0% (2.6 million workers) may have either a drug abuse or a drug dependence disorder. For the illicit use of prescription drugs, 0.3% of the workforce (0.4 million workers) may have a drug abuse disorder, 0.4% (0.5 million workers) may

TABLE 1.7

Prevalence of Illicit Drug Use in the Workforce During the Past 12 Months: Overall and by Frequency of Use

Dimension of illicit drug use and study		Frequency of illicit drug use				
	Never	Less than monthly	1–3 days per month	1–2 days per week	3 or more days per week	Overall prevalence
Use of illegal drugs[a]						
NSWHS	88.8%	5.8%	2.1%	1.0%	2.3%	11.2%
NSDUH	86.9%	4.6%	2.6%	2.3%	3.5%	13.1%
NCS-R	88.3%	5.3%	1.9%	1.5%	2.9%	11.7%
Average prevalence[b]	87.1%	4.7%	2.5%	2.2%	3.4%	12.9%
Estimated population[c]	112,149,021	6,051,669	3,218,973	2,832,696	4,377,803	16,609,901
Illicit use of prescription drugs[d]						
NSWHS	95.2%	2.6%	0.8%	0.5%	0.9%	4.8%
NSDUH	93.1%	3.7%	1.4%	1.1%	0.6%	6.8%
NCS-R	97.2%	2.0%	0.6%	0.2%	0.1%	2.8%
Average prevalence[b]	93.5%	3.5%	1.3%	1.1%	0.6%	6.5%
Estimated population[c]	120,389,592	4,506,562	1,673,866	1,416,348	772,553	8,369,330
Any illicit use of drugs[e]						
NSWHS	86.1%	6.9%	2.5%	1.2%	3.2%	13.9%
NSDUH	83.7%	6.2%	3.2%	2.9%	3.7%	16.3%
NCS-R	87.3%	5.9%	2.2%	1.6%	3.0%	12.7%
Average prevalence[b]	84.1%	6.2%	3.1%	2.7%	3.6%	15.9%
Estimated population[c]	108,286,253	7,983,053	3,991,526	3,476,490	4,635,321	20,472,669

Note. The National Survey of Workplace Health and Safety (NSWHS; $N = 2,783$) was conducted during 2002–2003. The National Survey on Drug Use and Health (NSDUH; $N = 46,271$) was conducted during 2002–2003. The National Comorbidity Survey Replication (NCS-R; $N = 3,590$) was conducted during 2001–2003. All prevalence estimates are weighted using the appropriate sampling weights for each study. Data from the National Epidemiologic Survey on Alcohol and Related Conditions (NESARC) are not reported because there is evidence that it substantially underestimated the 12-month use of marijuana, the most frequently used illicit drug. The marijuana prevalence estimate from the NESARC is 4.5%, which is less than half the size of the estimate from the other three studies. Including the NESARC estimate would lead to underestimates of the use of marijuana, illicit drugs, and any illicit drug use. The principal investigator of the NESARC recognizes this issue and does not know why the estimate is so low (B.G. Grant, personal communication, August 3, 2007). [a]*Use of illegal drugs* refers to the use of marijuana, cocaine, hallucinogens, heroin, or inhalants. [b]The average prevalence is the weighted average of estimates across studies. [c]The estimated population sizes were based on an overall estimate of 128,758,922 workers in the U.S. workforce during 2001–2003. See note in Table 1.3 for more details. [d]*Illicit use of prescription drugs* refers to the use of sedatives, tranquilizers, stimulants, or narcotic analgesics. [e]*Any illicit use of drugs* refers to the use of marijuana, cocaine, hallucinogens, heroin, inhalants, sedatives, tranquilizers, stimulants, or narcotic analgesics.

TABLE 1.8

Prevalence of Illicit Drug Impairment in the Workforce During the Past 12 Months: Overall and by Frequency of Use

Dimension of illicit drug use: NSWHS	Never	Frequency of drug use				Overall prevalence
		Less than monthly	1–3 days per month	1–2 days per week	3 or more days per week	
Intoxication from use of illegal drugs[a]	89.6% 115,367,994	5.4% 6,952,982	1.8% 2,317,661	1.0% 1,287,589	2.2% 2,832,696	10.4% 13,390,928
Intoxication from illicit use of prescription drugs[b]	97.8% 128,758,922	1.3% 1,673,866	0.3% 386,277	0.3% 386,277	0.3% 386,277	2.2% 2,832,696
Intoxication from any illicit use of drugs[c]	89.0% 114,595,441	5.5% 7,081,741	2.0% 2,575,178	1.1% 1,416,348	2.4% 3,090,214	11.0% 14,163,481

Note. For each dimension of illicit drug impairment, the top number is the prevalence of impairment and the bottom number is the estimated population total. The estimated population sizes were based on an overall estimate of 128,758,922 workers in the U.S. workforce during 2001–2003. See note in Table 1.3 for more details. The National Survey of Workplace Health and Safety (NSWHS; $N = 2,783$) was conducted during 2002–2003. All prevalence estimates are weighted using the appropriate sampling weights for the study.
[a]Use of illegal drugs refers to the use of marijuana or cocaine. [b]Illicit use of prescription drugs refers to the use of sedatives, tranquilizers, stimulants, or narcotic analgesics.
[c]Any illicit use of drugs refers to the use of marijuana, cocaine, sedatives, tranquilizers, stimulants, or narcotic analgesics.

TABLE 1.9
Prevalence of Estimates for *DSM–IV–TR* Drug Use Disorders
in the Workforce During the Past 12 Months

Substance and study	No disorder	Drug abuse	Drug dependence	Either disorder
Use of illegal drugs				
NESARC	98.3%	1.2%	0.4%	1.7%
NSDUH	97.7%	0.8%	1.4%	2.3%
Average prevalence[a]	97.9%	0.9%	1.0%	2.0%
Estimated population[b]	126,054,985	1,158,830	1,287,589	2,575,178
Illicit use of prescription drugs				
NESARC	99.4%	0.4%	0.2%	0.6%
NSDUH	99.2%	0.3%	0.5%	0.8%
Average prevalence[a]	99.3%	0.3%	0.4%	0.7%
Estimated population[b]	127,857,609	386,276	515,035	901,312
Any illicit use of drugs				
NESARC	97.9%	1.5%	0.6%	2.1%
NSDUH	97.2%	1.0%	1.8%	2.8%
NCS-R	98.4%	1.1%	0.5%	1.6%
Average prevalence[a]	97.3%	1.2%	1.4%	2.5%
Estimated population[b]	127,827,819	1,545,107	1,802,625	3,218,973

Note. The National Epidemiologic Survey on Alcohol and Related Conditions (NESARC; *N* = 25,026) was conducted during 2001–2002. The National Survey on Drug Use and Health (NSDUH; *N* = 46,271) was conducted during 2002–2003. The National Comorbidity Survey Replication (NCS-R, *N* = 3,590) was conducted during 2001–2003. All prevalence estimates are weighted using the appropriate sampling weights for each study. *DSM–IV–TR* = *Diagnostic and Statistical Manual of Mental Disorders* (4th ed., text revision). [a]The average prevalence is the weighted average of estimates across relevant studies. [b]The estimated population sizes were based on an overall estimate of 128,758,922 workers in the U.S. workforce during 2001–2003. See note in Table 1.3 for more details.

have a drug dependence disorder, and 0.7% (0.9 million workers) may have either a drug abuse or a drug dependence disorder. For any illicit use of drugs, 1.2% of the workforce (1.5 million workers) may have a drug abuse disorder, 1.4% (1.8 million workers) may have a drug dependence disorder, and 2.5% of the workforce (3.2 million workers) may have a drug abuse or a drug dependence disorder. Finally, the prevalence rate for having an abuse or dependence disorder from the use of illegal drugs is higher than that for having an abuse or dependence disorder from the illegal use of prescription drugs.

International Workforce

Some data exist for overall workforce substance involvement in other countries. On the basis of a large probability sample of the Australian workforce, J. G. Berry, Pidd, Roche, and Harrison (2007) and Pidd et al. (2006) reported that 89.4% of Australian workers used alcohol in the past 12 months and 43.9% drank at levels defined as risky at least once per year. Australian workers who drank during the past year reported the number of drinks they consumed on a typical drinking day as follows: 1 to 2 (48.2%), 3 to 4 (29.3%),

5 to 6 (12.6%), 7 to 9 (6.3%), 11 to 12 (1.7%), and 13 or more (1.9%). Illicit drug use during the prior 12 months was reported by 17.3% of the Australian workforce (Bywood, Pidd, & Roche, 2006), and 4% reported using amphetamines or methamphetamine (Roche, Pidd, Bywood, & Freeman, 2008).

Smith, Wadsworth, Moss, and Simpson (2004), using a large regional probability sample from the United Kingdom, reported that 13.0% of the workforce had used an illicit drug during the preceding 12 months and 7% reported use during the preceding month. Marijuana was the most prevalent drug used (11% of workers), followed by ecstasy (2.5%), amphetamines (2.3%), and cocaine (2.2%).

On the basis of a large probability sample of the workforce in Alberta, Canada (Alberta Alcohol and Drug Abuse Commission, 2003), 81% of Albertan workers reported using alcohol during the preceding 12 months, with 22% reporting alcohol use monthly or less, 40% reporting use 2 to 4 times per month, 13% reporting use 2 to 3 times per week, and 5% reporting use 4 or more times per week. Among Albertan workers who drank during the past year, the number of drinks consumed on a typical drinking day was reported as follows: 1 to 2 (59%), 3 to 4 (27%), 5 to 6 (9%), 7 to 9 (2%), and 10 or more (3%). Illicit drug use during the past 12 months was reported by 10% of Albertan workers. This primarily reflected marijuana use: 10% used marijuana, 1% used cocaine/crack, 1% used hallucinogens, 1% used amphetamines, 1% used narcotic analgesics, and 0.2% reported illicit use of some other drug.

Sterud, Hem, Ekeberg, and Lau (2007) explored the prevalence of hazardous alcohol use among a large national sample of Norwegian ambulance and police personnel. They reported that the prevalence of hazardous alcohol use was 17.7% for male police personnel, 16.6% for male ambulance personnel, 9.1% for female police personnel, and 7.4% for female ambulance personnel. A 2001 Norwegian study reported that 2.7% of employees reported using an illegal drug during the past 12 months (Gjerde et al., 2010).

Using a national sample of German physicians working in hospitals, Rosta (2008) reported that 90.6% drank alcohol during the past year, with 17.6% drinking once per month or less frequently, 31.9% drinking 2 to 4 times per month, 28.6% drinking 2 to 3 times per week, and 12.5% drinking 4 or more times per week. Among German physicians who drank during the past year, 82.6% reported consuming 1 to 2 drinks on a typical drinking day, 14.7% reported consuming 3 to 4 drinks, 2.2% reported consuming 5 to 6 drinks, and 0.5% reported consuming 7 or more drinks. With regard to heavy drinking (5 or more drinks per occasion), 52.5% reported drinking heavily during the past year, with 39.0% doing so less than monthly, 10.7% doing so about monthly, 2.7% doing so about weekly, and 0.1% doing so almost daily or daily.

PREVALENCE OF SUBSTANCE USE AND IMPAIRMENT IN THE WORKPLACE AND AFTER WORK

Given that representative national data exist on the overall prevalence of substance use among workers in the United States and in some other countries, what is known about the prevalence of substance use and impairment in the workplace or after work? Several sources of information have been used to estimate the extent of substance use in U.S. workplaces (Newcomb, 1994). The first source of information comes from samples of substance-using or substance-dependent workers. As noted previously, a common and misleading indirect method used to address the prevalence of workplace substance use is to report the employment rate among substance users. The employment rate among heavy drinkers and illicit drug users provides no actual information on the prevalence of substance use or impairment in the workplace. Even when substance users are asked if they use a substance at work, this information fails to provide an accurate estimate of workplace substance use and impairment. For example, one frequently cited figure comes from a study by Washton and Gold (1987). Based on reports from callers to the National Cocaine Hotline (1-800-COCAINE), Washton and Gold reported that 74% of callers in 1985 said they used cocaine at work. This prevalence rate confirmed Washton and Gold's initial speculation that "if most cocaine users are employed, then there must be a great deal of cocaine and other drug use occurring in the workplace" (p. 19). Although it is true that most cocaine users are employed, Washton and Gold ignored the equally accurate observation that most employees do not use cocaine (see Table 1.6). Given the self-selected sample and the fact that callers were likely to be cocaine dependent, the prevalence rate of 74% represented only the extent of workplace cocaine use among current cocaine users. To obtain an overall estimate of the prevalence of cocaine use in the workplace in 1985, one must multiply the rate reported by Washton and Gold by the overall rate of cocaine use in the employed population in 1985, which was approximately 3% (U.S. Department of Health and Human Services, 1998). Doing so leads to an estimated 12-month prevalence rate for cocaine use at work in 1985 of 2.2% ($.74 \times .03 \times 100$) rather than 74%. But even this estimate is probably high because callers were not representative of all cocaine users in 1985. In general, because samples of substance-using or substance-dependent individuals do not represent all employed individuals, they cannot be used to provide accurate estimates of the extent of illicit drug use and impairment in the workplace for the entire workforce.

The second source of information represents reports of workplace problems by union and management sources. For example, Schreier (1987) reported that 95% of the U.S. employers they surveyed reported that they had to deal with a drug problem among their workers. Such estimates, however, do not actually address the extent of illicit drug use in the workplace across the entire workforce. The reason is that the proportion of workers involved is unknown and may be small within and across these workplaces. For instance, using a national sample of 100 Israeli enterprises with 100 or more employees, Bamberger and Biron (2006) reported that 29% of the firms reported having dealt with at least one employee involved in workplace substance use during a 12-month period. Across all firms, however, there were only 53 cases among a total workforce of 32,500. Thus, the estimated prevalence of Israeli employees showing substance use problems in the workplace was actually 0.16% (53/32,500 × 100).

The third source of information is the proportion of positive drug screens. For example, based on more than 5.5 million urine drug tests conducted on the U.S. workforce during 2009, Quest Diagnostics Incorporated's (2010) Drug Testing Index reported that 3.6% of urine tests were positive for some form of illicit drug use. However, these drug screens cannot provide any information on the context of use (see Chapter 5 for more details). Thus, a positive drug screen primarily represents workforce drug use, not workplace drug use.

The fourth source of data comes from epidemiological surveys of employed adults that directly assess workplace substance use. In contrast to the first three sources of data, properly designed epidemiological surveys offer a more defensible method of obtaining estimates of alcohol and illicit drug use in the workplace—much like their longtime use in the United States and other countries to obtain overall estimates of alcohol and illicit drug use in the general population or workforce. The available epidemiological data on the prevalence of workplace and after work substance involvement are summarized for the United States and other countries.

U.S. Workplace and After Work Substance Involvement

Three reviews conducted in the mid-1990s summarized what was known about the prevalence of workplace substance use and impairment in the United States at that time (Ames, 1993; Newcomb, 1994; Normand et al., 1994). The prevalence rates revealed wide inconsistencies for workplace substance use or impairment, ranging from less than 1% to about 39%. These inconsistencies exist because the studies differed widely on several critical dimensions: (a) the nature and quality of the sample used (general samples vs. samples of specific subgroups; convenience samples vs. random probability samples); (b) the time frame evaluated (past month, past 6 months, past year); (c) the specific substance under investigation (e.g., alcohol, marijuana, cocaine); and (d) the dimension of workplace substance use and impairment assessed (e.g., use just before work, use during lunch, use while working, use during breaks, being at work impaired, or some unspecified combination). After summarizing the meager research on the prevalence of workplace alcohol and illicit drug use, Normand et al. (1994) concluded that there were insufficient credible scientific data regarding the prevalence of workplace alcohol and drug use. In an effort to address this issue, the NSWHS (described previously in the section on workforce substance use) explored the prevalence, frequency, and distribution of workplace and after work alcohol and illicit drug use in a national sample of the U.S. workforce. Relevant results from this study are summarized next.

Workplace and After Work Alcohol Use and Impairment

Table 1.10 provides 12-month prevalence data on workplace alcohol use (i.e., use within 2 hours before work or during the workday), workplace alcohol impairment, and initiation of alcohol use within 2 hours of leaving work. Table 1.11 provides information on the amount of alcohol consumed before work, during the workday, and after work. As shown in Table 1.10, alcohol use before work was reported by 1.7% of the workforce (2.2 million workers), with 1.6% (2.1 million workers) reporting doing so infrequently (less than weekly) and 0.1% (0.1 million workers) reporting doing so frequently (1 or more days per week). Table 1.11 shows that among those who drink before work, 66.7% (1.5 million workers) reported having 1 drink, 22.6% (0.5 million workers) reported having 2 drinks, and 10.7% (0.2 million workers) reported having 3 or more drinks.

Table 1.10 shows that alcohol use during the workday was reported by 7.0% of the workforce (9.0 million workers), with 6.1% (7.8 million workers) reporting doing so infrequently and 0.9% (1.2 million workers) reporting doing so frequently. The separate prevalence rates for alcohol use during work breaks, during lunch, and while working reveal that alcohol use during the workday primarily occurs during lunch breaks. Among those who drink during the workday, Table 1.11 shows, 77.7% (7.0 million workers) reported having 1 drink, 13.1% (1.2 million workers) reported having 2 drinks, and 9.3% (0.9 million workers) reported having 3 or more drinks. Any workplace alcohol use (see Table 1.10) was reported by 8.0% of the workforce (10.3 million workers), with 7.0% (9.0 million workers) reporting infrequent use and 1.0% (1.3 million workers) reporting frequent use.

Workplace impairment (intoxication or hangover) due to alcohol use was reported by 10.1% of the workforce (13.0 million workers), with 9.3% (12.0 million workers) experiencing impairment infrequently and 0.8% (1.0 million workers) experiencing impairment frequently. It is clear from Table 1.10 that employee alcohol impairment at work is primarily due to coming to work with a hangover and less likely due to being under the direct

TABLE 1.10
Prevalence of Alcohol Use and Impairment in the Workplace and Alcohol Use After Work During the Past 12 Months: Overall and by Frequency of Use (NSWHS)

Dimension of work-related alcohol use	Frequency of alcohol use				Overall prevalence
	Never	Less than monthly	1–3 days per month	1 or more days per week	
Workplace alcohol use					
Before work[a]	98.3% 126,570,020	1.2% 1,545,107	0.4% 515,036	0.1% 128,759	1.7% 2,188,902
During the workday[b]	93.0% 119,745,797	4.4% 5,665,393	1.7% 2,188,902	0.9% 1,158,830	7.0% 9,013,125
During work breaks	98.9% 127,342,574	0.6% 772,554	0.3% 386,277	0.2% 257,518	1.1% 1,416,348
During lunch	94.1% 121,162,146	3.7% 4,764,080	1.5% 1,931,384	0.7% 901,312	5.9% 7,596,776
While working	98.1% 126,312,502	1.0% 1,287,589	0.5% 643,795	0.4% 515,036	1.9% 2,446,420
Any workplace use[c]	92.0% 118,458,208	5.2% 6,695,464	1.8% 2,317,661	1.0% 1,287,589	8.0% 10,300,714
Workplace alcohol impairment[d]					
Being high on or under the influence of alcohol at work	98.3% 126,570,020	1.0% 1,287,589	0.4% 515,036	0.3% 386,277	1.7% 2,188,902
Hangover at work	90.9% 117,041,860	7.3% 9,399,401	1.3% 1,673,866	0.5% 643,795	9.1% 11,717,062
Any workplace impairment[d]	89.9% 115,754,271	7.7% 9,914,437	1.6% 2,060,143	0.8% 1,030,071	10.1% 13,004,651
Any workplace use or impairment[e]	84.8% 109,187,566	10.7% 13,777,205	2.9% 3,734,009	1.6% 2,060,143	15.2% 19,571,356
After work alcohol use[f]	62.3% 80,216,808	13.1% 16,867,419	11.9% 15,322,312	12.8% 16,481,142	37.8% 48,670,873

Note. The National Survey of Workplace Health and Safety (NSWHS; N = 2,783) was conducted during 2002–2003. All prevalence estimates are weighted. For each dimension of workplace alcohol use or impairment, the top number is the prevalence of use or impairment and the bottom number is the estimated population total. The estimated population sizes were based on an overall estimate of 128,758,922 workers in the U.S. workforce during 2001–2003. See note in Table 1.3 for more details. [a]*Alcohol use before work* means within 2 hours of starting work. [b]*Alcohol use during the workday* includes use during work breaks, lunch, or while working. [c]*Any workplace use* includes use during the workday or before work. [d]*Any workplace impairment* includes being at work under the influence of alcohol or with a hangover. [e]*Any workplace use or impairment* includes any workplace use or any workplace impairment. [f]*Alcohol use after work* represents initiation of drinking within 2 hours of leaving work.

TABLE 1.11
Amount of Alcohol Consumed Before Work, During the Workday, and After Work During the Past 12 Months Among Those Who Drink in Each Context (NSWHS)

Alcohol quantity: No. drinks per drinking occasion	Use before work	Use during the workday	Use after work
1	66.7%	77.7%	48.0%
	1,459,998	7,003,198	23,362,019
2	22.6%	13.1%	32.6%
	494,692	1,180,719	15,866,705
3/3 or more	10.7%	9.3%	13.8%
	234,213	883,221	6,716,580
4			2.8%
			1,362,784
5 or more			2.8%
			1,362,784

Note. The National Survey of Workplace Health and Safety (NSWHS; $N = 2,783$) was conducted during 2002–2003. All estimates are weighted. For each number of drinks per drinking occasion, the top number is the prevalence in each context and the bottom number is the estimated population total. The estimated overall population of employees drinking in each context was 2,188,902 for alcohol use before work, 9,013,125 for alcohol use during the workday, and 48,670,873 for alcohol use after work (see Table 1.10).

influence of alcohol at work. Combining across workplace alcohol use and impairment during the past year, 15.2% of the workforce (19.6 million) reported any alcohol involvement in the workplace, with 13.6% (17.5 million workers) reporting infrequent workplace alcohol involvement and 1.6% (2.1 million workers) reporting frequent workplace alcohol involvement.

Finally, Table 1.10 shows the prevalence of U.S. workers who engage in alcohol use within 2 hours of leaving work. Drinking after work was reported by 37.8% of the workforce (48.7 million workers), with 25.0% (32.2 million workers) reporting doing so infrequently and 12.8% (16.5 million workers) reporting doing so frequently. Among those who begin drinking shortly after work, Table 1.11 shows, 48.0% (23.4 million workers) reported having 1 drink, 32.6% (15.9 million workers) reported having 2 drinks, 13.8% (6.7 million workers) reported having 3 drinks, 2.8% (1.4 million workers) reported having 4 drinks, and 2.8% (1.4 million workers) reported having 5 or more drinks.

Workplace and After Work Illicit Drug Use and Impairment

Table 1.12 provides 12-month prevalence data on workplace illicit drug use (i.e., use within 2 hours before work or during the workday), workplace illicit drug impairment, and initiation of illicit drug use within 2 hours of leaving work. As shown in Table 1.12, illicit drug use before work was reported by 2.7% of the workforce (3.5 million workers), with 1.2% (1.5 million

TABLE 1.12

Prevalence of Illicit Drug Use and Impairment in the Workplace and Illicit Drug Use After Work During the Past 12 Months: Overall and by Frequency of Use (NSWHS)

Dimension of work-related illicit use of drugs	Never	Frequency of substance use			Overall prevalence
		Less than monthly	1–3 days per month	1 or more days per week	
Workplace illicit use of drugs					
Before work[a]	97.3% 125,282,431	0.8% 1,030,071	0.4% 515,036	1.5% 1,931,384	2.7% 3,476,491
During the workday[b]	97.6% 125,668,708	0.7% 901,312	0.3% 386,277	1.4% 1,802,625	2.4% 3,090,214
During work breaks	98.8% 127,213,815	0.3% 901,312	0.2% 386,277	0.7% 901,312	1.2% 1,545,107
During lunch	98.2% 126,441,261	0.5% 643,795	0.1% 257,518	1.2% 1,545,107	1.8% 2,317,661
While working	98.3% 126,570,020	0.6% 772,554	0.2% 128,759	0.9% 1,158,830	1.7% 2,188,902
Any workplace use[c]	96.9% 124,767,395	0.9% 1,158,830	0.5% 257,518	1.7% 1,158,830	3.1% 2,188,902
Workplace illicit drug impairment					
Being high on or under the influence of illicit drugs at work	97.2% 125,153,672	1.0% 1,287,589	0.7% 643,795	1.2% 2,188,902	2.8% 3,991,527
Any workplace use or impairment[d]	96.7% 124,509,878	0.9% 1,158,830	0.6% 901,312	1.8% 1,545,107	3.3% 3,605,250
After work illicit drug use[e]	94.3% 121,419,663	2.0% 2,575,178	1.1% 772,554	2.6% 2,317,661	5.7% 4,249,044

Note. The National Survey of Workplace Health and Safety (NSWHS; *N = 2,783*) was conducted during 2002–2003. All prevalence estimates are weighted. For each dimension of workplace alcohol use or impairment, the top number is the prevalence of use or impairment and the bottom number is the estimated population total. The estimated population sizes were based on an overall estimate of 128,758,922 workers in the U.S. workforce during 2001–2003. See note in Table 1.3 for more details. [a]*Illicit drug use before work* means any use of illicit drugs within 2 hours of starting work. [b]*Illicit drug use during the workday* includes any use of illicit drugs during work breaks, during lunch, or while working. [c]*Any workplace use* includes any use of illicit drugs during the workday or before work. [d]*Any workplace use or impairment* includes any workplace use or workplace impairment. [e]*After work illicit drug use* means any use of illicit drugs initiated within 2 hours of leaving work.

workers) reporting doing so infrequently and 1.5% (1.9 million workers) reporting doing so frequently. Illicit drug use during the workday was reported by 2.4% of the workforce (3.1 million workers), with 1.0% (1.3 million workers) reporting doing so infrequently and 1.4% (1.8 million workers) reporting doing so frequently. The separate prevalence rates for illicit drug use during work breaks, during lunch, and while working reveal that illicit drug use during the workday occurs roughly throughout the workday. Any workplace illicit drug use during the past year was reported by 3.1% of the workforce (4.0 million workers), with 1.4% (1.8 million workers) reporting doing so infrequently and 1.7% (2.2 million workers) reporting doing so frequently. Workplace impairment due to illicit drug use was reported by 2.8% of the workforce (3.6 million workers), with 1.7% (2.2 million workers) experiencing infrequent workplace impairment and 1.2% (1.5 million workers) experiencing frequent workplace impairment. Combining across illicit drug use and impairment, 3.3% of the workforce (4.2 million workers) reported illicit drug involvement in the workplace, with 1.5% (1.9 million workers) reporting infrequent workplace illicit drug involvement and 1.8% (2.3 million workers) reporting frequent workplace illicit drug involvement. Illicit drug use soon after leaving work was reported by 5.7% of the workforce (7.3 million workers), with 3.1% (4.0 million workers) reporting doing so infrequently and 2.6% (3.3 million workers) reporting doing so frequently.

Finally, Table 1.13 shows the breakdown of type of illicit drug use by workplace context. With regard to the use of illicit drugs, only marijuana use is shown because there were too few cocaine users to report separate estimates. Similarly, only the overall prevalence of illicit use of prescription drugs is shown because there were too few users when tranquilizers, sedatives, stimulants, and narcotic analgesics were considered separately. As shown in Table 1.13, the prevalence rates for marijuana and illicit prescription drug use are low across the various contexts. In terms of patterns, the prevalence of marijuana use and the prevalence of illicit prescription drug use were similar before work, during the workday, and for any workplace use, though marijuana was somewhat more likely to be used than prescription drugs after work.

International Workplace and After Work Substance Involvement

Some data from Israel, Australia, Canada, and New Zealand exist on substance use in the workplace and after work. On the basis of reports from 100 Israeli employers with a total workforce of 32,500 employees, Bamberger and Biron (2006) reported a 12-month prevalence rate for workplace substance use (alcohol or drugs) problems of 0.16%.

Pidd et al. (2006) summarized several published and unpublished findings on Australian workers. Among 337 Australian urban train drivers, 3.1% drank

TABLE 1.13
Prevalence of Illicit Drug Use in the Workplace and After Work
During the Past 12 Months by Type of Drug (NSWHS)

Context of use of work-related illicit use of drugs	Marijuana	Prescription drugs[a]
Before work[b]	1.4%	1.5%
	1,802,625	1,931,383
During the workday[c]	1.2%	1.3%
	1,545,107	1,673,866
Any workplace use[d]	1.6%	1.8%
	2,060143	2,317,660
After work[e]	4.5%	2.0%
	5,794,151	2,575,178

Note. The National Survey of Workplace Health and Safety (NSWHS; N = 2,783) was conducted during 2002–2003. All prevalence estimates are weighted. For each context of illicit drug use, the top number is prevalence of using a specific substance and the bottom number is the estimated population total. The estimated population sizes were based on an overall estimate of 128,758,922 workers in the U.S. workforce during 2001–2003. See note in Table 1.3 for more details.
[a]Illicit use of prescription drugs refers to the use of sedatives, tranquilizers, stimulants, or narcotic analgesics. [b]Illicit drug use before work means within 2 hours of starting work. [c]Illicit drug use during the workday includes use during work breaks, during lunch, or while working. [d]Any workplace illicit drug use includes use during the workday or before work. [e]Illicit drug use after work represents initiation of illicit drug use within 2 hours of leaving work.

within 3 hours of coming to work and 2% drank during actual work hours. Among 4,193 Australian police officers, 26% reported occasional drinking at work and 48% reported drinking with colleagues after work. Among 319 Australian construction apprentices, 29.3% drank during work hours, with 26.7% doing so less than weekly and 2.6% doing so at least weekly. Further, 72.1% of construction apprentices reported drinking after work but before they went home, with 51.7% reporting doing so less than weekly and 20.4% reporting doing so at least weekly. A regional study of 1,200 Australian workers found that 4% reported drinking at work. Finally, using data from a large probability sample of the Australian workforce, Bywood et al. (2006) reported that 2.5% reported going to work under the influence of illicit drugs during the past 12 months.

A study of the workforce in Alberta, Canada (Alberta Alcohol and Drug Abuse Commission, 2003; N = 2,836) found that during the past 12 months, 4.0% of workers reported drinking alcohol within 4 hours of coming to work, with 4.0% reporting doing so less than weekly and 1.3% reporting doing so weekly (in this report, the percentages across frequency of use add up to more than the reported overall prevalence). Also, 11.0% of Albertan workers reported drinking while at work, with 9.0% reporting doing so less than weekly and 2.3% reporting doing so weekly. In the same study of Albertan workers, 2.0% of workers reported using an illicit drug within 4 hours of coming to work, with 1.2% reporting doing so less than weekly and

0.7% reporting doing so weekly. Illicit drug use while at work was reported by 1.0% of the workforce, with 0.6% reporting doing so less than weekly and 0.5% reporting doing so weekly.

Population research shows that of New Zealanders (ages 12–65), 26.0% reported consuming some alcohol at their workplace and 0.5% reported heavy drinking (more than 6 drinks on an occasion for men and more than 4 drinks on an occasion for women) at their workplace during the past year (Ministry of Health, 2007). However, it is not clear whether this alcohol consumption occurred at a work-sponsored social event or during the workday. Also, 9.5% of New Zealanders (ages 16–64) reported that they worked while feeling under the influence of alcohol (Ministry of Health, 2009).

DEMOGRAPHIC DISTRIBUTION OF SUBSTANCE USE AND IMPAIRMENT IN THE WORKFORCE AND WORKPLACE

The prevalence rates for employee substance use presented so far might be taken as applying to all groups of workers and employers. For example, in Table 1.10 it was reported that the 12-month prevalence of any workplace alcohol use or impairment in the United States was 15.2%. However, this does not mean that 15.2% of employees in every company engage in these behaviors. Research suggests that the use of psychoactive substances is not distributed uniformly across the workforce or employers. In other words, the prevalence of substance use and impairment may be substantially greater in some segments of the workforce and substantially lower in others. Past research suggests that the prevalence of employee substance use varies across several general and workplace demographic characteristics, but the three most consistent and influential characteristics are gender, age, and occupation (e.g., Frone, 2006a, 2006b; Normand et al., 1994).

Prior research consistently demonstrates that workforce substance use is more common among men than women. Compared with employed women, employed men are more likely to drink and use illicit drugs, use alcohol and illicit drugs more frequently, engage in heavier use, experience intoxication more frequently, or be diagnosed with an alcohol or illicit drug use disorder (i.e., abuse or dependence; e.g., Alberta Alcohol and Drug Abuse Commission, 2003; Bacharach, Bamberger, & Sonnenstuhl, 2002; Bywood et al., 2006; Frone, 2003, 2006b; Frone, Russell, & Barnes, 1996; Frone, Russell, & Cooper, 1995; Hoffmann, Larison, & Sanderson, 1997; Larson et al., 2007; Mazas et al., 2006; R. S. Moore, Cunradi, Duke, & Ames, 2009; Newcomb, 1994; Pidd et al., 2006; Roche & Pidd, 2006; Rosta, 2008; Sterud et al., 2007; Wadsworth, Moss, Simpson, & Smith, 2004). Although fewer studies have examined gender differences in workplace substance use, past research reveals that employed men are more likely than employed women to engage in alcohol and illicit drug use before work and during the workday and to go to work impaired by alcohol or illicit drugs (e.g., Frone, 2003, 2006a, 2006b; Ministry of Health, 2009; Newcomb, 1994; Pidd et al., 2006).

Research on age and substance use among general populations, which include employed and nonemployed individuals, shows that the overall use of alcohol and illicit drug use increases from early adolescence until it peaks and begins to drop during the latter part of early adulthood (e.g., Anthony & Arria, 1999; O'Malley, Johnston, & Bachman, 1999). Little research has explored the relation of age to workforce and workplace substance use among adolescents. But consistent with the broader substance use literature, research has found that the level of workforce and workplace alcohol and illicit drug use increases with age among employed adolescents (Frone, 2003; R. S. Moore et al., 2009). In contrast, several studies of employed adults have consistently shown that alcohol and illicit drug involvement in the workforce and workplace decreases with age (e.g., Alberta Alcohol and Drug Abuse Commission, 2003; Bacharach et al., 2002; Bywood et al., 2006; Frone, 2006a, 2006b; Hoffmann et al., 1997; Larson et al., 2007; Mazas et al., 2006; Roche & Pidd, 2006; Roche, Pidd, Bywood, & Freeman, 2008; Sterud et al., 2007; Wadsworth et al., 2004).

Occupations are made up of clusters of work activities and work environments. Although there are some inconsistencies across studies, prior research generally suggests that heavy alcohol use, illicit drug use, and substance use disorders are more prevalent in the following broad occupation categories: arts/entertainment/sports/media; sales; food preparation and serving/hospitality; construction/extraction; building and grounds maintenance; and transportation and material moving (e.g., Anthony, Eaton, Mandell, & Garrison, 1992; J. G. Berry et al., 2007; Bywood et al., 2006; Frone, 2006a, 2006b; Hoffmann et al., 1996; Larson et al., 2007; Roche, Pidd, Bywood, & Freeman, 2008).

Despite the findings just summarized, the individual relations of gender, age, and occupation to workforce and workplace alcohol and illicit drug use may not tell the whole story. Certain combinations of the three characteristics may be associated with higher levels of workforce and workplace substance involvement than might be expected from their individual relations. For example, although women tend to report lower levels of alcohol and illicit drug use than men do, this does not mean that all women are at a relatively low risk of using these substances. Therefore, it may be more useful to examine the joint influence of these three variables on the prevalence of workforce and workplace substance use in the population of employed adults.

To explore the joint influence of gender, age, and occupation using data from the NSWHS, I created eight groups of employees by crossing gender (men vs. women), age (18–30 vs. 31–65), and occupation (low risk for sub-stance use vs. high risk for substance use). Age was split into two groups—ages 18 to 30 and ages 31 to 65—because the prevalence of illicit drug use and, to some extent, that of heavy drinking tend to drop after age 30. Also, occupations were split into two groups—low risk and high risk—using 22 major occupation groups based on the standard occupation classification (SOC) codes (U.S. Office of Management and Budget, 2000). To classify the 22 occupation groups into high- and low-risk occupations, I used data presented in Hoffmann et al. (1996), as well as additional analyses conducted with the NSWHS (for more details, see Frone, 2006a, 2006b).

The high-risk occupations for alcohol and illicit drug use were simi-lar but not identical. The high-risk occupational groups for alcohol use and impairment were (a) management occupations (management and business/financial operations managers); (b) arts, design, entertainment, sports, and media occupations; (c) food preparation and serving-related occupations; (d) building and grounds cleaning and maintenance occupations; and (e) sales occupations. The remaining 16 major SOC occupation groups were combined into a low-risk occupation category for alcohol use and impair-ment. The high-risk occupation groups for illicit drug use and impairment were (a) legal occupations; (b) arts, design, entertainment, sports, and media occupations; (c) food preparation and serving-related occupations; and (d) building and grounds cleaning and maintenance occupations. The remaining 18 major SOC occupation groups were combined into a low-risk occupation category for illicit drug use.

Table 1.14 presents subgroup prevalence rates for alcohol use and impairment in the workforce, in the workplace, and after work. The prevalence rates in the subgroups were considered *high* if they were at least 50% greater than the prevalence rate for the overall sample and were considered *low* if they were at least 50% smaller than the rate for the overall sample. The high and low prevalence rates are shown in boldface in Table 1.14. Young women in high-risk occupation groups (Group 2) have substantially elevated prevalence rates on three of the five alcohol use variables. Also, women over 30 years old in low-risk occupation groups (Group 3) have substantially lower prevalence rates on three of the five alcohol use variables. With one exception, young men (Groups 5 and 6) have substantially elevated prevalence rates on the workforce and workplace alcohol use variables regardless of being in low- or high-risk occupations. These patterns of results suggest that age and occupa-tional risk influenced rates of alcohol use and impairment among women. In contrast, among men, age but not occupational risk influenced differences in alcohol use.

Table 1.15 presents subgroup prevalence rates for illicit drug use and impairment in the workforce, in the workplace, and after work. As shown in

TABLE 1.14
Prevalence of Alcohol Use and Impairment in the Workforce, in the Workplace, and After Work During the Past 12 Months for Combinations of Gender, Age, and Occupation

Leading risk factor	Heavy alcohol use in the workforce[a]	Alcohol impairment in the workforce[b]	Any workplace alcohol use[c]	Any workplace alcohol impairment[d]	Alcohol use after work[e]
Overall sample	29.3% 37,726,364	33.3% 42,876,721	8.0% 10,300,714	10.1% 13,004,65	37.8% 48,670,873
Group 1 Gender: women Age: 18–30 OCC: low risk	31.8% 3,480,354	46.2% 5,056,363	3.6% 394,002	10.2% 1,116,340	32.0% 3,502,243
Group 2 Gender: women Age: 18–30 OCC: high risk	34.1% 1,712,365	52.2% 2,621,274	13.0% 657,829	22.8% 1,114,924	41.0% 2,058,855
Group 3 Gender: women Age: 31–65 OCC: low risk	12.9% 4,434,844	19.9% 6,841,348	3.7% 1,272,009	2.8% 962,602	30.7% 10,554,240
Group 4 Gender: women Age: 31–65 OCC: high risk	20.5% 2,085,251	28.6% 2,909,179	8.8% 895,132	11.2% 1,139,259	38.0% 3,865,343
Group 5 Gender: men Age: 18–30 OCC: low risk	55.0% 7,789,915	57.5% 8,144,002	7.7% 1,005,607	22.0% 3,115,966	36.3% 5,141,344
Group 6 Gender: men Age: 18–30 OCC: high risk	54.5% 3,017,466	55.7% 3,083,905	22.1% 1,223,596	26.1% 1,445,061	47.5% 2,629,901

(continues)

TABLE 1.14

Prevalence of Alcohol Use and Impairment in the Workforce, in the Workplace, and After Work During the Past 12 Months for Combinations of Gender, Age, and Occupation (*Continued*)

Leading risk factor	Heavy alcohol use in the workforce[a]	Alcohol impairment in the workforce[b]	Any workplace alcohol use[c]	Any workplace alcohol impairment[d]	Alcohol use after work[e]
Group 7 Gender: men Age: 31–65 OCC: low risk	31.8% 11,546,585	29.8% 10,820,385	6.9% 2,505,391	7.4% 2,686,941	40.8% 14,814,487
Group 8 Gender: men Age: 31–65 OCC: high risk	30.4% 3,718,558	28.0% 3,424,987	**18.3%** **2,238,474**	11.5% 1,406,691	49.1% 6,005,960

Note. The National Survey of Workplace Health and Safety (NSWHS; *N* = 2,783) was conducted during 2002–2003. All prevalence estimates are weighted. For each group, the top number is the prevalence of alcohol use or impairment and the bottom number is the estimated population total. Boldface type indicates high and low prevalence rates. The estimated population sizes were based on an overall estimate of 128,758,922 workers in the U.S. workforce during 2001–2003. See note in Table 1.3 for more details. OCC = occupations at low and high risk for alcohol use and impairment. [a]*Heavy alcohol use in the workforce* refers to consuming 5 or more drinks in a day. [b]*Alcohol impairment in the workforce* refers to any reported intoxication or hangover from using alcohol. [c]*Any workplace alcohol use* refers to using any alcohol during the workday (lunch, work breaks, while working) or before work. [d]*Any workplace alcohol impairment* refers to being at work impaired (intoxication or hangover) by the use of alcohol. [e]*Alcohol use after work* represents initiation of alcohol use within 2 hours of leaving work.

TABLE 1.15

Prevalence of Illicit Drug Use and Impairment in the Workforce, in the Workplace, and After Work During the Past 12 Months, for Combinations of Gender, Ages, and Occupation

Leading risk factor	Illicit drug use in the workforce[a]	Illicit drug impairment in the workforce[b]	Any workplace illicit drug use[c]	Any workplace illicit drug impairment[d]	Illicit drug use after work[e]
Overall sample	13.9% 17,897,490	11.0% 14,163,481	3.1% 3,991,527	2.8% 3,605,250	5.7% 7,339,259
Group 1 Gender: women Age: 18–30 OCC: low risk	19.6% 2,599,385	13.2% 1,750,606	2.1% 278,506	0.9% 119,360	5.3% 702,895
Group 2 Gender: women Age: 18–30 OCC: high risk	43.4% 1,173,509	42.6% 1,151,877	10.6% 286,617	11.4% 308,249	25.3% 684,096
Group 3 Gender: women Age: 31–65 OCC: low risk	6.7% 2,717,457	4.9% 1,987,394	0.8% 324,472	0.8% 324,472	2.4% 973,417
Group 4 Gender: women Age: 31–65 OCC: high risk	16.8% 692,208	14.2% 585,081	4.6% 189,533	3.8% 156,571	10.0% 412,029
Group 5 Gender: men Age: 18–30 OCC: low risk	23.6% 3,919,937	19.6% 3,255,541	7.9% 1,312,182	6.8% 1,129,473	8.4% 1,395,232
Group 6 Gender: men Age: 18–30 OCC: high risk	56.7% 1,752,151	37.2% 1,149,560	27.5% 849,809	25.7% 794,185	33.9% 1,047,583

(continues)

TABLE 1.15
Prevalence of Illicit Drug Use and Impairment in the Workforce, in the Workplace, and After Work During the Past 12 Months, for Combinations of Gender, Ages, and Occupation (Continued)

Leading risk factor	Illicit drug use in the workforce[a]	Illicit drug impairment in the workforce[b]	Any workplace illicit drug use[c]	Any workplace illicit drug impairment[d]	Illicit drug use after work[e]
Group 7					
Gender: men	10.3%	8.8%	**1.5%**	1.7%	4.2%
Age: 31–65	4,694,808	4,011,098	**683,710**	774,871	1,914,388
OCC: low risk					
Group 8					
Gender: men	12.0%	11.1%	2.5%	2.5%	8.4%
Age: 31–65	339,924	314,429	70,817	70,817	237,946
OCC: high risk					

Note. The National Survey of Workplace Health and Safety (NSWHS; *N* = 2,783) was conducted during 2002–2003. All prevalence estimates are weighted. For each group, the top number is the prevalence of illicit drug use or impairment, and the bottom number is the estimated population total. The estimated population sizes were based on an overall estimate of 128,758,922 workers in the U.S. workforce during 2001–2003. See note in Table 1.3 for more details. OCC = occupations at low and high risk for illicit drug use. [a]*Illicit drug use in the workforce* refers to any use of marijuana, cocaine, sedative, tranquilizers, stimulants, or narcotic analgesics. [b]*Illicit drug impairment in the workforce* refers to any reported intoxication from using any of the six types of drugs described above. [c]*Any workplace illicit drug use* refers to using any of the six types of drugs during the workday (lunch, work breaks, while working) or before work. [d]*Any workplace illicit drug impairment* refers to being at work impaired by the use of any of the six drugs mentioned above. [e]*Illicit drug use after work* represents initiation of illicit drug use (see six drugs noted above) within 2 hours of leaving work.

this table, young women in high-risk occupation groups (Group 2) have substantially elevated prevalence rates on all five illicit drug use variables. Also, women over 30 years old in low-risk occupation groups (Group 3) have substantially lower prevalence rates on all five illicit drug use variables. Young men (Groups 5 and 6) have substantially elevated prevalence on the illicit drug use variables, but the prevalence rates are especially high if these young men work in high-risk occupations (Group 6). These patterns of results suggest that age and occupational risk influenced rates of illicit drug use among women. Among men, age and, to a lesser extent, occupational risk influenced differences in the rates of illicit drug use and impairment.

FUTURE RESEARCH

Additional information is needed on the prevalence of workforce and workplace substance involvement in specific occupations. Most high-quality research on the prevalence of workforce and workplace substance involvement is based on national or regional probability samples. Despite the size of such samples, their heterogeneity usually limits the study of employee substance use to broad occupational categories. Exploring the prevalence of workforce, workplace, and after work substance involvement within specific occupations will help focus research on causes and outcomes in those occupations that show the highest risk, which may lead to more focused and effective workplace interventions. Also, research is needed on the prevalence of workforce, workplace, and after work substance involvement in multiple national contexts. Although relatively few detailed data exist on the prevalence of employee substance involvement in the United States, much less is known about such use in other countries. There also is a need for repeated cross-sectional surveys of employee substance use over time in national samples and in specific occupations. Repeated epidemiological surveys targeting the same population (e.g., Firebaugh, 1997) can be used to track changes in the prevalence of employee substance involvement, as well as changes in the demographic characteristics of users.

In the United States, data from the NSDUH provide several decades of information on overall alcohol and illicit drug use in the U.S. workforce. However, no national study in the United States has tracked workplace and after work substance involvement over time. Also, no published research has tracked the prevalence of workforce, workplace, and after work substance involvement outside the United States. The proposed prevalence studies should be broad with regard to the samples and measures used. And it is important to note that making comparisons of prevalence rates across nations, occupations, or time will require using similar methods, definitions, and measures to make such comparisons valid.

Additional prevalence research in specific occupations and national contexts is important because workplace policies are likely to be most successful when developed and implemented in specific and sometimes narrow contexts (Anglin, Caulkins, & Hser, 1993; Reuter, 1993). Moreover, such research may be useful in terms of assessing needs and resource allocation regarding prevention and treatment and evaluating the effectiveness of prevention and treatment interventions (Anglin et al., 1993; Reuter, 1993). As noted by Reuter (1993), "For conscientious policymakers, dealing with drug problems at the national and local levels, prevalence estimation ought to be a fundamental element of sensible decision making, which is impossible without knowing the scale of the drug problem and how it is changing" (p. 167).

GENERAL SUMMARY AND CONCLUSIONS

Alcohol use in the U.S. workforce is prevalent. Approximately three quarters of workers use alcohol at least once during a 12-month period, though frequent alcohol use is reported by only 37.2% of the workforce. On days that workers drink, the average number of drinks consumed was 3. Compared with that of alcohol consumption per se, the prevalence of heavy drinking, impairment, and drinking disorders is much lower. Approximately one quarter of workers reported heavy drinking (5 or more drinks per day), drinking to intoxication, or drinking enough to experience a hangover at least once during a 12-month period. But there is little evidence that heavy drinking and impairment occur frequently—only 9.2% of workers reported consuming 5 or more drinks, 3.6% reported drinking to intoxication, and 1.4% reported drinking enough to experience a hangover 1 or more days per week. Also, only 5.4% of workers may have an alcohol abuse disorder, and only 3.9% may have an alcohol dependence disorder during a 12-month period.

Illicit drug use in the U.S. workforce is not highly prevalent or frequent. Only 15.9% of workers report any illicit drug use, and 6.3% report engaging in any illicit drug use 1 or more days per week. The prevalence of any illicit drug use disorders is low (2.5%). The prevalence of use, impairment, and having a substance use disorder is higher for illegal drugs than for the illicit use of prescription drugs. Also, the use of illegal drugs predominantly reflects the use of marijuana.

Workplace alcohol use is not prevalent. Approximately 92% of the workforce does not report any alcohol use before or during the workday during the past year, and among those who do, it occurs infrequently. The most likely context for workplace alcohol use is during lunch. However, the amount of alcohol consumed during lunch is low (1 to 2 drinks). Reports of alcohol impairment at work during the past year are also rare (89.9% of workers report never being impaired at work) and infrequent (only 0.8% of employees report being under the influence of alcohol or experiencing an alcohol hangover at work 1 or more days per week). Although alcohol use within 2 hours of leaving work during the past year is more prevalent (37.8% of workers), it does not occur frequently, with 12.8% of workers doing so 1 or more days per week.

Workplace illicit drug use during the past year is not prevalent. Approximately 96.7% of the workforce does not report any illicit drug use or impairment before or during the workday. Also, workplace illicit drug use and impairment does not occur frequently—only 1.8% of the workforce reported illicit drug use or impairment at work 1 or more days per week. Illicit drug use within 2 hours of leaving work is also rare—only 5.7% of workers reported doing so during a 12-month period and only 2.6% reported doing so 1 or more days per week. The use of marijuana and the illicit use of prescription drugs before and during the workday were equally prevalent, whereas the use of marijuana was somewhat more prevalent after work.

The prevalence of workforce and workplace substance use is not distributed evenly across the U.S. workforce. For most employers, heavy drinking and illicit drug use in the workforce and workplace should not be a major concern. There are three segments of the workforce in which the prevalence of workforce and workplace substance use and impairment is substantially higher: young men and young women in high-risk occupations and young men in low-risk occupations. However, it is important to put these elevated prevalence rates into perspective. In these three high-risk groups, the proportion of individuals reporting overall alcohol impairment represents 10.7% of the overall U.S. workforce, and the proportion of individuals reporting workplace alcohol impairment represents 4.4% of the overall U.S. workforce. Also, in these three high-risk groups, the proportion of individuals reporting overall illicit drug use represents 5.3% of the overall U.S. workforce, and the proportion of individuals reporting workplace illicit drug use represents 1.9% of the overall U.S. workforce. Nonetheless, these segments of the workforce should be of some concern for those employers whose employees heavily comprise such individuals. Finally, women 30 years of age or older who work in low-risk occupations have the lowest rates of workforce and workplace alcohol and illicit drug use.

The prevalence of national estimates of workforce alcohol and illicit drug use across Australia, the United Kingdom, Norway, Canada, Germany, and the United States were surprisingly similar, given the cultural variation. However, there were differences in the frequency of heavy or risky drinking and in the usual amount of alcohol consumed per day. Discrepancies also existed regarding the prevalence of workplace alcohol and illicit drug use across Israel, Australia, New Zealand, Canada, and the United States.

However, it is difficult to tell if these differences are due to cultural norms, differing demographic makeup of the samples, or differences in the definitions and measurement of workplace alcohol and illicit drug involvement.

Finally, in the United States and other countries, alcohol should be more salient than illicit drugs for employers. For example, in the United States, the use of alcohol in the workforce is more prevalent than any use of illicit drugs. Alcohol intoxication in the workforce is more prevalent than illicit drug intoxication. Alcohol abuse or dependence is more prevalent than illicit drug use or dependence. Also, any workplace alcohol use or impairment is more prevalent than any workplace illicit drug use or impairment.

2

ETIOLOGY OF EMPLOYEE SUBSTANCE INVOLVEMENT

Etiology is the study of causes. So in this chapter, the key question of interest is why do employed individuals use psychoactive substances? The answer to this seemingly simple question is complex and has not yet been fully determined. What is certain though is that the complexity of the answer stems from the fact that there is more than one cause of substance involvement, and the causes are not necessarily homogeneous (e.g., they may differ across users of the same substance; they may differ across different substances for the same user; and they may differ for substance use, impairment, abuse, and dependence). Nonetheless, a starting point for thinking about the potential causes of employee substance involvement comes from an equation in which Lewin (1936) proposed that $B = f(PE)$. That is, behavior (B) is a function (f) of the person (P) and his or her environment (E). This equation is deceptively simple because it represents a general heuristic or perspective. With regard to the causes of employee substance involvement, we need to determine (a) which characteristics of the person are important, (b) which

DOI: 10.1037/13944-003
Alcohol and Illicit Drug Use in the Workforce and Workplace, by M. R. Frone
Copyright © 2013 by the American Psychological Association. All rights reserved.

characteristics of the person's environment are important, and (c) how these person and environmental characteristics combine to influence substance involvement. Further complicating things is the fact that multiple person and environmental characteristics might be in play simultaneously (Frone, 1999; Kraemer, Stice, Kazdin, Offord, & Kupfer, 2001). These issues are explored in this chapter.

CAUSES AND CORRELATES OF WORKFORCE AND WORKPLACE SUBSTANCE INVOLVEMENT

The literature on the possible person and environmental causes of substance use, impairment, abuse, and dependence is too large to summarize in this chapter. Therefore, my goal is to explore three main categories of person characteristics and three main categories of workplace environmental characteristics that are relevant to workforce and workplace substance involvement. The specific categories of person and workplace environmental characteristics are presented in Figure 2.1. Consistent with Lewin's notion that behavior is a function of the person and environment and the idea that person and environmental characteristics can combine to affect behavior, several possible ways that person and workplace environmental characteristics might influence workforce and workplace substance involvement are shown in Figure 2.1.

Lines 1 and 2 collectively show that person and workplace environmental characteristics may have independent and additive (i.e., simultaneous) effects on employee substance involvement. Line 3 shows that person and environmental characteristics may combine to have an interactive or synergistic effect on substance involvement. Multiple person characteristics may interact, multiple workplace characteristics may interact, and person and workplace characteristics may interact to cause employee substance involvement. That is, not everyone who manifests a certain person characteristic will behave in the same way, and not everyone exposed to a similar workplace environment will behave in the same way. An example of a Person × Workplace interaction would be if alcohol use during the workday is more likely to occur when a person has a specific personality disposition (e.g., intolerance of rules) and is exposed to a specific workplace environment (e.g., low levels of supervision). Also, an example of a Workplace Characteristic × Workplace Characteristic interaction would be if the frequency of overall employee marijuana use is elevated among workers who experienced frequent exposure to abusive supervision and exposure to coworkers who support marijuana use. Line 4 refers to a person–environment correlation or effect. For example, people with certain person characteristics (e.g., impulsive, aggressive) may gravitate toward or be

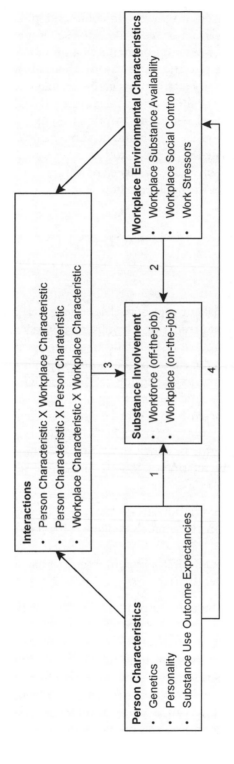

Figure 2.1. Predictors of employee substance use. Adapted from "Predictors of Overall and On-the-Job Substance Use Among Young Workers," by M. R. Frone, 2003, *Journal of Occupational Health Psychology, 8*, p. 41. Copyright 2003 by the American Psychological Association.

selected into certain work environments. In combination, Lines 4 and 2 suggest that certain individuals may be more likely to use substances because they seek out or are exposed to work environments that promote or at least do not inhibit substance use. Despite the various ways that person and workplace environmental characteristics may come together to influence an individual's involvement with alcohol or illicit drugs, most research to date has explored the independent relations of person and workplace environmental characteristics to employee substance involvement. Thus, this chapter primarily summarizes evidence related to Lines 1 and 2. Nonetheless, more complex relations between the person and workplace environment likely exist and are presented when allowed by available research.

PERSON CHARACTERISTICS

Genetics

A person's genetic makeup represents his or her *genotype* and is the most fundamental of person characteristics. The observed physical and behavioral characteristics——broadly defined to include cognition and emotion—of an individual that result from the effects of genotype and environment are called *phenotypes*. For instance, marijuana use and alcohol dependence are examples of specific phenotypes. Genetic theory, when applied to substance involvement, posits that substance use and disorder phenotypes are at least partly a function of a person's genotype (i.e., genetic makeup; e.g., Carey, 2003; Plomin, DeFries, McClearn, & McGuffin, 2008; Posthuma et al., 2003). Researchers exploring the relation of genetic makeup to substance involvement ask two general questions:

1. How much of the variation in substance involvement is due to genetic makeup and how much is due to characteristics of the environment?
2. If the risk for substance involvement is at least partly inherited, which genes confer the risk?

Each of these questions broadly corresponds, respectively, to two general areas of genetics research: quantitative genetics and molecular genetics. Before these two areas of genetics research are explored, it useful to point out that in the effort to document and understand the impact of genetics on human behavior, genetic studies provide some of the most compelling evidence that human behavior, such as substance involvement, results from environmental influences as well as genetic influences. After summarizing the general findings of quantitative and molecular genetics research on substance involvement, I discuss their implications for workforce and workplace substance involvement.

Quantitative Genetics

The general goal of quantitative genetics research is to estimate the overall relative effects of genetics and environments on individual differences in behavioral phenotypes. Two types of studies are conducted to address this issue: twin and adoption studies. In twin studies, concordance in levels of substance involvement is compared across monozygotic (identical) and dizygotic (fraternal) twins who have been raised together (e.g., Foroud, Edenberg, & Crabbe, 2010; Plomin et al., 2008). In contrast, adoption studies compare the substance involvement among adoptees with the same behaviors in their biological parents, who did not raise them, and with the same behaviors in their adoptive (nonbiological) parents, who did raise them (e.g., Agrawal & Lynskey, 2006; Plomin et al., 2008). Adoption studies may also involve comparisons involving twins reared together and apart as well as comparisons involving genetically related siblings and adoptive (genetically unrelated) siblings reared in the same family (e.g., Plomin et al., 2008).

Given certain assumptions, twin and adoption studies provide a general breakdown in terms of the relative contribution of individual differences in genetics (heritability) and individual differences in environmental exposure (*environmentability*; Carey, 2003) to individual differences in substance use and disorders. The contribution of the environment can be further broken down into that due to the shared environment (*shared environmentability*) and that due to the nonshared environment (*nonshared environmentability*). The shared environment refers to all nongenetic influences common to members of a single family that make them similar to one another and different from members of other families. Shared environmental characteristics can include family environment; social class; neighborhood characteristics; schools, and, among twins, the intrauterine environment (Prescott, 2002). In contrast, the nonshared environment refers to all other nongenetic influences unique to individual family members that make them different from one another. For most individuals, the workplace environment would represent one aspect of the nonshared environment.

A number of twin and adoption studies have been completed in several countries (Australia, Finland, Sweden, the Netherlands, the United Kingdom, and the United States). Most of this research has focused on substance use disorders rather than substance use per se, and more studies have focused on alcohol than on illicit drugs. In general, past research and literature reviews looking at individual differences in substance involvement support several findings. First, both genetic makeup and environment play important roles in vulnerability to substance use disorders (abuse and dependence). When one looks at substance use disorders among adults, roughly 50% (ranging from 40% to 60%) of the variability in having an alcohol or illicit drug use disorder is due to genetics and 50% (ranging from 60% to 40%) of such variability is due to the environment. However, the impact of the environment on individual differences in vulnerability to substance use disorders is largely due to the nonshared environment rather than the shared environment (e.g., Agrawal & Lynskey, 2006; Enoch & Goldman, 2002; Foroud et al., 2010; D. Goldman, Oroszi, & Ducci, 2005; Hansell et al., 2008; Heath et al., 1999; Kendler, Myers, & Prescott, 2007; Lachman, 2006; Mustanski, Viken, Kaprio, & Rose, 2003; Neale, Harvey, Maes, Sullivan, & Kendler, 2006; Pagan et al., 2006; Plomin et al., 2008; Prescott, Madden, & Stallings, 2006; Uhl, 2004).

Second, although less research has investigated substance use per se, as with substance use disorders, both genetics and environment play important roles in vulnerability to using alcohol or an illicit substance. The estimates of heritability and environmentability differ widely across these studies depending on the dimension of substance use examined and the specific substances explored. In general, the impact of genetics and environmental characteristics on heavy use of alcohol or drugs looks similar to that for substance use disorders, in that roughly 50% of variation in heavy substance use is due to genetics, roughly 50% of such variation is due to the nonshared environmental characteristics, and the shared environment has little impact (e.g., J. D. Grant et al., 2009; Kendler, Karkowski, Neale, & Prescott, 2000). In contrast, studies exploring whether or not someone has used alcohol or illicit drugs or exploring the usual frequency and quantity of use suggest that, for variation in substance use, roughly 33% to 50% is due to genetics, 33% to 25% is due to the shared environment, and 33% to 25% is due to the nonshared environment. So, unlike that for substance use disorders and heavy substance use, variation in substance use status and usual frequency and quantity of use is affected by the shared environment in addition to the nonshared environment (e.g., Agrawal & Lynskey, 2006; Agrawal et al., 2007; Hansell et al., 2008; Kendler, Gardner, Jacobson, Neale, & Prescott, 2005; Kendler et al., 2000; Lessem et al., 2006; Merikangas, 1990; Neale et al., 2006; Pagan et al., 2006; Swan, Carmelli, & Cardon, 1996; Young, Rhee, Stallings, Corley, & Hewitt, 2006).

Third, the findings summarized here suggest that the familial transmission of heavy substance use and substance use disorders is due primarily to heredity. The other factor that can explain familial transmission of heavy substance use and disorders—the shared family environment—plays little or no role. In contrast, the familial transmission of usual substance use is due both to heredity and to a shared family environment, perhaps because of shared access to substances. Although the nonshared environment cannot explain the familial transmission of substance involvement among family members, it nonetheless plays an important role in substance use and disorders. Later in this chapter, I explore the relation of the work environment, which partly comprises the nonshared environment, to workforce and workplace substance involvement.

Fourth, the research summarized previously shows that genetic makeup has a stronger impact on more severe substance involvement. For example, the impact of genetics on having a substance use disorder is stronger than its impact on merely having used alcohol or an illicit drug or on relatively infrequent use of substances. Fifth, the relative impact of genetics and environment on the risk of having used alcohol or drugs or having an alcohol or illicit drug use disorder is roughly equivalent for men and women (e.g., Ducci & Goldman, 2008; Enoch & Goldman, 2002; Kendler et al., 2007; Plomin et al., 2008; Prescott, 2002; Prescott et al., 2006). Finally, although quantitative genetics studies have shed light on how much of the overall variation in substance use and substance use disorders may be related to heredity, this research does not shed light on which genes play a role in these behaviors. Different research designs are required to do so.

Molecular Genetics

The general goal of molecular genetics research is to identify variation in specific genes or locations on chromosomes that explain variation in specific phenotypes, such as marijuana use or alcohol dependence. Genes can influence various processes related to substance use that increase or decrease the likelihood of heavy consumption or development of a substance use disorder. For example, genes may influence the way in which alcohol and drugs are metabolized or their reward properties. Although it is well established through the twin and adoption studies discussed previously that individual differences in substance involvement have a genetic component, with a few exceptions, the research on links involving specific genes has been largely inconsistent and inconclusive to date (e.g., Buckland, 2001; Science of Genetics Review Group, 2010). The lack of conclusive findings is likely due to a number of methodological challenges that must be overcome (e.g., Baker, 2004; Burmeister, McInnis, & Zöllner, 2008; Carey, 2003; Pearson & Manolio, 2008; Plomin et al., 2008; Romero, Kuivaniemi, Tromp, & Olson, 2002; Uhl, 2004). For example, substance use and disorders are complex phenotypes because they result from the small effects of many genes. Therefore, molecular genetics studies examining substance use and disorders require statistical methods that can detect small effects.

Nonetheless, some progress has been made related to alcohol metabolism and neurotransmitter systems that influence the effects of alcohol. For example, gamma-aminobutyric acid (GABA) is a major neurotransmitter in the brain that mediates several effects of alcohol, such as tolerance, sedation, anxiety reduction, and impaired motor control. Research has discovered that individuals with a specific variant of the GABRA2 gene are more likely to be become dependent on alcohol. The increased risk of alcohol dependence due to genetic effects on GABA and other neurotransmitters is likely due to decreasing sensitivity to the adverse effects of alcohol and increasing sensitivity to its rewarding properties (e.g., Dick & Agrawal, 2008; Foroud et al., 2010; D. Goldman et al., 2005; Hasin & Katz, 2010).

Gene–Environment Interplay

The genetics research summarized so far has assumed that the effects of genetics and environments on substance involvement are independent and additive, as reflected in Figure 2.1, Lines 1 and 2. However, a relatively new focus in genetics research is based on the growing realization that genetic and environmental characteristics work together rather than independently to affect behavior. More generally, this has been labeled gene–environment interplay (e.g., Carey, 2003; Moffitt, Caspi, & Rutter, 2006; Plomin et al., 2008; Rutter, Moffitt, & Caspi, 2006). One important form of interplay between genes and environment is the Gene × Environment (G × E) interaction, which reflects the fact that the effect of genotype on substance involvement may differ across levels of some environmental characteristic or, equivalently, that the effect of an environmental characteristic on substance involvement differs as a function of variation in people's genotype. G × E interaction is portrayed by Line 3 in Figure 2.1.

Both quantitative and molecular genetics research can explore G × E interaction. In quantitative genetics studies, the relation of overall genetic variation to substance involvement can be explored across levels of a specific environmental variable (e.g., Moffitt et al., 2006). For example, research by Agrawal et al. (2010) found that exposure to friends who have high levels of substance use (e.g., social environment) increases the effect of genotype on substance use among young twin women. In contrast, molecular genetics research can (a) test whether a specific environmental characteristic affects the relation between a specific gene and substance involvement or (b) test whether a specific gene can affect the relation between a specific environmental characteristic and substance involvement. For example, Dick et al. (2006) explored the effect of the interaction between variation in the GABRA2 gene (discussed previously) and marital status on alcohol dependence. There was no relation of GABRA2 genotypes to the prevalence of alcohol dependence among unmarried individuals (51% alcohol dependent with the low-risk genotype and 52% alcohol dependent with the high-risk genotype), whereas there was a relation between GABRA2 genotypes and the prevalence of alcohol dependence among married individuals (29% alcohol dependent with the low-risk genotype and 49% alcohol dependent in the high-risk genotype). Thus, the likelihood of being alcohol dependent was lowest among those who were married and who had the low-risk genotype.

The second type of gene–environment interplay is called *gene–environment correlation* (rGE), which represents genetic influences on variation in people's exposure to various types of environments (e.g., Carey, 2003; Plomin et al., 2008; Rutter et al., 2006). The rGE is represented by Line 4 in Figure 2.1 and may help to explain how genes eventually influence substance use and disorders. For example, quantitative genetics research suggests that individual differences in overall genetic makeup are associated with exposure to stressful life events and to substance-using peer groups (e.g., Harden, Hill, Turkheimer, & Emery, 2008; Kendler & Baker, 2007). This type of interplay may seem surprising because environments exist outside the individual, and therefore genes do not directly "code for specific environments" (Kendler & Baker, 2007, p. 624). Rather, the relation of genetic makeup to exposure to various environments may be indirect through "person" phenotypes that result from specific genotypes.

Two sets of person phenotypes that might mediate or explain the influence of genetics on environmental exposures are discussed in more detail next in this chapter—personality and substance use outcome expectancies (i.e., beliefs about the negative and positive effects of substance use). For example, quantitative genetics research suggests that about 40% to 50% of individual variation in various personality traits may be due to genetic influences (e.g., Bouchard, 2004). And molecular genetics research has found that variation in a gene related to serotonin (a neurotransmitter) function is related to higher levels of a personality trait called negative emotionality (i.e., chronic experience of negative mood; Plomin & Caspi, 1999). Further, stress research has found that relative to individuals with low levels of negative emotionality, those with high levels of negative emotionality are more likely to report exposure to negative events in their environment, such as work and family problems, because they either self-select into such environments or create problems because of their behaviors (e.g., Spector, Zapf, Chen, & Frese, 2000). As I discuss later, stressful environments may be related to higher levels of substance involvement among those exposed to them. Taken together, the present discussion of rGE suggests that an indirect path may exist from genes to substance use and disorders through person phenotypes and associated environmental exposures (i.e., Lines 4 and 2 in Figure 2.1).

Relevance of Genetics Research to Workforce and Workplace Substance Use and Disorders

Although the genetics research just summarized is intriguing, the relevance of these findings for workforce and workplace substance use may be unclear. The employment status of individuals in quantitative and molecular genetics studies is rarely provided, but it is likely that a large proportion of the study participants were employed. Thus, the quantitative genetics research regarding the overall effects of heritability and environmentability and the molecular genetics research into the effect of specific genes likely generalize to overall workforce substance involvement. However, because no genetics research on substance use has explicitly explored substance use in the workplace, there is no explicit information on the relative contribution of genetics, shared environment, and nonshared environment to variability in substance use before work, during the workday, and immediately after work. It is possible that the context of use (off the job vs. on the job) may influence the impact of genetics on employee substance use.

Quantitative genetics research also provides compelling evidence that the nonshared environment is just as important as genetic makeup in explaining variation in overall (i.e., workforce) substance use and disorders. Thus, research in quantitative genetics provides support for exploring the link of the work environment to employee substance involvement because the work environment is an important component of the nonshared environment. Genetics researchers, however, have not explicitly explored the role of workplace characteristics in relation to substance use and disorders, despite the fact that most adults spend a large portion of their time in the work environment. Nonetheless, as discussed later in this chapter, other researchers have begun to explore the relation of the work environment to employee substance use, though they have not explicitly considered the independent or joint role of genetics. Finally, although research on gene–environment interplay is just beginning and none of this research has explored specific characteristics of the work environment, the early findings suggest that research on the relation of the work environment to employee substance use should explore the interplay ($G \times E$; rGE) between employee genotypes, work environments, and other person phenotypes that have a documented genetic basis (e.g., personality characteristics, substance use outcome expectancies).

Final Caveats

Before leaving the discussion of genetics, it is important to highlight several general points regarding the interpretation of genetics research. First, the context for the measurement of heritability and environmentability is the population and not the individual (e.g., Agrawal & Lynskey, 2008; Carey,

2003; Plomin et al., 2008). Therefore, heritability and environmentability in a specific individual are undefined. What this means is that although researchers can estimate the proportion of variance in a complex phenotype (e.g., alcohol use or illicit drug dependence) due to heritability and environmentability across members of a population, we cannot know the relative effects of heredity and environment for a specific individual who manifests the same phenotype (e.g., illicit drug use or dependence). Second, it is incorrect and misleading to talk about a gene for substance use or disorders. Substance use and disorders are not the result of a single gene. These phenotypes are complex and multidetermined, which means they result from complex, though often weak, effects of multiple genes (e.g., Plomin et al., 2008; Rutter et al., 2006). Third, heritability does not lead to genetic determinism or essentialism (Dar-Nimrod & Heine, 2011; Plomin et al., 2008). In other words, if an individual's genotype contains a variant of a gene (or genes) that is associated with a higher vulnerability to problematic substance involvement in the population, this does not mean that the individual will necessarily exhibit problematic substance involvement. Fourth, as noted previously, complex behaviors and behavioral disorders are an outcome of the interplay between genetic and environmental influences (Carey, 2003; Plomin et al., 2008). Taken together, these four points suggest that just because genetics plays a role in a specific behavior, it does not follow that little can be done to change the behavior. A person's environment and environmental interventions inside and outside the workplace may alter the impact of heredity (e.g., Plomin et al., 2008).

Personality

Personality represents "the characteristic manner in which one thinks, feels, behaves, and relates to others" (Widiger, Verheul, & van den Brink, 1999, p. 347). As such, personality is composed of various dimensions called *personality traits* that are considered to be relatively stable across time and context, that differ across individuals, and that can affect future behavior. Researchers have assessed many personality traits—in fact, too many to list here. However, taxonomies of personality have been developed that group similar personality traits into a few broad categories (for reviews, see Dindo, McDade-Montez, Sharma, Watson, & Clark, 2009; John & Srivastava, 1999; Kotov, Gamez, Schmidt, & Watson, 2010; Markon, Krueger, & Watson, 2005; McCrae & Costa, 1997). Two prominent taxonomies of adult personality are the five-factor model (i.e., Big Five model) and the three-factor model (i.e., Big Three model). As the name implies, the five-factor model posits that personality comprises five broad traits: neuroticism, extraversion, agreeableness, conscientiousness, and openness. Neuroticism (vs. emotional stability) is the tendency to experience negative emotions (e.g., anger, anxiety, or depression) and general psychological distress. Extraversion (vs. introversion) is the tendency to experience positive emotions and to seek out stimulation and the company of others. Agreeableness (vs. antagonism) is the tendency to be compassionate and cooperative rather than suspicious and antagonistic. Conscientiousness (vs. lack of direction) is the tendency to show self-discipline, act dutifully, and aim for achievement. Openness (vs. closed to experience) is the tendency to appreciate art, adventure, unusual ideas, imagination, and variety of experience.

The three-factor model posits that personality comprises three broad traits: negative emotionality, positive emotionality, and behavioral disinhibition. Negative emotionality and positive emotionality from the three-factor model are essentially the same as neuroticism and extraversion, respectively, from the five-factor model. The third trait in the three-factor model, behavioral disinhibition (vs. constraint), reflects the tendency to focus on short-term incentives and ignore long-term consequences. Research suggests that behavioral disinhibition is related to the five-factor model because it, in part, represents low levels of agreeableness and conscientiousness (e.g., Dindo et al., 2009; Kotov et al., 2010; Markon et al., 2005). Other specific dimensions of personality that reflect the broad trait of behavioral disinhibition include impulsivity, intolerance of rules, and risk-taking propensity.

Based on two theoretical perspectives, the most likely broad personality traits related to substance involvement are neuroticism/negative emotionality and behavioral disinhibition, the latter including low agreeableness and low conscientiousness. The first theoretical perspective represents affect regulation (e.g., Conger, 1956; Cooper, Frone, Russell, & Mudar, 1995; Peirce, Frone, Russell, Cooper, & Mudar, 2000). This perspective posits that individuals use a psychoactive substance because of the substance's ability to reduce negative moods (e.g., depression, anxiety). Because individuals high in neuroticism/negative emotionality experience negative affect more frequently than those low in neuroticism/negative emotionality do, the former individuals are expected to engage in more frequent and heavier use of alcohol and illicit drugs to manage or regulate these negative emotions.

The second theoretical perspective is Gray's (1987; Pickering & Gray, 1999) reinforcement sensitivity theory, which provides a basis for the relation of behavioral disinhibition to substance involvement. Gray proposed that two neurological systems are at the heart of much of our personality and behavior. The role of the behavioral inhibition system (BIS) is to prevent or stop behavior that is expected to result in punishment or loss of reward. In contrast, the role of the behavioral activation system (BAS) is to energize behavior aimed at acquiring rewards or reducing punishment. Thus, individuals with high BIS sensitivity are expected to be more sensitive to cues associated with potential punishments, whereas individuals who are high in BAS sensitivity are expected to be more sensitive to cues associated with potential rewards. Consistent with Gray's theory, research has found that relative to individuals low in BAS sensitivity, individuals high in BAS sensitivity report higher levels of alcohol consumption, alcohol-related problems, and elevated levels of alcohol dependence and are more likely to use illicit drugs (e.g., Franken & Muris, 2006; Lyvers, Czerczyk, Follent, & Lodge, 2009; Pardo, Aguilar, Molinuevo, & Torrubia, 2007). The reason is that high BAS individuals are more sensitive to the potential rewards resulting from substance use and intoxication (e.g., reduced negative moods, increased relaxation). In contrast, relative to individuals low in BIS sensitivity, individuals high in BIS sensitivity report lower levels of alcohol consumption and are less likely to use illicit drugs (e.g., Franken & Muris, 2006; Pardo et al., 2007). The reason for this is that high-BIS individuals are more sensitive to the potential punishments resulting from substance use and intoxication (e.g., hangover, arrest, impaired ability to perform various tasks). Given such findings, individuals who are high in behavioral disinhibition (and low in agreeableness and conscientiousness) are expected to be more likely to use alcohol and illicit drugs because, as discussed previously, behavioral disinhibition reflects the tendency to be sensitive to potential rewards (high BAS sensitivity) and insensitive to potential punishments (low BIS sensitivity).

The expected relations of neuroticism/negative emotionality and behavioral disinhibition to substance involvement have received a fair amount of support. For example, a recent meta-analytic review by Kotov et al. (2010) examined the extent to which the traits from the five-factor model and the trait of behavioral disinhibition from the three-factor model were associated with having a substance use disorder (i.e., diagnosis of abuse or dependence).[1] Kotov et al. reported that higher levels of both neuroticism and behavioral disinhibition were associated with having any substance use disorder, an alcohol use disorder, or a drug use disorder. As noted previously, to the extent that low levels of conscientiousness and agreeableness reflect behavioral disinhibition, it is not surprising that low levels of conscientiousness also were associated with having any substance use disorder, an alcohol use disorder, or a drug use disorder and that low agreeableness was associated with having a drug use disorder. With regard to the other two traits in the five-factor model, there was no evidence that extraversion/positive emotionality or openness to experience were related to having a substance use disorder. Some research suggests that the relation of personality to substance use disorders is causal (e.g., Sher, Bartholow, & Wood, 2000; Sher, Trull, Bartholow,

---

[1] A *meta-analysis* is a set of statistical procedures to combine the results from several studies examining the same relation. For more information, see Hunter and Schmidt (2004).

& Vieth, 1999). Other research has explored the relation of neuroticism/ negative emotionality and behavioral disinhibition to substance use rather than having a substance use disorder, which was the focus of Kotov et al.'s meta-analysis. The results of this cross-sectional and longitudinal research suggest that both personality traits are positively related to elevated rates of alcohol and illicit drug use in general samples of adolescents and adults (e.g., Colder & Chassin, 1997; Cooper et al., 1995; Elkins, King, McGue, & Iacono, 2006; K. M. Jackson & Sher, 2003; Kashdan, Vetter, & Collins, 2005; King & Chassin, 2004; Terracciano, Löckenhoff, Crum, Bienvenu, & Costa, 2008).

Despite these prior findings, few studies have explored directly the relations of neuroticism/negative emotionality and behavioral disinhibition to workforce or workplace substance use. Using a sample of 211 Australian managers, Grant and Langan-Fox (2007) found that when the five-factor model traits were examined simultaneously, only neuroticism predicted workforce substance use. Using a national sample of 2,372 ambulance and 1,096 police personnel in Norway, Sterud et al. (2007) found that neuroticism was unrelated to workforce alcohol use, though it was positively related to reports of alcohol-related problems. Using a sample of 319 young U.S. workers (ages 16–19), Frone (2003) failed to find a relation of negative emotionality to workforce and workplace alcohol or marijuana use. However, several dimensions of behavioral disinhibition were related to employee substance use. Impulsivity and risk taking were positively related to workforce alcohol and marijuana use, and intolerance of rules was positively related to workplace alcohol use. Finally, using a sample of 1,473 U.S. blue-collar workers, Bamberger and Bacharach (2006) found that when the five-factor model traits were examined individually and simultaneously in relation to workforce substance use, low levels of agreeableness and conscientiousness (representing behavioral disinhibition) were related to being a problem drinker. They also found that extraversion was positively related to problem drinking. The other two traits (neuroticism and openness) were not related to problem drinking.

Substance Use Outcome Expectancies

Social learning theory (Bandura, 1977) posits that (a) humans learn, by direct experience or vicariously, that certain behaviors lead to certain outcomes; (b) humans learn to anticipate or "expect" the outcomes of behavior before the behavior occurs; and (c) these expectations of future outcomes become motivators of current behavior. Likewise, building from social learning theory, expectancy theorists have defined outcome expectancies as "anticipations of one's own automatic reactions to various situations and behaviors" (Kirsch, 1999, p. 4). As such, expectancy theories posit that outcome expectancies act as determinants of behavior (e.g., Kirsch, 1999; Roese & Sherman, 2007). Because substance use is a behavior that results in various outcomes that people learn to anticipate, either through direct experience or vicariously, it is not surprising that people hold expectancies regarding the various outcomes of substance use and that these expectancies motivate individuals to use or not use various substances (see Patel & Fromme, 2010, for a general review).

Researchers have found that individuals hold a number of specific expectancies regarding the outcomes of using psychoactive substances. For instance, alcohol and drugs are regarded as powerful transforming agents that might enhance or impede social behavior, cognitive and motor functioning, sexuality, arousal, and relaxation (e.g., George et al., 1995; M. S. Goldman, Brown, & Christiansen, 1987; Labbe & Maisto, 2010; Schafer & Brown, 1991). Of the various anticipated outcomes of substance use, two are particularly relevant to workforce and workplace substance use: affect regulation and performance regulation. Expectancies regarding affect regulation can range from being very positive to very negative. People who hold positive affect regulation expectancies anticipate that substance use will reduce negative emotions and/or increase positive emotions, whereas people who hold negative affect regulation expectancies anticipate that substance use will increase negative emotions and/or decrease positive emotions (e.g., Cooper et al., 1995; M. S. Goldman et al., 1987; Schafer & Brown, 1991). Thus, it is not surprising that cross-sectional and longitudinal studies have found that positive expectancies regarding affect regulation are related to higher levels of alcohol use and illicit drug use in general samples of adolescents and adults (e.g., Cooper et al., 1995; Grube & Agostinelli, 1999; Hayaki et al., 2010; B.C. Leigh & Stacy, 2004; Patrick, Wray-Lake, Finlay, & Maggs, 2010; Sher, Wood, Wood, & Raskin, 1996; Spada, Moneta, & Wells, 2007; Torrealday et al., 2008).

Although few outcome expectancy studies have focused explicitly on the substance use of employed individuals, research shows that positive affect regulation expectancies are related to higher levels of overall alcohol and marijuana use in the workforce (Frone, 2003; Frone, Russell, & Cooper, 1993). In addition to workforce substance use, two studies explored the relation of positive affect regulation expectancies to workplace substance use. One study found that positive affect regulation expectancies predicted higher levels of alcohol use during the workday but were unrelated to alcohol use before work in a sample of adult (mean age = 43 years) manufacturing employees (Grube, Ames, & Delaney, 1994). The other study failed to find a relation between positive affect regulation expectancies and either workplace alcohol or workplace marijuana use and impairment in a sample of young workers (mean age = 18 years) holding a variety of jobs (Frone, 2003).

A second but less studied anticipated effect of psychoactive substances with relevance to employee substance use is regulation of behavioral, cognitive, and motor performance. People who hold positive performance regulation expectancies anticipate that substance use will not impair performance and/or will improve performance, whereas people who hold negative performance regulation expectancies anticipate that substance use will not improve performance and/or will impair performance (e.g., M. S. Goldman et al., 1987; Hayaki et al., 2010; Labbe & Maisto, 2010; Schafer & Brown, 1991). Cross-sectional research with general samples of adolescents and adults has shown that individuals who believe that alcohol will not impair or will improve their ability to think and function are more likely to report heavy drinking (e.g., Christiansen & Goldman, 1983; Hayaki et al., 2010; B. C. Leigh & Stacy, 2004; Spada et al., 2007).

With regard to employee substance involvement, one cross-sectional study explored the link between performance regulation expectancies and overall workforce substance use (Frone, 2003). This study found that positive performance regulation expectancies were related to higher levels of workforce alcohol and marijuana use. Two cross-sectional studies explored the relation of positive performance regulation expectancies to workplace substance use. One study found that positive performance regulation expectancies predicted higher levels of alcohol use before work and during the workday (Grube et al., 1994). The second study found that positive performance regulation expectancies regarding alcohol and marijuana use were related to higher levels of workplace alcohol use and impairment and higher levels of workplace marijuana use and impairment, respectively (Frone, 2003).

WORKPLACE ENVIRONMENT

Workplace Substance Availability

A key proposition from general availability theory of substance use is that with increasing availability of a substance in a society come increasing levels of consumption in the population (e.g., Single, 1988). Applied to the workplace, availability theory suggests that work settings in which substances are more available may promote substance use among employees. Ames and colleagues (Ames & Grube, 1999; Ames & Janes, 1992) proposed two general dimensions of substance availability relevant to the workplace. The first general dimension is the physical availability of alcohol and drugs at work. This dimension represents the ease of obtaining alcohol or other drugs at work and the ease of using them during work hours and during breaks. The second general dimension represents social availability, which comprises two subdimensions: descriptive norms and injunctive norms. *Descriptive norms*, also known as *behavioral norms*, represent the extent to which members of an individual's workplace social network use or work while under the influence of alcohol or drugs at work. *Injunctive norms*, also known as *attitudinal norms*, represent the extent to which members of an individual's workplace social network approve of using or working under the influence of alcohol or drugs at work. The notion that social availability of substances (i.e., injunctive and descriptive norms) may act as a cause of substance use also derives from theories of social norms and social influence (e.g., Cialdini & Trost, 1998) and sociocultural theories of alcohol use (e.g., Trice & Sonnenstuhl, 1990). The relation of the two general dimensions of workplace substance availability to employee substance involvement is summarized next.

Workplace Physical Availability and Employee Substance Involvement

There are two types of evidence that address the potential relation between physical availability of substances at work and employee substance use. The first type of evidence is the finding that aggregate rates and levels of substance use or substance use disorders are higher within certain occupations that have, relative to other occupations, greater physical access to various substances. For example, as discussed in Chapter 1 and elsewhere (Dimich-Ward, Gallagher, Spinelli, Threlfall, & Band, 1988; Harford & Brooks, 1992; J. P. Leigh & Jiang, 1993; Mandell, Eaton, Anthony, & Garrison, 1992, Zhang & Snizek, 2003), alcohol use and disorders are higher among individuals in food service and hospitality occupations, who include bartenders and waitstaff. Also, opioid use and disorders are elevated among anesthesiologists compared with those in other medical specialties and other occupations (Gold et al., 2006). Two studies provided some support for a reciprocal relation between occupation and employee substance involvement (e.g., Plant, 1978; Zhu, Tews, Stafford, & George, 2011). In other words, although physical availability might cause increases in employee substance involvement, it is also likely that heavy alcohol and illicit drug users self-select into jobs and occupations where substances are physically available and where coworkers are more likely to support the use of alcohol or illicit drugs. Nonetheless, it is unlikely that individuals will self-select into occupations (e.g., nursing, anesthesiology) requiring many years of postsecondary education so that they will have access to various prescription drugs.

The second type of evidence regarding the relation between the physical availability of substances at work and employee substance involvement comes from survey research that asks employees directly about their access and ability to use various substances at work as well as their level of substance involvement. This approach provides a more direct assessment of physical availability. Although a study by Ames and Grube (1999) failed to find a relation between physical availability of alcohol at work and drinking at work, several other studies support a relation between workplace physical availability of substances and employee substance use. For example, using a random sample of adults in Ontario, Canada, Macdonald, Wells, and Wild (1999) found that reports of illicit drugs being easily available from coworkers were related to having an alcohol use problem. Farid, Lucas, and Williams (1994), using a clinical sample of individuals with liver disease due either to alcohol or to some other cause, found a positive association between reports of alcohol being freely available at work and having a liver disease due to heavy drinking. Hodgins, Williams, and Munro (2009), using a random sample of employed adults in Alberta, Canada, found a positive association between reports that alcohol was allowed on work premises and having an alcohol use disorder. Using a national sample of registered nurses in the United States, Trinkoff and colleagues (Trinkoff, Storr, & Wall, 1999; Trinkoff, Zhou, Storr, & Soeken, 2000) reported that availability and frequency of administration of controlled substances at work were positively related to overall illicit use of prescription drugs, use of illegal drugs, and heavy alcohol use among nurses. A review of literature related to health care professionals concluded that increased access to drugs at work was an important risk factor for illicit drug use (Kenna, Baldwin, Trinkoff, & Lewis, 2011). Finally, using a national sample of U.S. workers, Frone and Trinidad (2011) found that workplace physical availability of alcohol was positively related to employee alcohol use and impairment away from work and during the workday. Likewise, workplace physical availability of illicit drugs was positively related to employee illicit drug use and impairment away from work and during the workday.

Workplace Social Availability and Employee Substance Involvement

As discussed previously, workplace social availability has two components: use of substances at work by members of one's workplace social network (i.e., descriptive norms) and normative approval of substance use at work by members of one's workplace social network (i.e., injunctive norms). Although few studies have explored workplace social availability, their results generally support a positive relation to overall and workplace substance involvement. For example, Ames, Grube, and Moore (2000) found that injunctive workplace alcohol norms were positively related to alcohol use at work, and descriptive workplace alcohol norms were positively related to alcohol use before work, alcohol use at work, and having a hangover at work. Moore, Ames, Duke, and Cunradi (2012) reported that workplace descriptive norms regarding coming to work with a hangover were positively related to working with a hangover. Frone (2003) found that workplace descriptive marijuana norms were positively related to overall marijuana use but workplace descriptive alcohol norms were not related to overall alcohol use. In addition, workplace descriptive alcohol and marijuana norms were positively related to alcohol and marijuana use in the workplace, respectively. Macdonald et al. (1999) found that workplace descriptive norms regarding alcohol use were positively related to having an alcohol use problem. Finally, Bennett and Lehman (1998) found a positive relation between workplace descriptive norms regarding alcohol use and employee alcohol use, heavy drinking, and having problems with alcohol.

Frone and Brown (2010) used a national sample of U.S. workers to explore more broadly the relations of workplace injunctive and descriptive norms regarding both alcohol and illicit drug use to workforce and workplace alcohol and illicit drug use. This study extended past research by assessing (a) both alcohol use and illicit drug use, (b) both workforce and workplace substance use, and (c) both descriptive and injunctive workplace norms. The results revealed that workplace descriptive norms for alcohol and illicit drug use were related to workplace alcohol and illicit drug use but not to workforce alcohol and illicit drug use, respectively. In contrast, workplace injunctive norms for alcohol and illicit drug use were related to workplace alcohol and illicit drug use, as well as workforce alcohol and illicit drug use, respectively.

Workplace Social Control

Workplace social control is "exercised through socialization, patterns of reward distribution, and efforts to identify and control deviant behavior" (Roman, 1980, p. 407). The workplace social control perspective posits that substance use may be lower among employees who are integrated into or regulated by the work organization (e.g., Ames et al., 2000; Trice & Sonnenstuhl, 1990). Four broad categories of workplace social control exist: formal or informal substance use policies, supervisor control, visibility of job performance, and high levels of commitment. Although workforce substance use testing represents another form of social control, this issue is discussed separately in Chapter 5. The first category of workplace social control represents the existence of formal or informal policies regarding substance use and disciplinary outcomes. Using a national sample of U.S. workers, Larson et al. (2007) found no evidence that merely working for an employer who had a written policy on workplace alcohol and drug use was related to past month use of illicit drugs or heavy alcohol use.

The second category of workplace social control is supervisor social control. Supervisor social control consists of two dimensions (Bacharach et al., 2002; Harris & Heft, 1992). The first dimension is supervisor contact, which represents opportunities for substance use problem detection through normal contact between employees and their supervisor. The second dimension is supervisor enforcement, which represents the ability of supervisors to identify employee substance use problems, as well as their willingness to apply company policies and directly address employee substance use problems. Three studies failed to support a relation between supervisor contact and workforce alcohol use or illicit drug use (Bacharach et al., 2002; Macdonald et al., 1999; Parker & Farmer, 1988). In contrast, two studies found a negative relation between supervisor enforcement and workplace alcohol use or hangover (Ames et al., 2000; Moore et al., 2012).

Frone and Trinidad (2012) used a national sample of U.S. workers to explore more broadly the relations of supervisor social control to workforce and workplace alcohol and illicit drug use. They hypothesized that the relation between supervisor social control and employee substance use depends on (a) the dimension of supervisor social control (contact vs. enforcement), (b) the context of substance use (workforce use vs. workplace use), and (c) substance legality (alcohol vs. illicit drugs). Frone and Trinidad found that consistent with prior research, mere supervisor contact was unrelated to alcohol and illicit drug use in the workforce and in the workplace. In contrast, supervisor enforcement was negatively related to workplace alcohol use but not workforce alcohol use. Supervisor enforcement also was positively related to both workplace and workforce illicit drug use. Supervisor enforcement was likely related to both workplace alcohol and illicit drug use because any substance use and impairment at work is prohibited by most workplace substance use policies. Supervisor enforcement was likely unrelated to workforce alcohol use because alcohol use is legal and most workplace policies do address alcohol use outside of work. In contrast, workforce illicit drug use may be responsive to supervisor enforcement because it is often proscribed by workplace policy and many employers sanction job applicants and current employees for off-the-job illicit drug use (see discussion of drug testing in Chapter 5).

The third category of workplace social control is high visibility of job performance, which includes low mobility during work hours, contact with coworkers or customers, and work roles with high levels of interdependency. Of three studies exploring the relation of job visibility to employee substance involvement, all supported a negative relation. Frone (2003) found that the extent to which individuals performed their work duties in public or had to work closely with others was related to lower levels of workforce marijuana use and workplace alcohol use. Macdonald et al. (1999) found that less frequent travel was related to lower levels of problematic alcohol use in the workforce. Finally, Trinkoff et al. (1999) assessed job visibility regarding access to workplace prescription drugs among registered nurses. This study found that to the extent there was witnessing of wastage (i.e., proper disposal of prescription drugs) and written documentation of administration of prescription drugs, nurses were less likely to report illicitly using prescription drugs themselves.

The fourth category of workplace social control is high levels of commitment to one's employer and high levels of personal investment in one's job. Frone et al. (1995) explored the relation of psychological job involvement to heavy alcohol use in the workforce. No relation was found to exist between the psychological importance of work and heavy drinking when work stress was low (i.e., low work pressure and low job ambiguity), but there was a positive relation when work stress was high (i.e., high work pressure and high job ambiguity). These results suggest that employees who psychologically identified with their jobs drank more heavy after work because they may have been more sensitive to poor work conditions. This relation is opposite to what is predicted by the social control perspective, though it is consistent with the work stress perspective discussed in the next section. No research has examined the relation of high levels of organizational or job commitment to workplace substance use.

Workplace Stress

Stress has been defined in many ways. Two common approaches have been to define stress in terms of either stimulus or response (e.g., Jex, Beehr, & Roberts, 1992; Sayette, 1999). Stimulus definitions define stress in terms of exposure to aversive environmental stimuli that require adaptation. These aversive environmental stimuli are referred to as stressors. Thus, work stress would be synonymous with exposure to work stressors. Response definitions define stress in terms of the physiological, psychological, and behavioral responses resulting from exposure to aversive environmental stimuli. These responses are collectively referred to as *strains*. Thus, work stress would be synonymous with the experience of any number of strains that result from exposure to aversive workplace characteristics or events. In contrast, Lazarus (1985; Lazarus & Folkman, 1985) and Pearlin, Menaghan, Lieberman, and Mullan (1981) proposed that stress is best regarded as a rubric for a system of interdependent variables. It is this latter definition of "stress as process" that is used here. Therefore, the phrase *work stress* refers to a general process that involves work stressors, strains (e.g., alcohol or illicit drug use), and other variables that may affect the relation between work stressors and strains.

The notion that exposure to work stressors promotes employee substance use (i.e., one type of behavioral strain) is widely accepted and has been explored in many studies. Researchers have generated a large and growing literature devoted to understanding the relation of work stressors to employee substance involvement. For example, Cooper, Russell, and Frone

(1990) identified 17 such studies conducted during the 1980s; Frone (1999) identified 39 studies conducted during the 1990s; and a number of studies have been conducted subsequently. Although not every potential work stressor has been studied in relation to employee substance involvement, Figure 2.2 provides a framework to organize and highlight the types of work stressors considered in the work stress perspective (see also Barling, Kelloway, & Frone, 2005).

As shown in Figure 2.2, a distinction can be made between cross-role work stressors and within-role work stressors. The cross-role work stressors involve the extent to which the work demands interfere with meeting the responsibilities of one's family role (i.e., work-to-family conflict) and the extent to which family demands interfere with meeting responsibilities at work (i.e., family-to-work conflict). Although involving a nonwork role, cross-domain stressors, such as work-to-family conflict or family-to-work conflict, represent a type of work stressor because only employed individuals can experience these aversive environmental events. In contrast, within-role work stressors represent aversive conditions and events that derive solely from one's work role. Among the within-role work stressors, a basic distinction can be made between social stressors and nonsocial stressors. Social stressors at work represent aversive conditions involving workplace social relations, such as exposure to workplace aggression and other interpersonal conflicts, dysfunctional organizational politics, discrimination, or the lack of opportunity to develop friendships or interact with other individuals. The nonsocial work stressors can be further differentiated into three major categories. Work stressors related to financial security involve concerns such as a lack of job security, inadequate income, and lack of promotion opportunity. Work stressors related to the nature of one's job include aversive work conditions, such as a high level of work demands, repetitive work, exposure to noxious physical work environments, and overly simple or complex work. Finally, work stressors related to the organization of work represent aversive conditions, such as working night shifts, inadequate resources and staffing, inadequate supervision, and poor task-relevant communication.

The theoretical underpinning of research on work stress and employee substance use typically has been couched in the general conceptual framework of tension reduction or affect regulation (Conger, 1956; Cooper et al., 1995; Peirce et al., 2000). The general premise is that exposure to stressors will cause substance use as a means of mitigating experienced psychological tension and strain, which is referred to as *stress-induced substance use* (e.g., Frone, 1999; Sayette, 1999). In other words, frequent exposure to work stressors leads to more frequent experience of negative emotions and other forms of tension, which then causes more frequent and heavier use of alcohol and illicit drugs.

Most research has explored the overall relation of various work stressors to employee substance involvement. Several studies have explored the

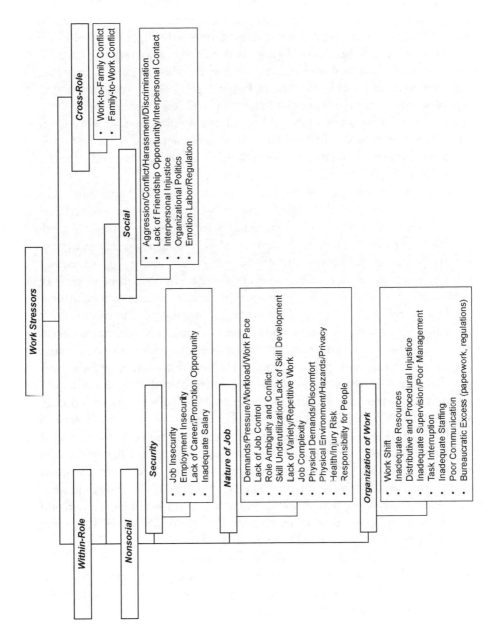

Figure 2.2. Taxonomy of work stressors.

cross-role work stressor of work–family conflict. Although one study failed to find such a relation to employee substance involvement (Steptoe et al., 1998), five cross-sectional studies (Bromet, Dew, & Parkinson, 1990; Frone, 2000; Frone et al., 1996; Roos, Lahelma, & Rahkonen, 2006; Vasse, Nijhuis, & Kok, 1998) and two longitudinal studies (Frone, Russell, & Cooper, 1997; Wang, Liu, Zhan, & Shi, 2010) support a positive association of work–family conflict to alcohol and illicit drug use and disorders. For example, using a regional sample of U.S. workers, Frone et al. (1997) found that higher levels of work-to-family conflict at baseline predicted more frequent overall heavy alcohol use 4 years later. Also, using a small sample of workers in China, Wang et al. (2010) found that daily assessments of work-to-family conflict were positively related to the amount of alcohol consumed later the same day over 5 weeks.

Turning to within-role stressors, several cross-sectional and longitudinal studies have examined social stressors at work. Among cross-sectional studies, Frone (2003) failed to find a relation of interpersonal conflict at work to overall alcohol use, overall marijuana use, workplace alcohol use, and workplace marijuana use. Bamberger and Bacharach (2006) found a positive association between exposure to abusive supervision and overall problem alcohol use. Marchand (2008) reported that workplace harassment was positively related to overall risky drinking. Rospenda, Richman, and Shannon (2009) reported cross-sectional findings on the associations of sexual harassment, generalized harassment, gender discrimination, racial discrimination, and other discrimination to alcohol intoxication and problem drinking. Rospenda et al. found that sexual harassment was positively related to drinking to intoxication and unrelated to problem drinking among men and that it had no relation to alcohol outcomes for women. Generalized harassment was positively related to problem drinking and unrelated to intoxication among women, and it was unrelated to both alcohol outcomes among men. Gender discrimination was positively related to problem drinking and intoxication among women and was unrelated to both alcohol outcomes among men. Racial discrimination was unrelated both to problem drinking and to intoxication among women and men. Discrimination based on other characteristics (not defined by Rospenda et al., 2009) was positively related to problem drinking and intoxication among women and was unrelated to both alcohol outcomes among men. Using a different sample, Richman et al. (1999) reported that sexual harassment and generalized harassment were positively related to the overall frequency of drinking among women and were unrelated to drinking among men.

In a longitudinal study, Madsen et al. (2011) found that among a sample of workers who did not use prescription drugs at baseline, exposure to physical violence at work was related to the use of psychoactive drugs (e.g., antidepressants and sedatives) during the subsequent 3.6 years.

Rospenda, Fujishiro, Shannon, and Richman (2008) explored the relation of sexual harassment and generalized harassment assessed in 2003 to reports of heavy drinking and intoxication in 2004. They found that among men, sexual harassment predicted more frequent heavy alcohol use and drinking to intoxication and generalized harassment predicted more frequent heavy alcohol use. Sexual harassment and generalized harassment did not predict either of the two alcohol outcomes for women. In another longitudinal study, Rospenda and colleagues (Rospenda, 2002; Rospenda, Richman, Wislar, & Flaherty, 2000) failed to find relations of sexual harassment and generalized harassment to overall alcohol use over time among both men and women.

A large number of studies have tested the overall relation of a wide range of nonsocial work stressors to employee substance involvement (see Cooper et al., 1990; Frone, 1999, for reviews). As noted by Frone (1999), this body of research provides little consistent support for such relations. For example, several cross-sectional and longitudinal studies reported that low levels of job complexity, high job demands, low job control, being unfairly rewarded, and general workplace problems were related to elevated levels of alcohol use, illicit drug use, or having an alcohol disorder (e.g., Chen & Cunradi, 2008; Crum, Muntaner, Eaton, & Anthony, 1995; Hemmingsson & Lundberg, 1998; Howard & Cordes, 2010; Liu, Wang, Zhan, & Shi, 2009; Pelfrene et al., 2004; Ragland, Greiner, Krause, Holman, & Fisher, 1995; Roxburgh, 1998; Storr, Trinkoff, & Anthony, 1999). Nonetheless, many other cross-sectional and longitudinal studies have failed to support relations involving these and other nonsocial work stressors in relation to workforce and workplace substance use (e.g., Cooper et al., 1990; Frone, 2003; Frone et al.,1995; Gimeno, Amick, Barrientos-Gutiérrez, & Mangione, 2009; Greenberg & Grunberg, 1995; Head, Stansfeld, & Siegrist, 2004; Kawakami, Araki, Haratani, & Hemmi, 1993; Kouvonen et al., 2005; Marchand, 2008; Rospenda, 2002; Rospenda et al., 2000; Trinkoff et al., 2000; Vasse et al., 1998; Wiesner, Windle, & Freeman, 2005; Zhang & Snizek, 2003).

Frone (2008) suggested that overall measures of workforce substance use primarily capture use that occurs at times and places far removed from the workday, such as days off work, and may be more likely to reflect substance use for reasons unrelated to work stressors, such as family-related stress or recreational socializing. Thus, one potential reason for the inconsistent relations between work stressors and employee substance use is that past research has failed to focus on substance use defined in terms of its temporal relation to the workday. Using data from a national sample of U.S. workers, Frone explored the relations of work overload and job insecurity to overall assessments of alcohol and illicit drug use in the workforce and to assessments of alcohol and illicit drug use during the workday and after work. Consistent with many prior studies, this study failed to support a relation between the two work stressors and workforce alcohol and illicit drug use. In contrast, both job insecurity and work overload were positively related to the frequency and quantity of alcohol use during the workday and the frequency of illicit drug use before work and during the workday. In addition, work overload was positively related to the frequency and quantity of alcohol use after work and the frequency of illicit drug use after work.

The inconsistent findings from past work stressor studies may also result from not considering individual differences in the relation between work stressors and employee substance involvement (Frone, 1999). Past research has implicitly assumed that work stressors cause substance use among all, or at least many, employees. However, as shown in Chapter 1, most employed adults do not use illicit drugs. Moreover, even though most employed adults consume alcohol, it is unlikely that most of them use alcohol in response to work stressors because there are alternate ways of dealing with work stress, many of which are more functional. Therefore, it may be more reasonable to expect that only employees who have certain vulnerabilities (e.g., holding the belief that alcohol or illicit drug use relieves negative emotions) will use substances to cope with work stressors. This perspective is depicted in Figure 2.1 as a Person Characteristic × Workplace Characteristic interaction and derives from various theoretical models, such as social learning and stress vulnerability models of substance use (e.g., Cooper, Russell, Skinner, Frone, & Mudar, 1992), diathesis–stress models of mental health (Belsky & Pluess, 2009; Monroe & Simons, 1991), and genetics research on G × E interactions that was discussed previously. If this presumption of individual differences in vulnerability to stress-induced substance involvement is true, research that fails to identify subgroups at risk for stress-induced drinking may produce inconsistent and weak findings.

Several studies provide support for the notion of individual differences in vulnerability to work-stress-induced alcohol use. Frone et al. (1993) found that a measure of work–family conflict was positively related to overall problem drinking only among employees with strong positive affect regulation expectancies. Wang et al. (2010) reported that work-to-family conflict was more strongly related to overall alcohol use when peer drinking norms supported the use of alcohol and when coworker and family social support were low. Seven studies tested and provided support for individual differences in vulnerability to stress-induced alcohol use in relation to within-role work stressors (Bacharach et al., 2002; Cooper et al., 1990; Frone et al., 1995; Grunberg, Moore, Anderson-Connolly, & Greenberg, 1999; Grunberg, Moore, & Greenberg, 1998; Liu et al., 2009; Parker & Harford, 1992). For example, building from identity theory, Frone et al. (1995) found that both job demands and role ambiguity were positively related to heavy drinking only among employees who defined themselves in terms of their work.

FUTURE RESEARCH

With regard to research on the causes of employee substance use, more attention to several issues is required. First, both workforce and workplace substance involvement must be assessed in the same study. The research discussed in this chapter suggests that there may be important differences in the predictors of these two dimensions of substance involvement. Second, more effort should be directed at the development of measures of workplace physical availability and social availability (i.e., descriptive and injunctive norms). The measures of these work characteristics often were developed for specific studies, and evidence of construct validity and cross-study comparisons of findings and conclusions therefore remain tenuous. Third, research has not assessed many dimensions of workplace social control. Moreover, rarely are multiple dimensions of social control explored simultaneously to see which dimensions are uniquely predictive of employee substance involvement. Fourth, studies of work stress have failed to explore systematically the various types of work stressors. Thus, we do not know which work stressors might be the most important causes of employee substance use. Also, there is a need for more research exploring the characteristics that make individuals vulnerable to work-stress-induced substance involvement. Finally, with Figure 2.1 used as a general framework, future research on the causes of employee substance involvement should take a more sophisticated and more integrated approach that includes (a) simultaneous overall (Lines 1 and 2), indirect (Lines 4 and 2), or interactive (Line 3) effects of several domains of predictors (e.g., genetics, personality, substance use expectancies, workplace availability, workplace social control, and work stressors); (b) a broader assessment of employee substance use that explores specific classes of substances (alcohol, marijuana, depressants, stimulants) and takes into account the temporal context of substance use (e.g., before work, during the workday, and after work); and (c) experimental and longitudinal research designs that can provide stronger evidence that observed relations are causal.

GENERAL SUMMARY AND CONCLUSIONS

The nearly 8-decade-old proposition by Lewin (1936) that human behavior is a joint function of person characteristics and characteristics of the environment is supported by modern genetics research, which provides consistent support for the heritability of substance use and disorders, as well as the impact of environmentability. Roughly, 50% of variation in heavy substance use and substance disorders is due to heredity and 50% of such variation is due to the nonshared environment. However, no research has explored the heritability of workplace substance involvement. In terms of other person characteristics, research suggests that two broad personality characteristics—negative emotionality and behavioral disinhibition—are associated with higher levels of substance use in the workforce and workplace. Also, substance use outcome expectancies regarding affect regulation are associated with higher levels of alcohol and illicit drug use in the workforce, though there is little evidence for an association with workplace substance use. Substance use outcome expectancies regarding performance regulation are associated with higher levels of alcohol and illicit drug use in the workforce and in the workplace.

The physical availability and social availability (i.e., social norms) of substances at work demonstrate consistent relations to workforce and workplace substance use. Some research suggests that two dimensions of social control—job visibility and supervisor enforcement—may be associated with lower levels of workforce and workplace substance use. However, just having frequent contact with a supervisor is unrelated to workforce and workplace substance involvement. Finally, the cross-role work stressor of work–family conflict is consistently associated with overall alcohol use. Within-role work stressors, such as job demands, low job control, and workplace harassment, are inconsistently related to overall alcohol and illicit drug use. More complex models of work stress that consider the temporal context of employee substance involvement and individual differences in vulnerability to work-stress-induced substance use may eventually provide more consistent support for and a better understanding of the relation between work stressors and employee substance involvement.

Although progress has been made in studying the association between a wide variety of putative causes of workforce and workplace substance involvement, the research is largely cross-sectional and many studies fail to control for important common causes. Thus, there is no strong evidence for causal effects involving the associations reviewed in this chapter. Also, it is unclear which of the many putative causes that were reviewed are the most important or how they might work together to cause employee substance involvement.

3

PERFORMANCE OUTCOMES: PSYCHOPHARMACOLOGY AND WORKPLACE SIMULATION RESEARCH

Human psychopharmacology can be defined, in part, as the study of the effects of psychoactive drugs on affective, cognitive, and psychomotor outcomes (Meyer & Quenzer, 2005; Patat, 2000). Affective outcomes represent things like elation, pleasure, anger, sadness, depression, anxiety, or impulse control. Cognitive outcomes represent attention (e.g., divided attention—simultaneously keeping track of more than one stimulus or engaging in more than one task), vigilance (e.g., detection of infrequent stimuli over a prolonged period), simple information processing (e.g., mental arithmetic), complex information processing (e.g., logical reasoning, mental rotation), and memory (recall, recognition). Psychomotor outcomes represent simple skills (e.g., tapping, aiming, balance, tracking) or complex skills (e.g., manual dexterity, two-dimensional coordination, complex simulator performance).[1]

DOI: 10.1037/13944-004
Alcohol and Illicit Drug Use in the Workforce and Workplace, by M. R. Frone
Copyright © 2013 by the American Psychological Association. All rights reserved.

[1]No attempt is made to describe the hundreds of measures, tests, and exercises devised to assess affective, cognitive, and psychomotor outcomes. The interested reader can consult Foltin and Evans (1993); Normand et al. (1994); Parrott (1991a); Patat (2000); Strauss, Sherman, and Spreen (2006); Wetherell (1996); Zacny (1995); and the various studies summarized.

My overall goal in this chapter is to summarize research on the relation of major classes of psychoactive substances to basic affective, cognitive, and psychomotor outcomes based on three types of research designs: experimental psychopharmacology, nonexperimental or observational psychopharmacology, and experimental workplace simulations. Although most of this research does not directly address worker productivity, the basic outcomes studied in all three types of research are important for work performance, and the results of this research are often cited to support the notion that various substances can affect productivity in work organizations. Therefore, the findings from this research must be understood, and they provide a baseline from which to understand research on employee productivity that is examined in Chapter 4. For each class of substances, experimental and observational psychopharmacological research are summarized, followed by workplace simulation research where it exists. After the results of psychopharmacological and workplace simulation research are summarized, the main strengths and limitations of this research are highlighted.

But before I turn to research on specific substances, several general observations that apply to most psychoactive substances can be summarized (e.g., Kerr & Hindmarch, 1998; Maisto et al., 2008; Martin, 2007; World Health Organization, 2004). In general, the acute effects of psychoactive substances are more pronounced with increasing dosage. Nonetheless, for a specific dose of a substance, marked variation can exist in the functioning of different people at a specific occasion of use, and variation can exist in the functioning of a specific person across different occasions of use. This inter- and intraindividual variation in the effect of a substance may be due to two processes. First, given the same dose of a substance, individuals will differ in the concentration of the substance in blood (this is discussed in Chapter 4 in more detail) and their level of tolerance to a substance. Second, many of the observed effects of a psychoactive substance are partly dependent on the context in which it is used, which may be a function of the psychological state of the person (happy vs. depressed), personality type (see Chapter 2), substance use outcome expectancies (see Chapter 2), or the environment in which use occurs.

DEPRESSANTS: ALCOHOL

Alcohol (ethanol or ethyl alcohol) is the most widely used psychoactive substance that can appreciably affect mood and cognitive and psycho-motor performance, and it is the most widely used depressant. The affective outcomes of acute alcohol intoxication at low to moderate blood alcohol content (BAC) of .01% to .08% are euphoria, relaxation, reduced anxiety, increased sociability, and lowered inhibitions (Meyer & Quenzer, 2005). At higher BAC, alcohol can lead to sedation and unconsciousness, feelings of depression, and social withdrawal. With regard to the effect of acute alcohol intoxication on cognitive and psychomotor performance, results are mixed at low ($\leq$.05%) to moderate (>.05% to .08%) BACs used in many experimental administration studies. Some studies have shown impairment, and other studies have not shown impairment. In terms of cognitive performance, low to moderate BAC may impair short-term memory and performance when several tasks are performed simultaneously and as the complexity of information processing increases (Glencross, 1990; Martin, 2007). With regard to psychomotor performance, evidence exists that low to moderate BAC does not affect performance on simple reaction time tasks, simple motor tasks, or simple choice reaction time tasks, but it may impair performance on more complex choice reaction time tasks and motor performance on tracking tasks (Glencross, 1990; Martin, 2007). In addition, cognitive and psychomotor impairment at low to moderate BAC may not be observed among individuals who have a broad history of alcohol and other drug use, because they have developed tolerance to the acute effects of this level of alcohol consumption (Zacny & Gutierrez, 2011). Although the psychopharmacological research summarized in this chapter refers to tolerance in its most general sense (see Chapter 1)—diminished response that occurs after repeated exposure to a fixed dose of a psychoactive substance—there are several types of tolerance (see discussion in Chapter 4). At higher BACs (>.08 to .12%), more consistency exists across experimental studies in gross impairment on a variety of cognitive and psychomotor outcomes (Glencross, 1990; Martin, 2007). In general, cognitive and psychomotor impairment increases as both the level of acute intoxication (BAC) and the complexity of the task increase (Jung, 2001).

Although ethical issues limit the amount of alcohol that can be administered in laboratory studies, most readers likely have seen firsthand that the high BACs reached in naturalistic settings (e.g., parties, bars, nightclubs) may lead to profound cognitive and psychomotor impairment. Nonetheless, the levels of BAC used in experimental studies may be more representative of levels of intoxication at work. To avoid detection, employees are unlikely to be at work profoundly impaired.

Some psychopharmacological research on the outcomes of alcohol use does not administer alcohol to individuals. Rather, these nonexperimental or observational studies compare the performance of long-term heavy drinkers with that of light drinkers or nondrinkers when individuals are unintoxicated (BAC = 0). However, as discussed subsequently, such studies are fraught with methodological problems that make firm conclusions difficult. Nonetheless, this research suggests that heavy alcohol consumption over many years may lead to severe and permanent brain damage in some people (Jung, 2001; Meyer & Quenzer, 2005). More generally, Oscar-Berman and Marinkovic (2007) reported that nearly half of the problem (abusive or dependent) drinkers in the United States are free of cognitive, sensory, or motor impairments when not under the influence of alcohol. Although a minority of alcohol-dependent individuals develop permanent debilitating conditions that require lifetime custodial care, most problem drinkers who develop cognitive and psychomotor problems have mild impairments that improve with long-term (1 year or more) abstinence (Fein, Torres, Price, & Di Sciafani, 2006; Maisto et al., 2008; Oscar-Berman & Marinkovic, 2007). Parsons and Nixon (1998) reviewed the literature since 1986 on the relation of drinking patterns to cognitive functioning in social drinkers with a BAC of zero. Despite various methodological issues with the reviewed studies, Parsons and Nixon (1998) speculated that "persons drinking five or six U.S. standard drinks per day over extended time periods [i.e., greater than 1 year] manifest some cognitive inefficiencies; at seven to nine drinks per day, mild cognitive deficits are present; and at 10 or more drinks per day, moderate cognitive deficits equivalent to those found in diagnosed alcoholics are present" (p. 180). Given this statement, it is important to point out that only 3.5% of the U.S. workforce reports drinking 5 or more drinks per day at least 3 days per week during the prior 12 months (see Table 1.3). The proportion consuming 5 or more drinks 6 to 7 days per week would be much smaller and even rarer for higher levels of daily alcohol intake over an extended period of time.

Hangover

The phenomenon of hangover was briefly defined in Chapter 1 and is usually associated with alcohol use. It refers to an adverse mental and physical state experienced after a heavy bout of drinking when BAC has returned to zero. The symptoms include such things as headache, nausea, drowsiness, dizziness, fatigue, tremulousness, sweating, and sensitivity to light and sound (e.g., Martin, 2007; Prat, Adan, Perez-Pamies, & Sanchez-Turet, 2008; Prat, Adan, & Sanchez-Turet, 2009; Verster, 2008). The exact causes of hangover are not well understood and are believed to involve acute withdrawal after heavy drinking, inability to properly metabolize alcohol, or effects related to congeners (other chemicals) contained in alcoholic beverages (e.g., Moore, 1998; Prat et al., 2008, 2009). Relative to research on the effects of acute alcohol intoxication and chronic heavy drinking, relatively little research has focused on the performance effects of alcohol hangover, especially in the workplace (Martin, 2007; Moore, 1998; Verster, 2008).

Before the putative effects of alcohol hangover are discussed, it is important to highlight three issues (Hesse & Tutenges, 2010; Howland et al., 2008; Prat et al., 2008, 2009; Verster, 2008). First, it is difficult to separate the effects of hangover from other states that result from heavy drinking, such as dehydration and sleep deprivation (Prat et al., 2008, 2009; Verster, 2008). Second, although most experimental studies of hangover document subjective symptoms of hangover among study participants, some drinkers are resistant to hangover symptoms. In experimental and field research, up to 25% to 30% of individuals do not report experiencing symptoms of a hangover after a specific night of heavy drinking (Howland et al., 2008). The proportion of individuals not showing signs of hangover may increase to 75% among alcohol-dependent individuals (Prat et al., 2009). Finally, among those who do experience a hangover, the severity is typically classified as mild or moderate (Howland et al., 2008).

Among psychopharmacological studies (experimental and non-experimental) that tested performance after BAC has returned to zero, some have found that there were no effects of alcohol hangover on cognitive or psychomotor performance (e.g., Chait & Perry, 1994; Finnigan, Hammersley, & Cooper, 1998; Lemon, Chesher, Fox, Greeley, & Nabke, 1993). Although other studies have reported some statistically significant effects of alcohol hangover on cognitive and psychomotor impairment, close inspection of the results reveals that (a) there is little consistency in the dimensions of cognitive and psychomotor performance that are presumably impaired by hangover, (b) the number of statistically significant effects is often small relative to the number of performance outcomes assessed, and (c) the size of the statistically significant effects is small (i.e., subtle) and may be of little practical importance (e.g., Finnigan, Schulze, Smallwood, & Helander, 2005; Howland et al., 2010; Kim, Yoon, Lee, Choi, & Go, 2003; McKinney & Coyle, 2004; Rohsenow et al., 2010; Verster, van Duin, Volkerts, Schreuder, & Verbaten, 2003). Finally, in a critical review of the hangover literature that considered laboratory studies and research in naturalistic settings, Stephens, Ling, Heffernan, Heather, and Jones (2008) concluded that

> currently there is little definitive empirical evidence determining what, if any, effects on performance arise as a result of the alcohol hangover. In this respect, the hangover and performance literature resembles the acute alcohol intoxication and performance literature, which has also yielded largely inconclusive data. Future research must overcome the shortcomings of previous research identified in this review if a full understanding of the performance effects of the alcohol hangover is to be gained. (p. 169)

Workplace Simulation Studies

A number of experimental workplace simulation studies have been conducted. In these studies, participants are randomly assigned to experimental conditions where they either consume a placebo drink that contains no alcohol or consume some predefined amount of alcohol in order to explore the effects of acute intoxication on various types of performance in a simulated work environment. A series of four simulation studies was conducted by Price and colleagues. Price and Hicks (1979) explored the effect of low levels of alcohol consumption (.01%, .02%, .03%, and .07% BAC) on assembling a common water faucet. In Phase 1 of the study, the six participants were skilled male workers from a university mechanical laboratory service. Individuals were pretrained to assemble six faucets in 3.2 minutes. Each participant then performed the assembly task under three alcohol conditions—after a placebo drink containing no alcohol, a drink containing a trace of alcohol (.01% BAC), and a drink containing a very light dose of alcohol (.02% BAC). The average time to assemble six facets in the three conditions was 3.1 minutes (0% BAC), 3.1 minutes (.01% BAC), and 3.2 minutes (.02% BAC). Although performance was statistically significantly slower in the .02% BAC condition than the other two conditions, the time differences across the three conditions were small, with the largest difference equal to 6 seconds. The number of errors in the three conditions was 0.5 (0% BAC), 1.0 (.01% BAC), and 1.5 (.02% BAC). Although the increasing trend in errors with increasing doses of alcohol was statistically significant, the differences were again small. Phase 2 of this study was a replication using six volunteer university students and employing three conditions with slightly higher doses of alcohol (0%, .03%, and .07% BAC). The time to assemble six faucets showed a statistically significantly increase with dose of alcohol: 3.1 minutes at 0% BAC, 3.2 minutes at .03% BAC, and 3.7 minutes at .07% BAC. The time differences across the three conditions in Phase 2 were larger than in Phase 1, with the largest difference equal to 36 seconds. A key difference was that relative to those in Phase 1, the participants in Phase 2 had less relevant work experience. In Phase 2, there were no statistically significant differences in the number of errors across the three alcohol conditions.

Price and Flax (1982) studied the effects of four doses of alcohol (0%, .03%, .06%, and .09% BAC) on hits and misses in a drill press operation task. Hits were defined as the number of drill probe strokes within a hole in a plate without touching the plate in 32 seconds, and misses were defined as drill probe strokes where the probe touched the plate. Participants were eight male university students. The number of hits in the four conditions was 15.2 (0% BAC), 15.0 (.03% BAC), 13.4 (.06% BAC), and 12.3 (.09% BAC). The number of hits did not differ in the 0% and .03% BAC conditions or in the .06% and .09% BAC conditions. However, the number of hits was statistically significantly lower in the .06% and .09% BAC conditions than in the 0% and .03% BAC conditions. The number of misses was not affected by the level of BAC.

Price and Liddle (1982) investigated the effects of three doses of alcohol (0%, .06%, and .09% BAC) on welding performance. Participants were 12 male experienced arc welders whose ages ranged from 26 to 41 years. Three outcomes were assessed: welding speed, variation in electrode angles, and current reversals. Level of BAC was unrelated to welding speed and variation in electrode angles but was statistically significantly related to current reversals. The number of current reversals was 62.9 at 0% BAC, 64.9 at .06% BAC, and 72.9 at .09% BAC. The number of current reversals did not differ in the 0% and .06% BAC conditions. However, the number of current reversals was statistically higher in the .09% BAC condition than in the 0% and .06% BAC conditions. Current reversals reduce the quality of the weld and are "believed to be caused by subjects' impaired ability to keep the electrode holder steady" (Price & Liddle, 1982, p. 19).

Price, Radwan, and Tergou (1986) explored the effects of four doses of alcohol (0%, .05%, .07%, and .09% BAC) on an electronics assembly task. Participants in this study were eight male and eight female university students who had to assemble resistors in specific locations on a grid board. Two primary outcomes were used: quantity of work, which represented the number of correctly completed units, and quality of work, which represented the total number of five different types of errors. The results revealed that level of BAC did not affect the work quantity and quality of the men. In contrast, among the women, the number of completed units decreased as BAC increased (12.3, 10.5, 8.8, and 7.4 units, respectively) and the number of errors increased as BAC increased (4.6, 8.6, 11.5, and 15.2 errors, respectively).

Streufert et al. (1994) investigated the effect of three levels of BAC (0%, .05%, and .10%) on managerial performance. Participants were 48 men with managerial training and experience who responded to newspaper advertisements. All managers participated in two elaborate managerial simulations that lasted an entire day (7:00 a.m. to 4:30 p.m.). On a given task day, participants were assigned to receive either a placebo (0% BAC) or one of the two alcohol conditions (.05% or .10% BAC). During the simulations, 13 dimensions of complex cognitive performance were assessed. The results revealed that relative to the 0% BAC condition, the .05% BAC condition was statistically significantly related to lower scores on three of the 13 outcomes, whereas the .10% alcohol condition was related to lower scores on eight of the 13 outcomes. Nonetheless, some of the differences did not seem large, and the translation of the outcomes to managerial performance in real-world jobs is not necessarily straightforward.

Howland and colleagues conducted two simulation studies exploring the effect of low-dose alcohol exposure on simulated merchant ship power plant operation and piloting. Howland, Rohsenow, Cote, Siegel, and Mangione (2000) explored the effect of two levels of BAC (0% and .05%) on merchant ship power plant operations. Participants were 18 male and female engineering students in their senior year of a maritime academy, at least 21 years old, who had previous experience on the diesel simulator and had volunteered to participate in the study. There were four simulation scenarios of equal difficulty—two involving malfunctions in a boiler and two involving malfunctions in a turbogenerator. After the malfunctions were introduced, participants were allowed 20 minutes to identify the problem, initiate remedial action, and bring the system back to normal operation. The outcome was the amount of time to complete the scenario correctly. The results revealed a statistically significant difference, where the time to restore system operations was 3.1 minutes in the 0% BAC condition and 5.8 minutes in the .05% BAC condition. Thus, a BAC of .05% increased time to restore systems by 2.7 minutes. Under normal vessel operations, this difference may not be practically important, though it might be in an emergency situation.

Howland et al. (2001) explored the relation of two levels of BAC (0% and .05%) on merchant ship piloting. Participants were 38 junior and senior students, at least 21 years old, who were enrolled in a maritime academy and had volunteered to participate in the study. Participants did not actually steer the ship; rather, they provided orders to an experienced helmsman. Various scenarios were similar with regard to location, type of ship, current, daylight, and wind conditions but differed with respect to other vessel traffic and weather (fog) conditions. Each participant was allowed 25 minutes to enter Halifax harbor to pick up a pilot at a specified time, without exiting the channel (grounding) or colliding with oncoming traffic. Participants were rated on a number of dimensions of ship handling, collision avoidance, communications, situational awareness, and timeliness of rendezvous with the pilot. All scores were combined into a single total outcome score. The results revealed that the total performance scores were 0.0 at 0% BAC and −0.91 at .05% BAC. Thus, a BAC of .05% led to a statistically significant decrease in total performance scores. However, the scoring system does not lend itself to ready interpretation regarding the practical importance of the difference between the two alcohol conditions.

Three studies looked at the relation of acute alcohol impairment to surgical performance. Kirby, Kapoor, Das-Purkayastha, and Harries (2012) examined the relation of alcohol use on simulated microlaryngoscopy with excision of a predetermined glottis lesion. Participants were four male ear, nose, and throat (ENT) surgeons. The simulated surgery involved a laryngeal training mannequin. The surgical procedure was performed four times over a period of 4 hours. The first procedure was performed without alcohol exposure. The subsequent procedures were performed 45 minutes after ingesting 1 glass (125 ml), 3 glasses, or 6 glasses of wine. The surgeons consumed the next glass of wine over a period of 10 minutes immediately after completing a procedure.

Participants were rated in terms of an overall surgical score that ranged from 0 to 100. Across all four alcohol conditions and all four surgeons, scores ranged from 75 to 100. But there was wide variability in overall performance across the surgeons. For example, Surgeon 1 had his lowest score (83) in the no alcohol condition, achieved his highest score (100) after 1 glass of wine, and achieved lower scores after 3 glasses (95) and 6 glasses (85) of wine. Surgeons 2 and 3 had scores of 98 to 100 in the no alcohol, 1-glass, and 3-glass conditions. It was not until 6 glasses of wine were consumed that scores dropped (75 for Surgeon 2 and 80 for Surgeon 3). Finally, Surgeon 4 had scores of 100 in the no alcohol and 1-glass conditions and scores of 83 in the 3- and 6-glass conditions. In general, overall performance did not show decrements until after consumption of 6 glasses of wine for three surgeons and 3 glasses of wine for one surgeon. The surgeons were rated on 14 specific surgical criteria (e.g., positioning patient correctly, choosing correct scope, correct manipulation of specimen). Several areas of surgical skills were unaffected by alcohol for all surgeons, such as positioning of patient, instrument selection, and laser setting. Increasing amount of alcohol had a detrimental effect on laser technique, scope insertion, and lip care (i.e., not traumatizing patients' lips).

Two ENT surgeons who reviewed video of the procedures found that the participating surgeons showed appropriate interaction with the scrub nurse in the no alcohol and 1 glass of wine conditions. However, they found that after 3 glasses of wine the participating surgeons began to use inappropriate language and showed delayed responses to communication, and after 6 glasses of wine, the participating surgeons began to forget the names of regularly used instruments and to show frustration. The two observers found no deleterious effects in surgical performance in the 1 glass of wine condition. However, after 3 and 6 glasses of wine, all participating surgeons were deemed to be unsafe, and the observers would have stopped the surgeon in a real-life setting. Nonetheless, it appears that performance decrements were larger for behaviors related to interpersonal interactions than for actual surgical skills per se. This study has a number of limitations to keep in mind: (a) It was based on only four surgeons; (b) no information was provided on the actual BAC experienced during each procedure; (c) the meaning of the surgical performance scores is not clear, in that no threshold was defined that would represent inadequate performance; and (d) there was no attempt to show that the performance scores were related to actual surgical performance.

Dorafshar, O'Boyle, and McCloy (2002) studied the effect of a single dose of alcohol on laparoscopic cholecystectomy (i.e., minimally invasive gallbladder removal) using a virtual reality laparoscopic surgical simulator. The participants were 28 male medical students with no laparoscopic surgery experience. The participants were randomly assigned to a placebo or alcohol condition. In the alcohol condition, participants reached an average peak BAC of .085%. In both conditions, the surgical procedure was conducted 30 minutes before, 60 minutes after, and 10 hours after (next morning) beverage (placebo or alcohol) consumption. Results for performance under intoxication are discussed here, and the results for next day (e.g., hangover) performance are discussed subsequently. Four performance measures were derived: (a) mean number of errors (rod–rod contact, rod–object contact, tip–object contact, or an outside bounding error), (b) average time taken to complete the experimental procedure, (c) mean economy of movement, and (d) excessive burn time with the diathermy. The results revealed a statistically significant decrement in performance for the alcohol group compared with the placebo group 60 minutes after beverage consumption. The mean number of errors was 4.0 in the placebo condition and 6.8 in the alcohol condition, representing a difference of 2.8 errors. The mean time to complete the procedure was 34.5 seconds in the placebo condition and 37.8 seconds in the alcohol condition, representing a difference of 3.3 seconds. The economy of movement score was 4.3 in the placebo condition and 5.3 in the alcohol condition, representing a difference of 1.0 points. Finally, the excessive use of diathermy score was 1.35 in the placebo condition and 1.51 in the alcohol condition, representing a difference of 0.16 points. Despite these statistically significant differences, Dorafshar et al. (2002) commented that errors on this simulator procedure "cannot be validated as surgical errors, but they do provide an index of the accuracy of psychomotor performance" (p. 1754). However, Dorafshar et al. failed to discuss whether the observed psychomotor effects due to alcohol were sufficiently large to be of clinical importance.

Kocher, Warwick, Al-Ghnaniem, and Patel (2006) studied the effect of naturalistic alcohol use on a laparoscopic surgical procedure using a virtual reality surgical simulator. The participants were five male surgeons. The surgeons performed the surgical procedure under three conditions: (a) after a control night with no alcohol and a full night of sleep (control condition), (b) after a sham night out (sleep deprived) without alcohol (sham condition), and (c) after a night out where the participants could consume alcohol ad libitum (alcohol condition). In each of these conditions, the surgeons performed the surgical procedure at three different times: (a) during the workday, (b) at midnight, and (c) the following morning. In the alcohol condition, the surgeons reached a mean BAC of .043% (range = .035% to .055%). Results for performance under intoxication (i.e., at midnight) compared with performance during the workday are discussed here, and the results for next day (e.g., hangover) performance are discussed subsequently. Four performance measures were derived: (a) average time taken to complete the experimental procedure, (b) mean number of errors, (c) mean diathermy time, and (d) average time of diathermy damage. The results revealed a statistically significant increase in time taken to complete the procedure in the alcohol condition (108 seconds) compared with the control condition (61 seconds). The number of errors was statistically significantly higher in the alcohol condition (4 errors) than in the control condition (2 errors). The mean diathermy time was statistically significantly higher in the alcohol condition (26 seconds) than in the control condition (18 seconds). Alcohol was unrelated to average time of diathermy damage. Despite these statistically significant differences, the study was based on only five surgeons, and Kocher et al. failed to discuss whether the effects were sufficiently large to be of clinical importance and the conditions under which they might be of importance (e.g., performance under routine conditions vs. a crisis).

Finally, five simulation studies explored the effect of alcohol hangover. The first two studies assessed managerial effectiveness (Streufert et al., 1995) and maritime ship power plant operation (Rohsenow, Howland, Minsky, & Arnedt, 2006). These studies compared the next-day performance of individuals who were randomly assigned to a placebo condition (0% BAC) or a high-dose alcohol condition (.10%–.12% BAC) the night before participation in the simulations. Neither study provided evidence of alcohol hangover effects on performance. A third study by Wolkenberg, Gold, and Tichauer (1975) explored alcohol hangover on performance related to industrial production jobs. The study tested sober performance and performance the morning and afternoon after consuming enough alcohol to achieve BACs of .10%, .13%, and .16%. BACs had returned to zero by the time of morning testing. However, this study has a number of major problems. It included only nine participants—three participants per alcohol condition. Also, the manipulation of BACs failed. Instead of the three intended levels of BAC, the observed BACs revealed a continuous range from .065% to .17%. Although this study reported a few statistically significant performance decrements, the vast majority of comparisons were not statistically significant and few data were provided on the size of the effects. The remaining two studies, discussed earlier, assessed laparoscopic surgical performance. Dorafshar et al. (2002) failed to find an alcohol hangover effect on any of the four outcome variables. Kocher et al. (2006) found some evidence that alcohol hangover increased the amount of time taken to complete the procedure (80 seconds for the alcohol condition compared with 58 seconds for the control condition), but no evidence of hangover effects was shown on the remaining three outcomes.

Discussion

Relative to the other psychoactive drugs discussed later in this chapter, alcohol is the most widely used drug by employed adults (see Chapter 1) and therefore is the most salient drug with regard to cognitive and psychomotor performance. The experimental psychopharmacology literature summarized earlier suggests that low to moderate levels of acute alcohol intoxication (i.e., BAC ≤ .08%) have little if any consistent impairing effect on cognitive and psychomotor performance. This has been confirmed in experimental studies that used various tests of cognitive and psychomotor performance and in studies that assessed performance in a number of simulated work environments. There is somewhat more evidence of performance decrements with BAC ≤ .08 in the three surgical simulations, though the meaning of the performance scores is not clear. In contrast, the same types of studies have shown that high levels of alcohol intoxication (BAC ≥ .09%) can lead to cognitive and psychomotor impairment, and the impairment is greater as the complexity of the task increases. In contrast to experimental studies of acute alcohol intoxication, nonexperimental studies provide little evidence that, when a person is not under the influence of alcohol, his or her typical pattern of alcohol consumption affects cognitive and psychomotor performance when compared with that of nondrinkers, unless the pattern of alcohol use is long term and heavy. And among most long-term heavy drinkers, impairment relative to nondrinkers is often mild and reversible with long-term abstinence. Finally, little evidence exists that alcohol hangover has a consistent and robust effect on cognitive and psychomotor performance, and there is almost no evidence of statistically significant effects of hangover in several workplace simulation studies.

DEPRESSANTS: THERAPEUTIC

The main therapeutic depressants include barbiturates, benzodiazepines, other sedatives (nonbenzodiazepine hypnotics), and antipsychotics. In each group of therapeutic depressants, many variants exist that have different characteristics (short vs. fast onset and short vs. long duration) and various purposes: anxiolytic (reduce anxiety), sedative-hypnotic (induce sleep), antipsychotic (reduce delusions and hallucinations), muscle relaxant, or anesthetic. Among the depressants, barbiturates, the sedative methaqualone (Quaalude), and benzodiazepines have been most likely to be used illicitly. Barbiturates and methaqualone had a number of undesirable properties as therapeutic drugs, such as quickly developed tolerance, increased likelihood of dependence, and a significant risk of fatal overdose (Faupel et al., 2004;

Maisto et al., 2008). Thus, methaqualone became a Schedule 1 drug, and barbiturates are rarely used therapeutically (Maisto et al., 2008). Currently, the therapeutic depressants most often prescribed are the benzodiazepines. Although there are similarities among the depressants, this brief overview focuses on the more commonly used benzodiazepines.

The primary affective outcomes of benzodiazepines, used both therapeutically and recreationally, are euphoria, relaxation, and reduced anxiety. Research on the cognitive and psychomotor effects of benzodiazepines is limited because not all benzodiazepines have been evaluated to the same extent and many studies use different tests of the same type of performance, thereby making comparisons and general conclusions more difficult. Nonetheless, evidence exists from experimental research that single therapeutic doses of benzodiazepines given to healthy individuals having no experience with this type of drug (i.e., naive individuals) can impair various dimensions of cognitive and psychomotor performance. With regard to cognitive function, some dimensions of memory are impaired. For example, administration of benzodiazepines can impair the ability to learn new information but not the ability to learn new skills or procedures (Barbee, 1993; Ghoneim & Medwaldt, 1990; Verster & Volkerts, 2004). Benzodiazepines also may impair vigilance and effortful cognitive processes relative to automatic cognitive processes (Ghoneim & Medwaldt, 1990; Heishman & Meyers, 2007; Koelega, 1989).

In terms of psychomotor performance, inconsistencies exist across studies. It appears from experimental studies that therapeutic doses of benzodiazepines may impair performance after acute administration to naive individuals on simple tasks, such as finger tapping, and complex tasks, such as reaction time and tracking (Heishman & Meyers, 2007; Verster & Volkerts, 2004). However, one review concluded that simple motor skills are less likely than complex motor skills to show impairment (Kunsman, Manno, Manno, Kunsman, & Przekop, 1992), and another review concluded that simple motor tasks are impaired, whereas there is little evidence that "well established higher mental processes are adversely affected" (Wittenborn, 1979, p. 61S). As noted by Vermeeren and Coenen (2011), impairment varies according to a number of drug-related factors, such as the type of benzodiazepine, dosage, time of dosing (before bedtime vs. during the day), length of time since dosing, and frequency of dosing. Vermeeren and Coenen also noted that "increasing awareness of the risks associated with use of older benzodiazepines has changed the drugs prescribed. The majority of prescriptions nowadays are for relatively low doses of short half-life hypnotics, which have minor residual effects on daytime performance" (p. 99). Such changes in prescription practices are also likely to change the benzodiazepines available for illicit use, which may reduce the level of impairment among recreational users.

When treated daily with the same dose, individuals tend to develop tolerance to the impairing cognitive and psychomotor effects of benzodiazepines without developing tolerance to the positive affective outcomes. Thus, most cognitive and psychomotor impairment is observed after acute administration of therapeutic doses to nontolerant (naive) healthy individuals. In both patients who use benzodiazepines daily and frequent recreational users, tolerance develops such that impairment is less likely to be observed without increasing dosage (Barbee, 1993; Ghoneim & Medwaldt, 1990; Heishman & Meyers, 2007; Koelega, 1989; Kunsman et al., 1992; Roy-Byrne & Cowley, 1990; Vermeeren & Coenen, 2011; Verster & Volkerts, 2004). One meta-analysis is in disagreement with these conclusions, suggesting that long-term use of benzodiazepines is statistically significantly related to decreased cognitive and psychomotor performance (Barker, Greenwood, Jackson, & Crowe, 2004). However, the results of this review were based on a small number of studies for each outcome examined; did not address adequately whether or not impairment was affected by the drug-related factors highlighted earlier by Vermeeren and Coenen (2011); and cannot be used to discern whether or not the reported levels of impairment have any practical importance for functioning in daily life roles.

Workplace Stimulation Studies

In a laboratory simulation, Streufert et al. (1996) explored the acute effect of benzodiazepine administration, using moderate and high doses of alprazolam (trade names Xanax and Niravam), on complex cognitive functioning in a convenience sample of 16 male and five female managers recruited through newspaper advertisements. All managers participated in three elaborate managerial simulations that lasted an entire 9-hour day (7:00 a.m. to 4:00 p.m.). On a given task day, managers were assigned to receive a placebo, 0.5 mg alprazolam, or 1.0 mg alprazolam, which was administered twice during the task day. Six dimensions of complex cognitive performance were assessed during the simulations. The results revealed that relative to the placebo condition, drug treatment did not affect one outcome, diminished performance on two outcomes, and improved performance on three outcomes. On the basis of these results, Streufert et al. concluded that the use of alprazolam had diverse effects and that whether benzodiazepines and similar drugs would have positive or negative effects would depend on the current work environment and task conditions. It should be cautioned that the tasks used in this study may not generalize to real-world work situations, where decisions may be based on input from sources not available in these experimental simulations. Also, because the study used a very small convenience sample, the findings may not generalize to the broader population of managers and workers in general.

The results should be replicated in a larger and more representative sample of managers.

Hart and colleagues (Hart, Ward, Haney, & Foltin, 2003—Study 1; Hart, Haney, Nasser, & Foltin, 2005—Study 2) conducted workplace simulation studies to explore the possible beneficial effects of zolpidem (trade names Ambien, Edluar, Stilnox, and Zolpimist), which is a nonbenzodiazepine hypnotic, on psychomotor deficits due to shift work that might be the result of sleep disruptions. In Study 1, seven individuals completed a 23-day residential laboratory experiment. During this time, individuals worked alternating series of day and night shifts. During the day shift, individuals completed computerized psychomotor tasks from 8:30 a.m. to 5:30 p.m. and went to bed at midnight. During the night shift, individuals completed the psychomotor tasks from 12:30 a.m. to 9:30 a.m. and went to bed at 5:00 p.m. A placebo or one of two doses of oral zolpidem (5 mg or 10 mg) was administered 1 hour before going to bed. This study was replicated in Study 2 with eight participants over 21 days. The results of both studies showed that psychomotor performance declined during night shifts compared with day shifts and this performance decrement began to diminish after the third night shift in a row. In Study 1 both doses of zolpidem reduced the performance decrements due to the night shift, though the effects were small. In Study 2, the effects were mixed, with some performance outcomes improving and others worsening. Overall, the effect of zolpidem on shift-work-induced performance deficits was mixed and small. In terms of study limitations, the small convenience samples used in these two experiments limit the generalizability of the results to the broader population of shift workers, and the experimental paradigm may not generalize to actual shift work in various occupations.

Discussion

The research summarized here suggests that with the exception of acute intoxication in inexperienced users or due to increased dosage among frequent users, the illicit use of therapeutic depressants may not pose a large problem in the workforce or in the workplace. Further supporting this observation, Table 1.6 shows that only 0.4% to 1.1% of the general workforce reported illicit use of some form of sedative and 1.4% to 2.3% of the general workforce reported illicit use of a tranquilizer at least once during the past 12 months. Frequent use would be less prevalent. Moreover, additional analyses based on combined data from the National Survey on Drug Use and Health (NSDUH) and National Epidemiologic Survey on Alcohol and Related Conditions (NESARC) revealed that among U.S. employed adults, only 0.07% had a sedative use disorder (abuse or dependence) and 0.14% had a tranquilizer use disorder.

STIMULANTS

The primary stimulants include cocaine, amphetamine, and methamphetamine. Their main pharmacological effect is increased central nervous system stimulation that can counter the effects of fatigue. For recreational users who use low to moderate doses infrequently, the primary affect-related outcomes are feelings of exhilaration and euphoria, an increased sense of well-being, increased self-confidence, and heightened energy and alertness (Heishman & Meyers, 2007; Logan, 2002; Meyer & Quenzer, 2005). The typical findings of experimental studies of low to moderate acute doses of stimulants in naive users and abusers are either enhanced performance on many aspects of cognitive performance—including visuospatial perception, vigilance, selective attention, information processing speed, and memory—or no effects (Hart, Marvin, Silver, & Smith, 2012; Heishman & Meyers, 2007; Koelega, 1993; Meyer & Quenzer, 2005; Scott et al., 2007; Silber, Croft, Papafotiou, & Stough, 2006; Stough et al., 2012). Psychomotor effects of low to moderate acute doses include improved performance on simple, repetitive tasks; gross motor coordination; and sustained physical effort without rest or sleep (Heishman & Meyers, 2007; Meyer & Quenzer, 2005; Scott et al., 2007). Finally, no evidence exists of residual effects of methamphetamine use on early next day cognitive and psychomotor performance (Perez et al., 2008; Stough et al., 2012). In fact, the military has understood the value of using stimulants, such as amphetamines and more recently modafinil, to counteract performance deficits due to fatigue resulting from lack of sleep in ground troops and pilots since World War II (Eliyahu, Berlin, Hadad, Heled, & Moran, 2007; Logan, 2002). However, stimulants are administered to military personnel orally (slower onset of effect) in small, divided doses under medical supervision (Eliyahu et al., 2007; Logan, 2002), which differs from the unsupervised use of illicit users.

Despite potential benefits of proper use of stimulants, chronic and high-dose binge intake observed in many nonexperimental studies may be associated with irritability, anxiety, delusions of grandiosity, exhaustion, rapid flow of ideas, total insomnia, and fatigue (Cruickshank & Dyer, 2009; Heishman & Meyers, 2007; Logan, 2002; Meyer & Quenzer, 2005). However, when comparing the cognitive and psychomotor performance of chronic illicit users of stimulants who are not under the influence of stimulants to the performance of nonusers, several reviews have concluded that statistically significant impairments occur on a minority of outcomes, the size of these effects is typically small, and the scores for both chronic users and nonusers fall within a normal range of functioning (Cruickshank & Dyer, 2009; Hart et al., 2012; Scott et al., 2007). These findings suggest that few practically important performance differentials exist between nonusers and chronic stimulant users not taking stimulants.

Workplace Simulation Studies

Hart and colleagues (Hart, Ward, Haney, Nasser, & Foltin, 2003—Study 1; Hart et al., 2005—Study 2) conducted workplace simulation studies to explore the potential beneficial effect of methamphetamine on psychomotor deficits caused by shift work. In Study 1, seven individuals completed a 23-day residential laboratory experiment, and in Study 2, eight individuals completed a 21-day residential experiment. During these studies, individuals alternated between a series of day and night shifts. During the day shift, individuals completed computerized psychomotor tasks from 8:30 a.m. to 5:30 p.m. and went to bed at midnight. During the night shift, individuals completed the psychomotor tasks from 12:30 a.m. to 9:30 a.m. and went to bed at 5:00 p.m. A placebo or one of two doses of methamphetamine (5 mg or 10 mg) was administered 1 hour after waking. The results of both studies showed that psychomotor performance declined during night shifts compared with day shifts and that this performance decrement began to diminish after the third night shift in a row. Both doses of methamphetamine reduced the performance decrements due to the night shift in a dose-dependent manner. Moreover, methamphetamine improved performance on some outcomes that were not negatively affected by working a night shift per se. The performance improvements due to methamphetamine use were greatest on the first night shift and diminished across the second and third night shifts. The size of the beneficial effects on the night shift depended on the outcome and ranged from small to large. Methamphetamine had little effect on performance during day shifts. In terms of study limitations, these two experiments used small convenience samples, which limited the generalizability of the results to the broader population of shift workers, and the experimental paradigm may not generalize to actual shift work in various occupations.

Discussion

The research on stimulant use suggests that use of stimulants at a low to moderate dose has primarily positive results on cognitive and psychomotor performance. Also, when individuals are not under the influence of stimulants, the cognitive and psychomotor performance of chronic, high-dose users does not differ substantially from that of nonusers. High-dose binge intake of stimulants, however, may be associated with irritability, anxiety, insomnia, and fatigue. Nonetheless, these findings suggest that stimulant use may not have a substantial impact in the workforce or in the workplace. Further supporting this observation, Table 1.6 shows that approximately 1.2% to 2.1% of the adult U.S. workforce has reported using a stimulant at least once during the past 12 months. Rates of frequent high-dose bingeing use would be even lower. Moreover, additional analyses based on combined data from the NSDUH and NESARC revealed that among U.S. employed adults, only 0.13% had a prescription stimulant use disorder (abuse or dependence), and 0.51% had a cocaine use disorder.

MARIJUANA

Marijuana refers to the dried leaves and flowering tops from the hemp plant (*Cannabis sativa*). The primary psychoactive compound in marijuana is Δ^9-tetrahydrocannabinol (THC). Natural derivatives of marijuana are *hashish*, which is compressed resin extracted from the flowering tops that contains a higher concentration of THC than marijuana, and *hash oil*, which is a viscous liquid derived from hashish that contains a higher THC concentration than hashish. But the most popular form of use is smoking or eating marijuana, though this depends somewhat on the region of the world.

The primary motivation for using marijuana is for its psychological effects, which include a sense of well-being, feelings of relaxation, intensified sensory experiences, and increased sociability (Adams & Martin, 1996; Maisto et al., 2008; Mosher & Akins, 2007). Evidence suggests that many of the psychological effects of marijuana are learned, that they differ across individuals, and that they are shaped by the situation in which marijuana is used (Earleywine, 2002; Maisto et al., 2008; Mosher & Akins, 2007). With regard to cognitive effects, experimental administration studies suggest that acute intoxication is unlikely to affect simple learning and remote memory for things already learned (Earleywine, 2002). Nonetheless, acute intoxication may have detrimental effects on attention during long dull tasks but not during short dull tasks, speed of learning new material, short-term memory of things learned during intoxication, and mathematical ability (Adams & Martin, 1996; Earleywine, 2002; Huestis, 2002; Ranganathan, & D'Souza, 2006; Schwenk, 1998). Acute intoxication may also alter time perception, making intoxicated individuals perceive that time is passing more slowly (Adams & Martin, 1996; Earleywine, 2002).

Results for psychomotor performance are mixed. Experimental studies of acute intoxication and observational studies that compare nonintoxicated marijuana users and nonusers are about equally split between reporting impairment and finding no effects on various types of psychomotor performance, such as coordination and tracking (Earleywine, 2002; Schwenk, 1998). However, any cognitive and psychomotor impairments related to acute marijuana intoxication can (a) increase with dosage and the complexity of the task, (b) decrease with well-practiced (i.e., overlearned) tasks and skills, and (c) generally resolve after 3 to 4 hours (Earleywine, 2002; Huestis, 2002;

Schwenk, 1998). Tolerance may also play a role. For example, Hart, van Gorp, Haney, Foltin, and Fishman (2001) explored the acute effect of three doses of THC (0%, 1.8%, and 3.9%) on the cognitive performance of 18 experienced marijuana smokers who averaged 24 marijuana cigarettes per week. They concluded that "acute marijuana smoking produced minimal effects on complex cognitive task performance in experienced marijuana smokers" (Hart et al., 2001, p. 757).

Some research has explored the effects of chronic marijuana use by comparing individuals reporting long-term, heavy use (several months to 20 years) and individuals who had not used marijuana. As noted by Earleywine (2002) and Solowij and Battisti (2008) and as discussed subsequently, such studies are fraught with methodological problems that make firm conclusions difficult. Nonetheless, such research suggests that long-term, heavy use of marijuana does not produce statistically significant or practically relevant debilitating impairment of cognitive function (e.g., Coggans, Dalgarno, Johnson, & Shewan, 2004; Earleywine, 2002; Hall & Babor, 2000; Smith, Longo, Fried, Hogan, & Cameron, 2010; Solowij & Battisti, 2008; Tait, MacKinnin, & Christensen, 2011). This failure to find impairment may be the result of tolerance developed among chronic users (Adams & Martin, 1996; Ramaekers, Kauert, Theunissen, Toennes, & Moeller, 2009; Tait et al., 2011). Finally, any observed cognitive deficits due to long-term, chronic heavy use of marijuana are subtle; their meaning for performance in various life domains is unclear, and they may be reversible with lower levels of use (Tait et al., 2011). It is also important to consider that long-term chronic marijuana users would represent a small proportion of the workforce. For example, Frone (2006b) reported that only 1.5% of the U.S. workforce used marijuana daily or nearly daily over the preceding 12 months. Thus, the proportion of the workforce using marijuana chronically for many years likely would be smaller.

Workplace Simulation Study

A simulation study was conducted by Wadsworth et al. (2006) with a convenience sample of 85 U.K. workers (34 marijuana users and 85 nonusers) representing a variety of occupations. Each person completed a number of assessments of mood and took part in a number of tasks assessing various dimensions of psychomotor and cognitive performance. Some marijuana users may have used marijuana during this test week, though insufficient information was provided. The measures and tasks were completed immediately before and after the first day and last day of a workweek. During each workday, participants completed questionnaires assessing various outcomes that occurred during the day. The results of the daily reports are discussed in Chapter 4. The results of the beginning and end of week testing showed that compared with nonusers, marijuana users did not perform more poorly on recognition memory, simple reaction time, focus of attention, intrusion errors, semantic recall, immediate recall, speed of encoding new information, or ratings of anxiety. However, compared with nonusers, marijuana users showed lower levels of alertness and some deficits in psychomotor and cognitive performance. Although these relations were statistically significant, the size of the relations was not large and may be of little practical importance. For example, during a search task, the average speed of response for marijuana users was 22.18 milliseconds (i.e., 0.02 second) and that for nonusers was 29.89 milliseconds (i.e., 0.03 second). In other words, marijuana users' average speed of response was 0.01 second (i.e., 1/100th of a second) slower than the average speed of response among nonusers. Also, in a test of delayed recall before work, marijuana users correctly recalled an average of 5.8 words compared with an average of 6.3 words among nonusers. Not only is this statistically significant difference small, when one considers that the maximum number of words that could be recalled was 20, marijuana users and nonusers performed equally poorly. Thus, this study of employed marijuana users shows little evidence of noteworthy impairment on a number of affective, cognitive, and psychomotor laboratory measures and tasks.

Kagel, Battalio, and Miles (1980) conducted three elaborate simulation studies to explore the influence of marijuana use on work output and hours worked in an experimental economy. Studies 1 and 2 each had 20 male participants between 21 and 27 years of age, and Study 3 had 20 female participants between 18 and 25 years of age. The participants in each study represented a convenience sample of regular marijuana users. Those in the drug and placebo conditions resided continuously for 98 days in the simulated economic environment in separate wings of the hospital facilities of the Addiction Research Foundation. In each environment, income was earned by weaving sash belts on primitive, portable handlooms. The work could be done anywhere on the ward, at any hour of the day or night and for any length of time. This flexibility meant that the researchers were unable to explore the effects of marijuana on absenteeism and tardiness, and the simple job meant that injuries could not be explored. The ward included five bedrooms, four workrooms, four lounges, and a dining room. The floor also had a store, open 24 hours per day, where the participants could purchase consumable items with their income (e.g., tobacco cigarettes, soft drinks, candy, alcoholic beverages, toiletries).

Participants in each study were randomly assigned to an environment where they were provided marijuana cigarettes or placebo marijuana cigarettes that contained low levels of THC. In each condition, no marijuana was available during the first 17 days. In the drug condition of Study 1, after the no-drug period, participants could purchase unlimited numbers of marijuana cigarettes containing 8 milligrams of THC for the first week with no required smoking. During the next 27 days, participants were required to smoke 2 marijuana cigarettes (8 milligrams THC) consecutively at 8:15 each evening, and they could purchase unlimited number of marijuana cigarettes containing 8 milligrams of THC. During the last 15 days of Study 1, the THC content of the mandatory and purchased marijuana cigarettes was increased from 8 to 12 milligrams. In the drug condition of Studies 2 and 3, after the no drug period, participants were immediately required to smoke 2 marijuana cigarettes (8 milligrams THC) consecutively at 8:15 each evening, and they could purchase unlimited numbers of marijuana cigarettes containing 2 milligrams of THC.

In the control condition in Study 1, after the no drug period, participants were immediately required to smoke 2 placebo marijuana cigarettes (1 milligram THC) consecutively at 8:15 each evening, and they could purchase unlimited numbers of these placebo marijuana cigarettes. In the control condition in Studies 2 and 3, after the no drug period, participants were not required to smoke placebo marijuana cigarettes, although they could purchase unlimited numbers of these placebo marijuana cigarettes containing 2 milligrams of THC.

The findings indicate that average daily intake of THC in the drug condition ranged from 16.3 milligrams in Study 3 to 18.7 milligrams in Study 1. In all three studies, there was no statistically significant difference between the drug condition and the placebo condition in terms of overall daily production (number of belts made per person). The number of hours worked per day did not differ across conditions in Studies 1 and 2, but there was statistically significant reduction in work hours in the drug condition compared with the placebo condition in Study 3. Finally, there was no difference between conditions in output per hour in Studies 1 and 3. In Study 2, the output per hour was statistically significantly higher in the drug condition than in the placebo condition. To explore the effect of acute intoxication, Kagel et al. (1980) examined the number of hours worked in the 2.5 hours after smoking the mandatory marijuana cigarettes. The results indicate that there was a reduction in work hours. They also reported that this tendency to schedule work time away from the period of maximum intoxication showed interindividual variability, concluding that "the results reported here disprove any contention that the heavy use of marijuana is *inherently* incompatible with maintaining productivity levels . . . and the capacity to carry out vocational responsibilities" (Kagel et al., 1980, p. 390). Nonetheless, they clearly stated that it would be unwarranted to generalize the results of these studies to the effect of heavy, regular marijuana use on labor productivity in the general labor force. However, the results do suggest that any effects of marijuana on productivity are likely due to acute intoxication and not overall patterns of use per se.

Discussion

The importance of the relations described here for the workforce and the workplace is not easy to gauge. After alcohol, marijuana is the next most prevalent psychoactive substance used by the workforce, and it is substantially more prevalent than any of the other illicit drugs or illicitly used prescription drugs (see Table 1.6). Although marijuana is the most frequently used illicit substance among employees, additional analyses based on combined data from the NSDUH and NESARC revealed that among U.S. employed adults, only 1.6% had a marijuana use disorder (abuse or dependence). Consistent with this finding, Looby and Earleywine (2007) reported that most daily marijuana users are not dependent. Moreover, because unintoxicated marijuana users do not show gross impairment compared with nonusers, the key issue is the extent to which marijuana users are acutely impaired just before work or during work hours. Frone (2006b) estimated that only about 1% of the U.S. workforce used marijuana before work or during the workday or was impaired by marijuana during the workday at least 1 day per week. This further supports the idea that most regular marijuana users find intoxication incompatible with major life commitments and schedule use during times of leisure (Kagel et al., 1980).

NARCOTIC ANALGESICS

There are several classes of narcotic analgesics (Faupel et al., 2004). Opium is the dried sap that comes from the seed capsule of the opium poppy (*Papaver somniferum*). Opiates are alkaloids extracted from raw opium (e.g., codeine, morphine). Semisynthetic opioids do not occur naturally and are created from natural opiates (e.g., heroin, oxycodone, hydrocodone). Finally, synthetic opioids are artificially manufactured and have no origin in the poppy plant (e.g., methadone, fentanyl, Demerol, Darvon).

The primary pharmacological effect of all narcotic analgesics is to reduce pain, with some sedation as a side effect. Nonetheless, they are used recreationally for their affective effects, which include a sense of relaxation and euphoria (Maisto et al., 2008; Meyer & Quenzer, 2005). Several reviews have suggested that in terms of cognitive and psychomotor outcomes, narcotic analgesics produce little or no impairment in human performance (Fishbain, Cutler, Rosomoff, & Rosomoff, 2003; Heishman & Meyers, 2007; Zacny & Gutierrez, 2011). In contrast, other studies and reviews suggest that narcotic analgesics cause sedation and impairments in gross motor coordination, fine motor skills, focused attention, and perhaps memory (Heishman & Meyers,

2007; Kalant, 1997; Meyer & Quenzer, 2005; World Health Organization, 2004). Zacny (1995) stated that the answer to the question "Do opioids impair performance?" is a "guarded yes, depending on the particular opioid and dose involved, the population studied, and the length of opioid use" (p. 460).

Two key factors influence whether or not research shows cognitive and psychomotor impairment due to narcotic analgesics. First, acute administration impairs performance in a dose-dependent manner. The second and perhaps more important factor is tolerance (Fishbain et al., 2003; Heishman, 1998; Zacny, 1995, 1996). Acute performance impairments are sometimes found in experimental studies after administration of narcotic analgesics to naive healthy individuals. In contrast, little or no performance impairments are observed among occasional and frequent users, licit or illicit, who have developed tolerance to narcotic analgesics. Research also suggests that withdrawal among dependent opioid users produces little cognitive and psychomotor impairment (Zacny, 1995). In concluding his detailed review of narcotic analgesics and psychomotor and cognitive performance in humans, Zacny (1995) concluded that "for opioid users (dependent and nondependent), laboratory studies show little if any impairment, and most epidemiologic studies suggest no increased risk of accidents or impaired neuropsychological functioning" (p. 458). He further concluded that "individuals taking opioids at a stabilized dose for medically approved reasons should be allowed to work" (Zacny, 1996, p. 1583). Similarly, Heishman and Meyers (2007) concluded that "when administered to opioid-tolerant individuals, such as opioid abusers or patients with chronic pain, opioids typically produce little or no performance impairment, including impairment of skills related to driving" (p. 224). A similar conclusion was reached by Fishbain et al. (2003).

Discussion

These results suggest that with the exception of acute intoxication in inexperienced users or recreational users who increase their typical dose, narcotic analgesic use may not pose a general problem in the workforce or in the workplace. Further supporting this observation, Table 1.6 shows that only 0.1% of the workforce reported using heroin and 2.3% to 5.3% reported illicit use of a prescription narcotic analgesic at least once during the past 12 months in the overall workforce. Frequent use would be less prevalent. Moreover, additional analyses based on combined data from the NSDUH and NESARC revealed that among U.S. employed adults, only 0.06% had a heroin use disorder (abuse or dependence) and 0.52% had a narcotic analgesic use disorder.

HALLUCINOGENS

A number of substances have been grouped under the heading of hallucinogens. The serotonergic hallucinogens, such as LSD, mescaline, and psilocybin, cause perceptual distortions (hallucinations) in any sensory modality (e.g., hearing, sight, touch), impairment in psychomotor and cognitive performance, and a variety of emotional experiences (euphoria, depersonalization, anxiety, and fear; Faupel et al., 2004; Maisto et al., 2008; Meyer & Quenzer, 2005; World Health Organization, 2004). However, the exact constellation of symptoms and experiences differs across individuals and is affected by the state of the person and the context in which the drugs are used. Serotonergic hallucinogen use occurs infrequently because consistent use results in a loss of effect due to the quick onset of tolerance (e.g., World Health Organization, 2004). Unlike many other drugs, serotonergic hallucinogens do not lead to dependence or withdrawal (Meyer & Quenzer, 2005; Nichols, 2004).

Another group of substances classified as hallucinogens is methylated amphetamines, of which ecstasy (abbreviated as MDMA) is the best known. The effects of using ecstasy are similar to those of using stimulants (amphetamines, methamphetamine, and cocaine) and the serotonergic hallucinogen mescaline. Various reviews of user reports and experimental studies suggest that ecstasy leads to generally pleasurable affective effects, such as feelings of euphoria, increased emotional warmth and empathy, extraversion, lowered defensiveness, and increased emotional and physical energy. Although ecstasy can enhance sensory perceptions, it does not produce the hallucinations that may result from use of the serotonergic hallucinogens (e.g., Dumont & Verkes, 2006; Maisto et al., 2008; Mosher & Akins, 2007; Parrott, 2001; Teter & Guthrie, 2001; World Health Organization, 2004). Paradoxically, some evidence exists that ecstasy may increase anxiety as well (Dumont & Verkes, 2006). Also, there are retrospective reports by some heavy ecstasy users of "rebound effects" in which the initial positive affect turns to fatigue and negative mood in the days following use (e.g., Parrott, 2001). Reports of the effect of ecstasy on cognitive and psychomotor performance are inconsistent. Research suggests that there may be no effects, improvements, or deficits in various dimensions of cognitive and psychomotor performance, but the effects may be small. In nonexperimental studies, little impairment exists among the predominant group of infrequent and light users compared with individuals who do not use ecstasy, whereas deficits sometimes occur among heavy and chronic users (Fisk, Montgomery, Wareing, & Murphy, 2006; Golding, Groome, Rycroft, & Denton, 2007; Jager et al., 2007; Kalechstein, De La Garza, Mahoney, Fantegrossi, & Newton, 2007; Montoya, Sorrentino, Lukas, & Price, 2002; M. J. Morgan, 2000; Parrott, 2001; Teter & Guthrie, 2001; Verkes et al., 2001). In a review that focused solely on 29 experimental administration studies that used placebo control groups,

Dumont and Verkes (2006) found little evidence for the effects of ecstasy on cognitive and psychomotor performance. Also, an experimental study by Stough et al. (2012) found no evidence of next day residual effects of ecstasy administration on 15 measures of cognitive and psychomotor performance.

A final category of hallucinogens is dissociative anesthetics, such as phencyclidine (PCP, angel dust) and ketamine (Special K). PCP and ketamine were developed as anesthetics for humans and animals. The use of PCP as a human anesthetic was stopped because of a variety of negative postoperative side effects, such as hyperexcitability, hallucinations, delirium, dizziness, and visual disturbances, and it is no longer used as a veterinary anesthetic (Maisto et al., 2008; Meyer & Quenzer, 2005; C. J. Morgan & Curran, 2012; Mosher & Akins, 2007). Ketamine had less severe reactions and is still used for anesthesia and pain management in humans and for veterinary anesthesia (Maisto et al., 2008; Meyer & Quenzer, 2005; C. J. Morgan & Curran, 2012; Mosher & Akins, 2007). When PCP or ketamine are used recreationally, acute intoxication is related to feelings of euphoria; numbness; slurred speech; insensitivity to pain; feelings of being disconnected from one's body; distorted perception of time and space; and a dose-dependent elevated risk of cognitive impairment, psychomotor impairment, and accidents and injuries (Jansen, 2000; Maisto et al., 2008; Meyer & Quenzer, 2005; C. J. Morgan & Curran, 2012; Mosher & Akins, 2007). In terms of the chronic effects of general patterns of use when not intoxicated, a longitudinal observational study (C. J. A. Morgan, Muetzelfeldt, & Curran, 2010) found that when statistically significant cognitive deficits were observed, it was only among very frequent ketamine users (used drug more than 4 days per week) compared with less frequent ketamine users (used drug less than 4 days per week), abstinent ketamine users (abstinent for at least 1 month), polydrug users who did not use ketamine, and non–drug users. Morgan and Curran's (2012) review of the ketamine literature also reported that evidence of chronic cognitive and psychomotor impairment when not intoxicated was restricted to frequent ketamine users. Tolerance to the hallucinogenic properties of ketamine develops quickly (Jansen & Darracot-Cankovic, 2001; C. J. Morgan & Curran, 2012), leading some individuals to stop using the substance, though others continue to use it for effects that resemble those of other drugs (e.g., cocaine, opium, marijuana, and depressants; Jansen & Darracot-Cankovic, 2001).

Discussion

This research suggests that acute impairment from hallucinogens, as well as chronic use, can negatively affect cognitive and psychomotor performance. Despite these findings, hallucinogen use may not pose a major problem in the workforce or in the workplace. As shown in Table 1.6, less than 2% of the adult U.S. workforce reported using any hallucinogen at least once during the past 12 months. Frequent use would be less prevalent. Moreover, additional analyses based on combined data from the NSDUH and NESARC revealed that among U.S. employed adults, only 0.11% had a hallucinogen use disorder (abuse or dependence).

INHALANTS

Inhalants represent a broad set of volatile compounds that are grouped according to route of administration. The three types used for their psychoactive effects are volatile solvents (e.g., gasoline, lighter fluid, paint thinner, toluene), aerosols (e.g., spray paint, hair spray, vegetable oil spray for cooking, fabric protector spray), and gases (e.g., nitrous oxide, ether, chloroform, butane, propane, refrigerants). Relative to the other classes of psychoactive substances, less is known about the acute and chronic effects of inhalants (Balster, 1998). Research suggests that in low doses, the performance-related effects of inhalants mimic those of the central nervous system depressants, most notably alcohol (J. F. Williams & Storck, 2007). For example, the immediate affective effects associated with the use of inhalants are feelings of euphoria, excitation, and exhilaration, which usually last only a few minutes without repeated use (J. F. Williams & Storck, 2007). Higher doses can lead to affective, psychomotor, and cognitive deficits, such as depression, slurred speech, delusions, disorientation, sedation, and weakness (Kurtzman, Otsuka, & Wahl, 2001; Lubman, Yucel, & Lawrence, 2008; Meyer & Quenzer, 2005). With prolonged use, inhalants may have effects similar to those of hallucinogens (Kurtzman et al., 2001; Lubman et al., 2008; J. F. Williams & Storck, 2007).

Discussion

Despite their impairing effects, inhalants may not represent a major issue in the workforce or in the workplace because of their low rate of use among adults (J. F. Williams & Storck, 2007). Table 1.6 shows that 0.5% of the adult U.S. workforce reported using an inhalant at least once during the past year. Frequent use would be even less prevalent. Moreover, additional analyses based on combined data from the NSDUH and NESARC revealed that among U.S. employed adults, only 0.02% had an inhalant use disorder (abuse or dependence). The near-zero prevalence of inhalant use and disorders among employed adults is not surprising because inhalants are used primarily among children and adolescents worldwide, though most do not use them on a regular basis, and their use tapers off relatively quickly for most individuals (Lubman et al., 2008; J. F. Williams & Storck, 2007; Wu & Ringwalt, 2006). For instance, the 2008 NSDUH showed that in the general U.S. population, the past 12-month (past 30-day) prevalence rate declined from 3.0% (1.1%) among 12- to 17-year-olds to 1.1% (0.1%) among those 26 years or older (U.S. Department of Health and Human Services, 2009).

STRENGTHS AND LIMITATIONS OF PSYCHOPHARMACOLOGY AND WORKPLACE SIMULATION RESEARCH

Psychopharmacological research can be classified into two types of studies: experimental and nonexperimental or observational. The major strength of experimental studies, which include most workplace simulation studies, is that participants are randomly assigned to experimental conditions (i.e., levels of substance exposure). Random assignment of participants to conditions balances individual differences in personal characteristics and environmental exposures across the experimental conditions. This reduces the likelihood that the effect of substance use on some measure of performance is spurious, because of uncontrolled common causes, and increases our ability to conclude that different levels of substance exposure cause differences in the assessed outcomes (e.g., Fava, 1996; Meyer & Quenzer, 2005).

Because it is unethical to randomly expose individuals to certain substances, certain doses, or long-term use of a substance, nonexperimental designs are often used. In such studies, researchers typically compare naturally occurring groups of individuals who use a specific substance at different frequencies (e.g., infrequent users vs. daily users) among themselves and to a group of individuals who do not use the specific substance. However, nonexperimental studies do not have the same advantage as experimental studies, because individuals in the various user groups (nonusers, infrequent users, daily users) are likely to differ on a number of preexisting personal characteristics (personality, cognitive functioning, psychomotor functioning) and environmental exposures (work stress, coworkers and friends who use the substance), and the users of a given drug may use drugs other than the one under investigation (e.g., Falk, Yi, & Hiller-Sturmhofel, 2008; Lubman et al., 2008; Mintzer, 2007; Montoya et al., 2002; Swendsen et al., 2010). Therefore, unless all relevant causes of being in a particular user group and of performance levels on some outcome are assessed and controlled in the study design or statistical analyses, it is impossible to attribute an observed difference in performance across user groups to their substance use with any confidence (e.g., M. J. Morgan, 2000; Teter & Guthrie, 2001).

A strength of experimental and nonexperimental psychopharmacological studies is that researchers use objective measures of cognitive and psychomotor performance rather than rely on individuals' self-reports of how well they think they function. Although self-reports of behavior can be useful, they can have a number of deficiencies that make their use and interpretation more challenging (for more details, see Stone et al., 2000; Tourangeau, Rips, & Rasinski, 2000).

Regardless of whether or not experimental or nonexperimental designs are used in psychopharmacological studies, there are study design and researcher practice issues that can affect the conclusions drawn from any single study or set of studies. It is not my goal to summarize all possible research limitations. Rather, I focus on a few issues readily observed in the literature that affect the inferences that can be drawn regarding employee productivity from the results of psychopharmacological research. For more information, the interested reader should consult the review of methamphetamine use and cognitive performance by Hart et al. (2001). Their review provides an important discussion of how methodological issues in psychopharmacological research can result in unwarranted and misleading conclusions.

The first issue relates to the sampling of participants. The samples are often very small (fewer than 15 participants) and are not randomly drawn from any specific target population of interest. In other words, convenience samples are used where the participants are self-selected. Typically, volunteers are recruited by various nonsystematic means (e.g., newspaper advertisements). Thus, it is not possible to generalize findings beyond the sample of individuals participating in a given study. Also, information on the employment status of the participants is almost never reported, making it impossible to determine the extent to which the active workforce is represented in most of these studies. A final sampling issue relevant to workplace simulation studies is that participants are usually college students inexperienced with the job being simulated. The generalizability of the findings from simulation studies to real workplaces would be enhanced if study participants were randomly selected, employed, and experienced job holders with respect to the simulated job.

A second issue is that nonexperimental studies focus on length of using a substance or the frequency of use over some specified period of time. These studies pay little attention to the quantity or dose of substance use because, with the exception of alcohol, it is difficult to assess actual dose consumed and the likely concentration in blood because there are issues regarding substance quality and many alternate routes of administration. Therefore, in nonexperimental studies, higher frequency of use may be inappropriately used as a proxy for higher dosage (Temple, Brown, & Hine, 2011).

A third issue is related to the assessment of cognitive and psychomotor performance. Dozens of different tests are used across studies to assess various dimensions of psychomotor and cognitive performance. Some of these tests are validated, though the validity of others is unknown, and it may not be appropriate to equate the outcomes of different measures of the same performance dimension (Hart et al., 2012; Wittenborn, 1979). But more important, it is unknown how scores on these cognitive and psychomotor tests relate to performance in daily life, in particular performance at work. In other words, the tests may have low relevance to everyday functioning, making it difficult to determine if statistically significant differences found in psychopharmacological studies have any relevance to practically important impairment at work (Barbee, 1993; Hart et al., 2012; Heishman, 1998; Huestis, 2002; Parrott, 1991b; Stein & Strickland, 1998; Verster & Volkerts, 2004). There also may be a lack of correspondence between performance using simulators (driving, flight, ship piloting, surgery) and real-life performance (Dorafshar et al., 2002; Howland et al., 2001; Mayhew et al., 2011; Patat, 2000). Although Parrott (1991b) noted that it is very difficult to assess everyday performance, he advised psychopharmacological researchers to put more effort into doing so.

A fourth issue that has been mentioned several times is that the conclusions regarding performance impairment are based on the statistical significance of differences and relations. Little attempt is made to determine or discuss whether the statistically significant effects are practically important (Hart et al., 2012; Temple et al., 2011), even when the outcomes can be measured in meaningful metrics (e.g., milliseconds, number of words recalled). This issue is closely related to the third issue above. To determine the practical importance of statistically significant differences in cognitive and psychomotor tests for everyday life and the workplace, researchers should begin exploring the relation of these test scores to actual performance in various life roles. Statistically significant results are often used to argue for various changes regarding treatment, policy, and the like. Yet, in the absence of showing that an effect on a laboratory task is large and related to performance in everyday life, it is likely that proposed interventions and policies are not justified, may not have much impact, or may even have unanticipated negative consequences. The utility of evidence-based interventions or policy is a function both of the quality of the study design and of the practical importance of the effects.

Fifth, in many experimental studies researchers fail or do not attempt to disentangle pharmacological and expectancy effects. Individuals often are not blind to having or not having received a substance. Thus, any performance effects may be due to the pharmacological effects of a drug, individuals' expectations that they received the drug, or some combination of pharmacological and expectancy effects.

Finally, the focus of most psychopharmacology and workplace simulation research has been on tests of basic cognitive and psychomotor outcomes. Such research cannot explore certain outcomes of direct relevance to employers, such as attendance outcomes (absenteeism, tardiness, leaving work early), performance in specific jobs, and on-the-job injuries. Although such outcomes could be examined in nonexperimental psychopharmacological studies, this literature has not explored such outcomes. Nonetheless, nonexperimental organizational field research summarized in Chapter 4 has studied these and other, broader employee productivity outcomes.

FUTURE RESEARCH

Resolving key methodological issues highlighted earlier that limit the generalizability of psychopharmacological research to the workforce and workplace should receive more attention. For example, future studies should use samples that are larger and more directly representative of employed adults. More research should focus on the development and use of workplace simulations. However, such research should develop a link between (a) scores on cognitive/psychomotor tests and performance in workplace simulations and (b) actual employee performance and other workplace behavioral outcomes. Finally, more attention should be devoted to determining the practical importance of observed performance impairments for functioning in real-life roles.

GENERAL SUMMARY AND CONCLUSIONS

At low to moderate doses, all psychoactive substances initially cause positive emotional experiences, which motivate their use. However, high acute doses or frequent heavy use may be associated with negative emotional experiences. With the exception of stimulants, increasing levels of acute intoxication among inexperienced or naive users lead to greater cognitive and psychomotor impairment. The level of impairment is typically greater for complex tasks than for simple tasks. However, individuals taking fixed doses of most psychoactive substances develop tolerance to many of their effects on cognitive and psychomotor performance. Increasing dose among those who develop tolerance will lead to renewed impairment until tolerance is reestablished.

The substance most likely to present a problem in the workforce and workplace is alcohol. Acute alcohol intoxication is consistently related to statistically significant cognitive and psychomotor performance impairment at BACs $\geq$ .09%. Also, heavy alcohol use and drinking to intoxication are more prevalent than illicit drug use in the workforce, and the use of alcohol in the workplace is more prevalent than the use of illicit drugs (see Chapter 1). In contrast, studies of alcohol hangover provide little evidence of strong or consistent effects on cognitive or psychomotor performance. It may be that psychopharmacological research has not induced severe hangovers. Nonetheless, less severe hangovers may be more representative of the hangovers experienced at work. Those drinking to a level that induces a severe hangover are likely to be absent from work the next day.

Even among experimental psychopharmacological studies using naive individuals, the observed cognitive and psychomotor effects based on neuropsychological tests and workplace simulations are often not strong and may be of little practical importance. Among nonexperimental psychopharmacological studies, evidence exists for some impairment among unintoxicated users of alcohol and hallucinogens compared with nonusers. However such impairment is associated with heavy, long-term use, and impairment is likely to resolve with long-term abstinence. But, for most substances, comparisons of unintoxicated users with nonusers show little evidence that an individual's typical pattern of substance use affects cognitive and psychomotor performance. Where differences do exist, it is difficult to establish that a pattern of psychoactive substance use causes a particular outcome because it is difficult to rule out the possibility (a) that the relation is spurious due to common causes both of the substance use and of the outcome or (b) that the putative outcome is actually the cause of using the substance (i.e., reverse causality).

It is easy to determine if the relation between substance use and performance is greater or less than zero and is statistically significant. However, it is difficult to determine if the size of a statistically significant relation is clinically or practically important, and few researchers attempt to make this assessment. The development of interventions and policies must address effects that have practical relevance, or the policies and interventions will expend resources with little or no notable return on investment and may result in unanticipated negative outcomes.

4

PRODUCTIVITY OUTCOMES: ORGANIZATIONAL FIELD RESEARCH, COST-OF-ILLNESS STUDIES, AND AN INTEGRATIVE MODEL

The productivity outcomes of employee substance involvement and the cost of employee substance involvement to employers have received much attention and speculation in the research and trade literatures. The basic question underlying this interest and much research has been, can employee substance use impair work-related behaviors and outcomes? If this is the basic question of interest, the answer is a simple yes. In other words, it would be reasonable to assume that a large-enough dose of any psychoactive substance can lead to acute intoxication sufficient to interfere with employee attendance, performance, or safety. But this is not a useful question for those interested in employee productivity (e.g., Normand et al., 1994). Moreover, experimental psychopharmacology and workplace simulation research summarized in Chapter 3 supports the irrelevance of such a basic question. A broader and more relevant question is this: Given employees' typical patterns (e.g., prevalence, frequency, and quantity), contexts (e.g., outside the workplace and work hours or during the workday), and experience (e.g., tolerance) related

DOI: 10.1037/13944-005
Alcohol and Illicit Drug Use in the Workforce and Workplace, by M. R. Frone

to the use of psychoactive substances, as well as their personal and workplace characteristics, will their substance use lead to attendance, productivity, or safety problems? It can be anticipated that the answer to this question will not be a simple yes or no.

Thus, my first goal in this chapter is to summarize nonexperimental organizational field research on substance use and employee productivity outcomes. The following three categories of outcomes are considered: (a) attendance, (b) task performance and other on-the-job behaviors, and (c) job accidents and injuries.[1] The strengths and weaknesses of organizational field studies are then summarized. The second goal is to look at major cost-of-illness studies to see if they provide any useful information on the potential costs of employee substance involvement to employers. The final goal is to present a general model of employee substance involvement and workplace productivity that integrates prior research findings, highlights the complexity of these relations, and provides directions for future research.

ORGANIZATIONAL FIELD RESEARCH

Before I summarize research on productivity outcomes, four general issues must be considered. First, organizational field studies are similar to nonexperimental psychopharmacological studies in that the use of psychoactive substances is not manipulated and there is no random assignment of workers to levels of substance use. In organizational field studies, researchers typically compare naturally occurring groups of individuals who use a specific substance with those who do not use the substance or simply assess the frequency of using a substance for every participant in a study. Second, in contrast to psychopharmacological (experimental and observational) and workplace simulation research discussed previously, organizational field

---

[1]Several studies of productivity outcomes are not included in the review because of an important methodological flaw: measurement confounding the outcome variable with the putative cause variable (French, Zarkin, Hartwell, & Bray, 1995; Jones, Casswell, & Zhang, 1995). Two other studies reported both confounded and unconfounded measures of absenteeism (Roche, Pidd, Berry, & Harrison, 2008; Roche, Pidd, Bywood, & Harrison, 2008). Only the results for the latter measure are reported. As an illustration of the nature of the problem, consider the following example. With regard to absenteeism, the confounded outcome variable represents answers to a question such as "How often are you absent from work due to your drinking?" and the putative causal variable represents responses to a question such as "How often do you drink?" The outcome variable simultaneously assesses individual differences both in absence and in alcohol use. Therefore, both the cause and outcome variables are measures of the frequency of drinking. Because two measures of the same thing are expected to be related, assessing absenteeism this way (a) will inflate the size of the relation between alcohol use and absenteeism and (b) may create a spurious relation. A better way to assess absenteeism is to ask, "How often have you been absent from work?" without attribution to any possible cause. This problem occurs with other outcomes, such as reports of job performance or job injuries. Because measures are often not adequately described in published papers, it is possible that this problem may exist with some of the studies that are summarized.

research typically distinguishes only between alcohol use and any illicit drug use. In other words, when substances other than alcohol are studied, there are few attempts to explore the effects of specific drug classes on productivity outcomes. All psychoactive drug use is lumped together. For example, all illicit drug users are compared with those who report no illicit drug use, or a measure of the frequency of any illicit drug use may be used. Nonetheless, combining the use of all illicit drugs may not be as problematic as it might first appear. Based on the psychopharmacology literature, all drugs used illicitly, if they have any effect at all, are expected to have a negative effect on performance. One exception is the appropriate use of stimulants that can increase performance, though appropriate use may not characterize illicit use.

Third, organizational field research has focused more attention on alcohol use than illicit drug use. This may be surprising, given that the primary concern of the media, policymakers, and managers is the use of illicit drugs (see also Chapter 5). Nonetheless, this focus on alcohol is not misplaced because the use, impairment, and dependence associated with alcohol are much more prevalent than those associated with illicit drugs (see Chapter 1). Finally, the productivity outcomes that are the focus of organizational field studies (e.g., absenteeism, job injuries, task performance) are broader and more complex than the basic dimensions of cognitive performance (number of words recalled from a list) and psychomotor performance (i.e., amount of time in milliseconds to respond to a cue) assessed in psychopharmacological research. Although these productivity outcomes have greater direct relevance to employers, they are much more difficult to assess well than the outcomes in psychopharmacological research.

Attendance Outcomes

Employee attendance represents three different behaviors that are of interest when they occur without prior approval: full-day absence, tardiness, and leaving work early. Unscheduled time away from work is a key defining characteristic of attendance problems because it tends to be more costly and disruptive than scheduled time away from work (e.g., Cascio & Boudreau, 2008), and one might assume that unscheduled time away from work is more likely to be related to substance use. Of the three attendance outcomes, full-day absence has been the almost exclusive focus of past research. In the summary to follow, all attendance outcomes are assumed to be unscheduled, and *absenteeism* means full-day absence.

A consensus exists across several older literature reviews that absenteeism is the productivity outcome most consistently related to overall alcohol use (e.g., Martin, Kraft, & Roman, 1994; Normand et al., 1994; Zwerling, 1993). However, these conclusions were based on a few studies that used small, nonrandom samples of employees. Some studies looked at alcohol-dependent employees who were undergoing treatment and had no comparison group (e.g., non-alcohol-dependent employees or nondrinkers). The results, therefore, may not accurately represent the experiences of all alcohol-dependent workers and certainly do not represent the workforce at large. Other studies used broader but still unrepresentative samples; were unpublished and of unknown quality; or failed to control adequately for important common causes of both overall alcohol involvement and absenteeism, such as preexisting person characteristics (e.g., personality, affective disorders), environmental characteristics (e.g., stressful work environments, family problems), or the use of other drugs. Finally, this research often focused on whether or not a person was absent over some period of time and failed to consider the frequency of absenteeism or the length of each spell of absenteeism.

More recent research and reviews show more inconsistent relations between overall alcohol involvement and attendance. Many studies support a positive relation (e.g., Bacharach, Bamberger, & Biron, 2010; Cunradi, Greiner, Ragland, & Fisher, 2005; Laaksonen, Piha, Martikainen, Rahkonen, & Lahelma, 2009; Mangione et al., 1999; Marmot, North, Feeney, & Head, 1993; McFarlin & Fals-Stewart, 2002; Norström, 2006; Roche, Pidd, Berry, & Harrison, 2008; Salonsalmi, Laaksonen, Lahelma, & Rahkonen, 2009; Vahtera, Poikolainen, Kivimäki, Ala-Mursula, & Pentti, 2002), whereas many studies fail to support a relation (e.g., Ames et al., 1997; Blum, Roman, & Martin, 1993; Boles, Pelletier, & Lynch, 2004; Independent Inquiry Into Drug Testing at Work [IIDTW], 2004; Lim, Sanderson, & Andrews, 2000; Moore, Grunberg, & Greenberg, 2000; Peter & Siegrist, 1997; Stewart, Ricci, Chee, & Morganstein, 2003; Upmark, Moller, & Romelsjo, 1999; Vasse et al., 1998). Given this inconsistency, closer inspection of the research findings suggests two factors that may affect the relation between overall alcohol involvement and absenteeism. First and most important is the assessment of alcohol involvement. Studies that assessed frequency of heavy drinking, such as consuming five or more drinks per occasion, or that clearly separated out individuals with high levels of consumption or impairment from those with moderate or no consumption were more likely to find a relation between alcohol use and absenteeism. Second, one study reported that the relation between overall heavy alcohol use and absenteeism increased at higher levels of supervisor social support and decreased at higher levels of peer social support (Bacharach et al., 2010). This study suggests that workplace characteristics might influence the relation between heavy alcohol use and absenteeism.

With regard to overall illicit drug involvement, the few studies that have looked at absenteeism also have reported inconsistent results. Some research supports a statistically significant positive relation between overall illicit drug involvement and poor attendance, either absenteeism or tardiness (Bass et al., 1996; El-Bassel et al., 1997; Normand, Salyards, & Mahoney, 1990; Roche, Pidd, Bywood, & Freeman, 2008; Zwerling, Ryan, & Orav, 1990), and some research fails to support this relation (Lim et al., 2000). However, the studies supporting a relation between illicit drug involvement and attendance often used self-selected samples and failed to control adequately for preexisting person characteristics (e.g., personality, affective disorders), environmental characteristics (e.g., stressful work environments, family problems), or the use of alcohol. For example, Zwerling et al. (1990) warned that "we cannot exclude the possibility that the associations we found . . . were confounded by alcohol abuse" (p. 2643). Two U.S. studies support these concerns (Becker, Sullivan, Tetrault, Desai, & Fiellin, 2008; French, Zarkin, & Dunlap, 1998). These studies used large random samples and controlled for a wide range of demographic variables, coexisting mental and physical health problems, and in one case the use of alcohol. These studies failed to find a relation of any overall illicit drug use (French et al., 1998) or opioid use (Becker et al., 2008) to absenteeism.

Finally, one study addressed the practical importance of the relation of alcohol and illicit drug disorders to absenteeism. In other words, do alcohol and illicit drug use disorders play a major role in employee absence relative to other potential causes of absence? Using U.S. national data, Foster and Vaughan (2005) estimated that the cost of absenteeism due to combined alcohol or drug abuse and dependence represented 0.2% of U.S. payroll and 4.5% of lost wages due to all absences. On the basis of their results, they concluded that

> [substance] abuse-based absenteeism is, at best, an incidental cost to business and is insufficient to justify significant prophylactic or therapeutic investments of scarce human resource dollars to achieve an abuse and dependence free workplace. These findings force both public and private sector policymakers to turn to a "hazardous use"/"critical incident" rationale as the basis of their argument that American business should invest human resource dollars in specific programs and technologies to achieve a drug-free workplace. (Foster & Vaughan, 2005, p. 27)

Compared with other research on overall substance involvement and attendance, Foster and Vaughan (2005) broached an important and typically ignored issue. Rather than ask the typical question—are substance use disorders related to absenteeism?—it asked a more useful question: Relative to other possible causes of employee absenteeism, are substance use disorders a major cause that should be addressed or a minor cause with little practical importance? The latter question deserves much more attention among researchers exploring any putative productivity outcome of employee substance involvement.

Job Performance and Dysfunctional Workplace Behaviors

Researchers have examined the relation of overall alcohol involvement to several dimensions of job performance and dysfunctional work behaviors. Friedman, Granick, Utada, and Tomko (1992) found that current alcohol abuse and frequency of intoxication were negatively related to supervisory ratings of job performance. Boles et al. (2004) failed to find a relation between overall alcohol use and employee reports of presenteeism, which represents coming to work ill such that the quantity and quality of one's work were diminished. Lim et al. (2000) failed to find a relation of alcohol abuse or dependence to employee reports of presenteeism. Burton et al. (2005) failed to find a relation between overall alcohol use and self-reported productivity loss. Blum et al. (1993) failed to find a relation of overall alcohol use to employee self-ratings of job performance and provided little evidence of a relation involving collateral (coworker or supervisor) ratings of several dimensions of job performance. Two studies failed to find a relation between overall problem alcohol use and supervisory ratings of job performance among police officers (Lowmaster & Morey, 2012; P. A. Weiss, Hitchcock, Weiss, Rostow, & Davis, 2008). Finally, a meta-analytic review found that the relation of overall alcohol use to self-reports, supervisor reports, and archival records of job performance was very weak, and no research could support a causal effect (Ford, Cerasoli, Higgins, & Decesare, 2011).

Looking at overall alcohol involvement and other dysfunctional work behaviors, Moore et al. (2000) reported a weak but statistically significant positive relation between a measure of overall problem drinking and employee self-reports of the percentage of work time spent "goofing off" at work, but they reported no relation to the likelihood an employee would be retained (i.e., not fired). Lehman and Simpson (1992) explored the relation of overall alcohol use to general behavioral outcomes. They found statistically significant but small associations of overall alcohol use both to work-related psychological withdrawal (e.g., daydreaming, putting in less effort than should have, spent time on personal matters) and to physical withdrawal (falling asleep at work, taking longer lunch or rest breaks than allowed). However, alcohol use was not related to lower levels of positive work behaviors (e.g., did more than required, tried to think of ways to make job better) or higher levels of antagonistic behaviors (argued with coworkers, disobeyed supervisor's instructions).

Three studies found a statistically significant relation between overall alcohol use and the expression of various forms of aggression at work. McFarlin, Fals-Stewart, Major, and Justice (2001) found that alcohol use was positively related to the expression of both psychological and physical aggression at work. Greenberg and Barling (1999) reported that alcohol use was positively related to an overall measure of psychological and physical aggression against coworkers but was unrelated to aggression against subordinates or supervisors. Bacharach, Bamberger, and McKinney (2007) explored the relation of alcohol use among men and gender harassment reported by women across work groups. They found a positive association between the proportion of men in a work group identified as heavy drinkers and the probability that a female coworker would report that she had experienced gender harassment by her male coworkers. Moreover, this relation was stronger among groups that had social norms supporting alcohol use during lunch.

A few studies have examined the relation of overall illicit drug involvement to several performance outcomes. Zwerling et al. (1990) reported that that marijuana use was positively related, cocaine use was unrelated, and the use of other drugs was positively related to experiencing formal discipline because of inadequate job performance. Friedman et al. (1992) failed to find a relation between overall illicit drug use and supervisory ratings of job performance. Two studies failed to find a relation between overall problem drug use and supervisory rating of job performance among police officers (Lowmaster & Morey, 2012; P. A. Weiss et al., 2008). Lim et al. (2000) failed to find a relation of overall illicit drug abuse or dependence to self-reported job performance. Finally, Wadsworth et al. (2006) asked a sample of marijuana users and nonusers to provide daily reports regarding nine dimensions of work performance for 1 week. Marijuana users and nonusers did not differ on any of the nine measures: amount of effort devoted to work, productivity, inefficiency, making mistakes, loss of concentration, forgetting what one intended to do, trouble making decisions, forgetting where one put things, and getting sidetracked.

All the studies of job performance and dysfunctional work behaviors described so far assessed overall patterns of alcohol or illicit drug use in the workforce. In contrast, a study by Ames et al. (1997) examined the simultaneous relations of overall and workplace alcohol use and impairment to several dimension of dysfunctional work behaviors. Ames et al. found that overall alcohol use (usual and heavy) was unrelated to problems with supervisors, sleeping on the job, and problems with tasks and coworkers. Similarly, drinking before work was unrelated to all three outcomes. Drinking at work was positively related to problems with supervisors and sleeping on the job but not to problems with tasks and coworkers. Finally, having a hangover at work was positively related to sleeping at work and problems with tasks and coworkers but not to problems with supervisors.

A study by Mangione et al. (1999) simultaneously tested the relation of several dimensions of alcohol consumption to an overall measure of performance problems. Unfortunately, the outcome measure combined items assessing attendance, task performance, and job injuries, thereby making the meaning of the results unclear. Mangione et al. found that usual alcohol use was unrelated to the overall measure of performance problems. Overall frequency of intoxication had a weak positive relation to performance problems, and drinking on the job had a stronger positive relation to performance problems.

Lehman and Simpson (1992) explored the simultaneous relations of overall alcohol use, overall illicit drugs use, and workplace substance use (alcohol and illicit drug use combined) to four outcomes. The four outcomes, which are described in more detail in the discussion of alcohol use, were positive work behaviors, psychological withdrawal, physical withdrawal, and antagonistic behaviors. The results indicated that overall illicit drug use had a weak negative relation to positive work behaviors and was unrelated to the other three outcomes. In contrast, substance use at work had weak positive relations to psychological withdrawal, physical withdrawal, and antagonistic behaviors but was unrelated to positive work behaviors.

Accident and Injury Outcomes

Workplace safety—injuries and accidents—is the most widely researched productivity outcome, especially with respect to employee substance use. Two general sources of data address this relation. The first source of data comes from medical examiner records, emergency room visits, and large drug testing programs. Zwerling (1993) estimated that acute alcohol impairment is present in approximately 5% of nonfatal work injuries and 10% of fatal work injuries. Based on the average positivity rates for over 37.5 million urine tests for employee illicit drug use over a 5-year period (2005–2009), conducted by Quest Diagnostics Incorporated (2010), 2.6% of postaccident drug tests were positive for at least one illicit drug in the federally mandated safety-sensitive workforce, and 5.6% of postaccident drug tests were positive in the general workforce. However, to conclude that an accident or injury was "drug related" because some level of inactive metabolites is present in a person's urine is insufficient evidence that the substance is related to or even played a causal role in the accident or injury. The primary problems with studies that report the proportion of postaccident drug tests that are positive for an illicit drug are the lack of a control condition and the inability of urine tests to discern the timing of substance use relative to the injury or accident and the level of impairment (see Chapter 5).

Nonetheless, the relation between overall use of an illicit drug and job injuries can be addressed by comparing the positivity rate from postaccident urine drug tests to the positivity rate from random urine drug tests. If overall employee drug use is strongly related to workplace accidents and injuries, the positivity rate for postaccident urine drug tests (2.6% in the safety-sensitive workforce; 5.6% in the general workforce) should be substantially higher than the positivity rate for random urine drug tests (1.5% in the safety-sensitive workforce; 5.7% in the general workforce). However, these comparisons do not support a relation, causal or otherwise, between overall illicit drug use and workplace accidents and injuries. But this is not surprising because, as highlighted later in this chapter and suggested in Chapter 3, workplace injuries are the likely outcome of acute impairment at work at the time of injury, and urine drug testing provides evidence only of drug use that occurred sometime in the recent past and therefore does not assess acute impairment at the time of injury. Further supporting this conclusion, a study of commercial aviation accidents from 1995 to 2005 by Li et al. (2011) compared the prevalence of illicit drug test violations from random urine drug tests (0.64%) with the prevalence of postaccident urine drug tests (1.82%). Li et al. concluded that because of the very low prevalence of drug violations and the small relation between illicit drug use and being involved in an accident, only a small fraction of aviation accidents (1.2%) might be related to illicit drug use. It was not possible to determine if this small relation was causal because the study did not control for potential common causes of illicit drug use and being involved in an accident.

Although urine tests have been the standard for employee drug testing, other specimens are starting to be used (more is said about this in Chapter 5). In its most recent report, Quest Diagnostics Incorporated (2011) summarized the results of oral fluid testing for the years 2006 to 2009 for the general workforce. No data on oral fluid testing are reported for the safety-sensitive workforce because U.S. federal drug testing guidelines do not allow for the use of biological specimens other than urine. Compared with urine testing, oral fluid testing is argued to provide a more sensitive test for the presence of a drug at the time of testing (see Chapter 5). Thus, one might expect that oral fluid testing would provide stronger evidence for a relation between illicit drug use and job injuries or accidents. The average postaccident positivity rate in the general U.S. workforce was 3.2% based on oral fluids, whereas the positivity rate was 3.4% for random oral fluid tests. Therefore, as with urine tests, oral fluid testing provides no evidence of a link between overall illicit drug use and job accidents or injuries.

Quest Diagnostics does not report results for workplace alcohol testing, but the Federal Transit Administration (FTA) in the Department of Transportation publishes an annual report on the positivity rates for random and postaccident drug and alcohol tests among safety-sensitive job categories (i.e., vehicle operation, vehicle and equipment maintenance, vehicle control and dispatch, commercial driver's license holders, and armed security personnel). A look at combined results for 2006 to 2008 (FTA, 2008, 2009, 2010) reveals that the positivity rates for illicit drug use were 0.8% for random testing and 1.3% for postaccident testing. The positivity rates for alcohol use were 0.14% for random testing and 0.13% for postaccident testing. Thus, these comparisons do not support a relation of either illicit drug use or alcohol use to major workplace accidents and injuries. The results for alcohol are interesting because the confirmatory breath tests should be able to detect impairment at time of testing (i.e., on-the-job), whereas tests for illicit drug use largely capture off-the-job use and cannot be used to document on-the-job impairment. But an alcohol violation is defined by the FTA as having a blood alcohol content (BAC) $\geq .04\%$. The FTA reports do not provide information on the distribution of BAC for those with an alcohol violation. However, one explanation for the lack of relation between a positive alcohol test and driver accidents is that drivers with an FTA alcohol violation may have BACs clustered at the low end. In other words, if driver BACs were mostly in the range of $\geq .04\%$ to $\leq .07\%$, the psychopharmacology results presented in Chapter 3 would suggest that alcohol may not play a major contributory role in many accidents, especially if the drivers had developed tolerance to low levels of alcohol.

The second source of data on employee substance involvement and work-related accidents and injuries is epidemiologic and organizational field studies. Most of this research has compared individuals with various chronic patterns of overall alcohol or illicit drug use with nonusers or has compared those who have a substance abuse or dependence disorder with those who do not have such a disorder. Several reviews of this literature have been published (e.g., Beach, Ford, & Cherry, 2006; Feinauer, 1990; Frone, 1998, 2004; IIDTW, 2004; Macdonald, 1997; Macdonald et al., 2010; Normand et al., 1994; Ramchand, Pomeroy, & Arkes, 2009; Stallones & Kraus, 1993; Veazie & Smith, 2000; Webb et al., 1994; Zwerling, 1993). From these reviews, a set of conclusions can be derived: (a) The evidence for a relation between overall alcohol or illicit drug involvement and job injuries is mixed, with more studies failing to find a relation; (b) in the studies finding a statistically significant positive relation, the strength of the relation is weak; (c) most studies finding a statistically significant relation cannot support a causal effect of overall substance involvement on job injuries because the studies failed to account for the temporal order of substance use and injuries, they failed to control adequately for possible common causes of substance use and being injured, or they failed to do both; and (d) even if the relations were causal, the generally weak effects and the often typical low base rate of illicit drug use and heavy drinking suggest that only a small proportion of occupational injuries would be related to alcohol or illicit drug use.

The results from drug test positivity rates and organizational field studies summarized above are consistent in suggesting that little, if any, relation exists between overall alcohol or illicit drug use and job injuries. An examination of the general epidemiological literature on overall unintentional injury rates is instructive for understanding this lack of relation. This literature is largely based on studies of emergency room visits that used a variety of research designs, though some general survey studies also exist. The outcome represented in these studies is experiencing an unintentional injury in any context and largely represents injuries that occur away from work. As with the literature on substance use and work injuries, this literature suggests that typical overall patterns of alcohol use are not related or only weakly related to experiencing an unintentional injury (e.g., Cherpitel, 2007; Coghlan & Macdonald, 2010; Taylor et al., 2010).

Although epidemiologic research does not support a strong relation between typical patterns of overall alcohol use and experiencing an injury, this literature shows that injuries are consistently associated with a single occasion of heavy drinking (i.e., BAC > .08% for women and .10% for men) that occurs within 1 to 6 hours of being injured. Thus, consistent with research summarized in Chapter 3, acute alcohol intoxication, not one's typical pattern of drinking per se, is the likely operative cause of injuries (Bazargan-Hejazi, Gaines, Duan, & Cherpitel, 2007; Borges, Cherpitel, & Mittleman, 2004; Cherpitel, 2007; Cherpitel, Giesbrecht, & Macdonald, 1999; McLeod, Stockwell, Stevens, & Phillips, 1999; Taylor et al., 2010; Watt, Purdie, Roche, & McClure, 2004; M. Williams, Mohsin, Weber, Jalaludin, & Crozier, 2011). One emergency room study that looked at work and nonwork injuries separately found that any relation between alcohol use and both types of injuries was almost exclusively due to recent use, with chronic use playing a very minor role (Pidd et al., 2006). Furthermore, even the effect of acute intoxication may have to be qualified. A study by Borges et al. (2004) found that the relation of acute intoxication to experiencing an injury was much lower among individuals who frequently get intoxicated and those who are alcohol dependent. Consistent with research reviewed in Chapter 3, this finding suggests that acute intoxication is most likely to cause injury among those who have little tolerance to alcohol's effects on cognitive and psychomotor functioning. Finally, with regard to illicit drugs, it appears that both typical use of illicit drugs and the use of drugs within 6 hours of an injury may not predict injuries after controlling for acute alcohol intoxication (e.g., Bazargan-Hejazi et al., 2007; Cherpitel et al., 1999; Watt et al., 2004; M. Williams et al., 2011).

This epidemiological research suggests that because virtually all workplace injury research summarized in the reviews cited above has assessed employees' typical pattern of substance use away from work, it is not surprising that little evidence exists for a relation between employee substance use and job injuries. Research should assess substance impairment during the workday rather than typical patterns of overall use, and two studies have attempted to do so. Frone (1998) found that when examined separately, both overall substance impairment (alcohol and marijuana combined) and workplace substance impairment were positively associated with job injuries among working adolescents. However, when the measures were examined simultaneously, only workplace substance impairment was positively related to job injuries, even after controlling for a number of other demographic, personality, and health variables. In contrast, a study by Ames et al. (1997) failed to find a relation between drinking at work and having an accident at work. There is a clear need for more research on work injuries focusing on substance impairment during the workday. Yet even if future research supports a relation between workplace substance use and job injuries, it might be anticipated from the prevalence data in Chapter 1 (Tables 1.14 and 1.15) that workplace substance use will play only a minor causal role relative to other possible causes of workplace injuries and accidents.

Strengths and Limitations of Organizational Field Studies

Compared with the psychopharmacological studies (experimental, observational, and workplace simulations) discussed in Chapter 3, organizational field studies have two strengths. First, these studies examine the behavior of actual employees in naturalistic work settings. Second, rather than studying basic outcomes, such as reaction time or delayed recall, organizational field studies explore higher level productivity outcomes that are directly relevant to employers, such as attendance, job performance and dysfunctional workplace behaviors, and job injuries. Nonetheless, organizational field studies suffer from several major methodical problems. Researchers study patterns of typical substance use rather than experimentally manipulated levels of acute intoxication or impairment. However, one does not need to list the reasons why it would be unethical to randomly expose individuals to different substances or different levels of a substance in order to see if they make it to work or not (absenteeism) and, if they do go to work, whether their performance would suffer or they would experience an injury or accident. Also, most studies use research designs that cannot provide evidence of causal effects; they can provide only evidence of associations, and it is unclear whether or not many of these associations are spurious due to inadequate control of common causes of substance use and the various productivity outcomes. Even if the observed relations were causal, the research designs provide no information on the direction of causality. For example, being injured at work or having a job that one cannot perform well may be a source of stress that causes the use of alcohol or illicit drugs.

Most organizational field studies also suffer from several general problems shared by psychopharmacological studies and workplace simulations and described in Chapter 3: (a) failing to randomly sample study participants from a defined population and instead relying on nonrandom samples of self-selected volunteers; (b) paying much attention to the use or frequency of use of a substance, with little attention being paid to the quantity or dose of a used substance; (c) using many different measures to assess productivity, which makes comparisons across studies difficult; and (d) basing evidence for possible performance impairment due to substance use on the determination of the statistical significance of observed relations, with little emphasis paid to whether or not the size of the relations is practically important. A final problem of special importance to organizational field studies is the failure to consider the various contextual features of substance use, such as the distinction between use and impairment, the influence of tolerance on the effects of a substance, and the timing of use or impairment (off-the-job use vs. during the workday, including just before work and during breaks).

COST-OF-ILLNESS STUDIES

Past research has attempted to estimate the cost of employee alcohol and illicit drug involvement to employers using an economic analysis referred to as a *cost-of-illness* (COI) study.[2] COI studies assess many individual costs of an illness that are aggregated into broader categories, such as medical, nonmedical, productivity loss, and intangible. Such studies provide an estimate of the overall societal cost, along with aggregate costs associated with the various categories. For present purposes, the primary interest is in the cost of lost productivity. COI studies for alcohol or illicit drug use have been conducted in a number of countries other than the United States: Australia, Canada, Finland, France, Germany, Japan, the Netherlands, New Zealand, Portugal, Scotland, South Korea, Spain, Sweden, Thailand, and the United Kingdom (Baumberg, 2006; Collins & Lapsley, 2002; Fenoglio, Parel, & Kopp, 2003; García-Altés, Ollé, Antoñanzas, & Colom, 2002; Rehm et al., 2006; Thavorncharoensap, Teerawattananon, Yothasamut, Lertpitakpong, & Chaikledkaew, 2009). However, the present discussion is restricted to COI studies conducted in the United States because there are a larger number of such studies, and the issues that relate to them are relevant to many COI studies conducted outside the United States.

The following issues are considered in turn: (a) cost of lost productivity from the major COI studies in the United States, (b) the limitations of these cost estimates in terms of representing employer costs, (c) whether

---

[2]The details of conducting COI studies are beyond the scope of this chapter, but the interested reader is referred to Akobundu, Ju, Blatt, and Mullins (2006); French, Rachal, and Hubbard (1991); Segel (2006); and Single et al. (2001).

better estimates exist, and (d) the general limitations of COI studies. A number of estimates of the cost of lost productivity due to substance abuse/dependence have been presented over the years. With regard to alcohol abuse/dependence, Rice and colleagues (Rice, 1999; Rice, Kelman, Miller, & Dunmeyer, 1990) estimated the cost of lost productivity to be $51.3 billion in 1985 and $121.4 billion in 1995. Harwood and colleagues (Harwood, 2000; Harwood, Fountain, & Livermore, 1998) estimated the cost to be $107.0 billion in 1992 and $134.2.billion in 1998. These earlier estimates by Harwood and colleagues were updated by Bouchery, Harwood, Sacks, Simon, and Brewer (2011) to reflect the estimated cost of lost productivity due to excessive alcohol consumption (not alcohol abuse/dependence), which was $161.6 billion in 2006. With regard to illicit drug abuse/dependence, Rice and colleagues (Rice, 1999; Rice et al., 1990) estimated the cost of lost productivity to be $8.5 billion in 1985 and $38.1 billion in 1995. Although Harwood et al. (1998) provided an estimate of the productivity costs of illicit drug abuse/dependence for 1992, that estimate was updated by the Office of National Drug Control Policy (2004) and yearly estimates were provided from 1992 to 2002. The estimated cost of lost productivity due to illicit drug abuse/dependence was $77.4 billion in 1992, $107.3 billion in 1999, and $128.6 billion in 2002.

These COI study estimates suggest that alcohol and drug abuse/dependence potentially cost employers in the United States a staggering amount of money annually. Moreover, such estimates catch the attention of the media and are cited on web pages and in trade and scientific publications to make just this point. However, the estimated cost of lost productivity in these COI studies is not borne by employers. To understand the underlying issue, one needs to consider the definition of lost productivity in major COI studies. It might be assumed that the cost of lost productivity due to substance involvement represents the costs associated with outcomes like poor attendance (full- and partial-day absence), poor performance, and job injuries. In fact, assessing such dimensions of productivity is what COI guidelines recommend (e.g., Harwood & Reichman, 2000; Single et al., 2001). As noted by Single (2009), however, "there is a lack of data on the costs of specific substance-related productivity problems, such as absenteeism, job turnover, lower on-the-job productivity, substance-attributable disability and so forth" (p. 118). Because such outcomes are absent from the data sets used to estimate the substance-related productivity costs in the COI studies summarized previously, how was lost productivity defined? The COI studies used a human capital approach to assessing productivity costs and defined lost productivity in terms of potential lost wages due to substance-related premature death, incarceration, crime victimization, hospitalization for treatment, inability to perform household tasks, and, in the case of alcohol, being born with fetal-alcohol syndrome.

In other words, the lost productivity costs represented the present value of potential lost future earnings for work in the labor market and household that was never performed but might have been performed in the absence of a substance use disorder.

Putting aside the many arguable and unverifiable assumptions used to derive the actual costs (e.g., Baumberg, 2006; Larg & Moss, 2011), the potential forgone losses in wages do not represent costs to employers. Although the lost productivity costs they presented have been cited as employer costs due to alcohol and illicit drug abuse/dependence, Harwood et al. (1998) explicitly stated that "this study has not attempted to estimate the burden of drug and alcohol problems on work sites or employers, nor should the estimates in this study be interpreted in this manner" (Section 1.4). The reason is that the costs of lost productivity represented by potential lost earnings due to work not performed are borne primarily by the substance users and their families (Harwood et al., 1998; Heien & Pittman, 1989; Larg & Moss, 2011). Although other COI researchers have failed to address the issue of who bears the costs of their lost productivity estimates, the fact that it is not employers applies to all COI studies reviewed previously. As Harwood and Reichman (2000) commented, "The studies of the costs to society include important components of costs beyond the workplace, but they explicitly refrain from attributing specific amounts to workplaces and, in particular, to employers" (p. 50).

If the major COI studies reviewed above do not address the costs of employee substance involvement to employers, has any study done so? Using data from the 1990–1992 National Comorbidity Survey, Hertz and Baker (2002) estimated the costs of lost productivity to employers based on self-report measures of absenteeism and reduced work performance. Reporting costs in 1999 dollars, they estimated that the annual cost of lost productivity to employers was $6.1 billion for alcohol abuse/dependence and $2.5 billion for illicit drug abuse/dependence. Foster and Vaughan (2005) estimated the cost of absenteeism in 2000 dollars using data from the 2000 National Survey on Drug Abuse and the 2000 National Occupational Employment Statistical Survey. It was estimated that the combined cost of alcohol and illicit drug disorders (abuse and dependence) in terms of absenteeism was $8.1 billion.

As discussed previously, Foster and Vaughan (2005) estimated that the cost of absenteeism due to substance use disorders represented 0.20% of U.S. annual payroll. According to the U.S. payroll estimates of Foster and Vaughan, the 1999 absenteeism/performance costs reported by Hertz and Baker (2002) would represent 0.15% of U.S. payroll for alcohol disorders and 0.06% of U.S. payroll for illicit drug use disorders. Moreover, the estimated employers' costs due to substance use disorders provided by Hertz and Baker and Foster and Vaughan, which ranged from $2.5 billion to $8.1 billion in

1999 to 2000, are substantially smaller than the estimates from the earlier COI studies that represent the costs of substance use disorders to employees and their families, which were $134.2 billion for alcohol abuse/dependence in 1998 and $107.3 billion for illicit drug abuse/dependence in 1999.

Are Hertz and Baker's (2002) and Foster and Vaughan's (2005) estimates reasonable? It is impossible to know. They may be underestimates because not all potential productivity outcomes were assessed (e.g., job injuries, turnover). On the other hand, for absenteeism and reduced performance, they may be overestimates because, as with all other COI studies conducted to date, the costs were not estimated with actual causal effects of substance abuse/dependence on the productivity outcomes. The estimates were based on cross-sectional associations that (a) did not fully adjust for possible confounding due to common causes of substance abuse/dependence and the productivity outcomes and (b) did not adjust for potential reverse causation. Given this issue and the findings summarized in Chapter 3 and above in the present chapter, it cannot be overemphasized that Hertz and Baker and Foster and Vaughan may have overestimated the causal effect of substance abuse/dependence on their productivity outcomes and therefore overestimated the costs to employers. When studies cumulate over roughly 125 to 130 million workers, relatively small overestimates in the assumed causal effect of employee substance involvement on productivity outcomes can lead to large overestimates of overall employer costs.

The results summarized above suggest that we have no credible information on overall employer costs attributable to employee substance use disorders and no information on the cost of substance use per se. So, is it useful to conduct further COI studies? Such studies have been criticized by a number of researchers (e.g., Baumberg, 2006; Cohen, 1999; Hartman & Crow, 1993; Heien & Pittman, 1989; Kleiman, 1999; Kopp, 1999; Reuter, 1999). For example, Reuter (1999) pointed to the inherent uncertainties and inconsistencies in the results of such studies. He also stated that no strong substantive justification other than sheer curiosity is provided for such studies. After reviewing how such cost estimates have been cited in the past, Reuter (1999) noted that "in each instance it was a prop for a policy argument, which would hardly have been affected if the number had been only half as large or twice as large" (p. 637). On this issue, Larg and Moss (2011) noted that "large 'cost' estimates may simply be one-upmanship by disease advocates vying for greater funding" (p. 654). The critics have pointed to other important issues, such as a lack of direct estimates of many costs, many questionable and unverifiable assumptions underlying the cost estimates, and a lack of information regarding actual causal effects (Baumberg, 2006; Cohen, 1999; Hartman & Crow, 1993; Heien & Pittman, 1989; Larg & Moss, 2011; Reuter, 1999).

Although acknowledging the problems with COI studies, Single (2009) suggested that they should continue "even if we needn't pay undue attention to the bottom line" (p. 117). Single's hope was that COI studies will be refined over time and that they will become more useful for the design of prevention programs and policy. It is unclear when or if COI studies will improve in terms of the data used and the assumptions made, especially regarding costs to employers, but it is clear that they will continue. The conduct of COI studies has grown in popularity, and many are published addressing various health conditions, including substance involvement. This means, however, that those who cite the estimates from COI studies have an obligation to understand clearly how the costs were computed and the underlying assumptions and study design issues; otherwise, the inferences drawn from COI studies are likely to be incorrect and misleading. Toward this end, Larg and Moss (2011) provided a guide to critically evaluating COI studies so that the reader and user will understand the major issues and limitations.

AN INTEGRATIVE MODEL OF EMPLOYEE SUBSTANCE INVOLVEMENT AND PRODUCTIVITY

Inconsistency exists in research attempting to address the relation between employee substance use and various productivity outcomes. Some of the inconsistency is found across organizational field studies exploring different outcomes (e.g., injuries, attendance, task performance), and some is found in comparing experimental psychopharmacological and workplace simulation studies exploring cognitive and psychomotor impairment to organizational field studies of various broader productivity outcomes. These inconsistencies may not be surprising because, as noted at the beginning of this chapter, most organizational field research has set out to explore a simple research question: Can employee substance use impair work-related behaviors and outcomes? Those trying to answer this question often assume that the mere consumption of a psychoactive substance will have the same effect across all productivity outcomes for all employees. However, the relation between employee substance use and productivity is much more complex and may depend on a number of factors, such as consumption patterns (e.g., frequency and quantity of use), contexts (e.g., outside the workplace and work hours or during the workday), and experience (e.g., tolerance) related to the use of psychoactive substances, as well as personal and organizational characteristics. Failure to account for this complexity may explain inconsistencies and weak relations found in past organizational field research.

A detailed conceptual model has not guided past research on employee substance use and productivity. In an effort to account for past inconsistencies, highlight the underlying complexity in the relations between employee substance use and productivity, and provide guidance for future research, I developed an integrative conceptual model of employee substance use and productivity (Frone, 2004). A somewhat revised and expanded version of this model is presented in Figure 4.1. The major features of this model are summarized next.

Matching Context of Substance Use With Type of Productivity Outcome

One key issue is that past organizational field research has failed to match the context of substance use with the type of productivity outcome under study. With very few exceptions, researchers have assessed overall alcohol and drug use in the workforce, which largely reflects substance use off the job. The distinction between off-the-job substance use or impairment and on-the-job substance use or impairment is important. *Off-the-job substance use* represents the consumption of alcohol and other drugs at times and places that occur away from work and outside one's normal work shift. *Off-the-job substance impairment* represents impairment (i.e., intoxication and withdrawal) due to alcohol and illicit drug use experienced at times that occur away from work and outside one's normal work shift. In contrast, *on-the-job substance use* represents the consumption of alcohol and illicit drugs at times that occur just before or during a person's workday. *On-the-job substance impairment* represents impairment due to alcohol and illicit drug use experienced during a person's workday.

Further inspection of past organizational field research reveals a general failure to distinguish between several types of productivity outcomes. Two types of attendance outcomes can be distinguished. The first type represents not arriving at work on time (*tardiness*) or not arriving at work at all (*absenteeism*). The second type represents leaving work early. Finally, performance outcomes represent behaviors and outcomes that occur on the job, such as task performance, contextual performance (i.e., working extra hours or helping coworkers), counterproductive behaviors (aggression, damaging company property, sleeping at work), and job accidents and injuries.

As shown in Figure 4.1, it is proposed that a correspondence exists between the context of employee substance use and impairment and the type of productivity outcome affected. Off-the-job substance use and impairment are the sole cause of tardiness and absenteeism. After all, if an employee is late for or absent from work because of recent substance use and impairment, the substance use and impairment must have occurred off the job. In contrast, on-the-job substance use and impairment are the primary causes of leaving work early and performance outcomes. Nonetheless, off-the-job substance

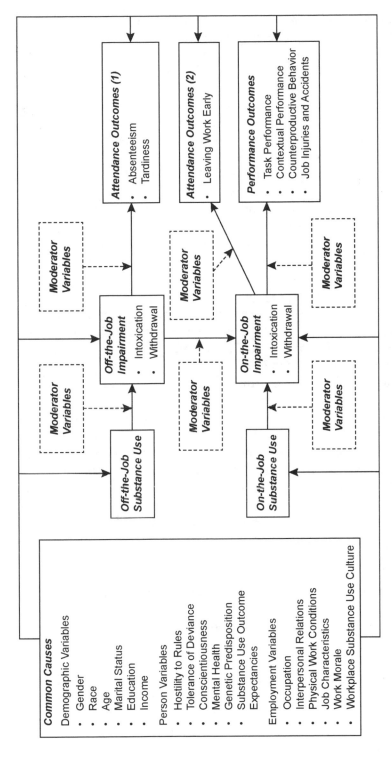

Figure 4.1. An integrative model of employee substance use and productivity. Adapted from *The Psychology of Workplace Safety* (p. 135), by J. Barling and M. R. Frone (Eds.), 2004, Washington, DC, American Psychological Association. Copyright 2004 by the American Psychological Association.

use may indirectly affect performance outcomes to the extent that it causes off-the-job substance impairment, which when carried into the workplace becomes workplace impairment. For example, a night of heavy drinking may lead to intoxication that has not subsided before the person arrives at work, or it may lead to coming to work with a hangover, even if the person's BAC returned to zero before he or she arrived at work. Off-the-job impairment, therefore, is not expected to directly cause leaving work early or employee performance outcomes unless the impaired person comes to work, thereby leading to on-the-job impairment.

The inability of many organizational field studies to document a relation between employee substance use and injuries or accidents at work, as well as poor task performance and other dysfunctional behaviors at work, may result from a failure to differentiate between off-the-job and on-the-job substance use and impairment. The distinction between off-the-job and on-the-job substance use and impairment may also explain prior inconsistencies when looking across organizational field studies and experimental psychopharmacological and workplace simulation studies. Past organizational field studies have provided little evidence for a relation of employee substance use to job performance. In contrast, experimental psychopharmacology and workplace simulations provide more consistent evidence showing that acute intoxication from alcohol and many drugs can impair performance on many cognitive and psychomotor performance tests among naive (i.e., intolerant) individuals, even if many effects are not strong. A fundamental difference between organizational field research and experimental psychopharmacological research is that the former has largely focused on substance use and impairment off the job by using measures of overall substance use, whereas the latter has focused on substance impairment while performing a task. This underscores the importance of explicitly considering the context of substance use. More consistent relations between employee substance use and workplace injuries and accidents, leaving work early, and other performance outcomes might be expected if organizational researchers begin to assess on-the-job substance use and impairment.

Distinguishing Between Substance Use and Substance Impairment

Another major issue represented in the model is the distinction between substance use and substance impairment (intoxication and withdrawal; see definitions provided in Chapter 1). Research generally shows that an increasing dose of alcohol and illicit drugs is associated with higher levels of intoxication and more severe withdrawal when use ceases (see research summarized in Chapter 3; Caetano, Clark, & Greenfield; 1998; Saitz, 1998; Swift & Davidson, 1998). Further, the experimental psychopharmacological research discussed in Chapter 3 suggests that acute intoxication affects cognitive and psychomotor performance, and there is some evidence that substance withdrawal may have negative effects on various physical, cognitive, and affective outcomes as well (e.g., Saitz, 1998; Swift & Davidson, 1998; Wiese et al., 2000). However, with the exception of general reports of alcohol hangover, no organizational research has explored the impact of acute substance withdrawal on employee productivity.

Given the distinction between substance use and substance impairment, it is expected that substance impairment is a proximal cause of poor productivity outcomes and that it mediates the more distal effect of substance use. That is, increasing levels of off-the-job substance use are expected to cause higher levels of off-the-job impairment, which then cause tardiness and absenteeism. Likewise, higher levels of on-the-job substance use are expected to cause higher levels of on-the-job impairment. In turn, on-the-job impairment is expected to increase the likelihood of leaving work early and negatively affect performance outcomes. In addition, off-the-job substance impairment may lead to on-the-job impairment because individuals may still have nonzero blood concentrations of a substance when they arrive at work, and withdrawal symptoms experienced outside work may be taken into the workplace if dependent individuals do not consume the substance before or during their workday. To date, however, little organizational field research has directly tested the relation of off-the-job substance impairment to tardiness and absenteeism. Likewise, little research has tested the relation of on-the-job substance impairment to leaving work early and the various performance outcomes. Finally, no research has tested whether context-specific substance impairment mediates the effect of context-specific substance use on the three categories of productivity outcomes.

Future research should address these issues. For example, as discussed in this chapter, early literature reviews concluded that employee alcohol use had the most consistent relation to absenteeism. However, more recent research has shown a fair amount of inconsistency regarding this relation. To understand this inconsistency, recall that early research focused on employees who were alcohol-dependent heavy drinkers. Many more recent studies have merely compared the attendance behaviors of alcohol users and nonusers. Even studies that used measures of overall frequency and quantity of alcohol use may have differed substantially in the proportion of participants at the higher end of the frequency and quantity distributions. As noted previously, the extent to which past studies differentiated those who drank heavily off the job from those who did not drink heavily explained some of the between-study variation in support for a relation between employee alcohol use and absenteeism.

Control for Common Causes and Consideration of Temporal Order

The discussion until now has tried to show how the model might help explain why past research failed to document consistent relations between employee substance use and productivity outcomes. Nonetheless, many of the studies that have supported such relations should be interpreted with caution because they lacked adequate controls for common causes of substance use, substance impairment, and productivity outcomes. The conceptual model in Figure 4.1 shows that off-the-job substance use, off-the-job substance impairment, on-the-job substance use, on-the-job substance impairment, attendance outcomes, and performance outcomes may share a set of common causes. For example, Normand et al. (1994) speculated that substance use and poor productivity may be related, at least in part, because both constructs reflect individuals' general predisposition to engage in deviant behaviors. Prior findings also should be interpreted cautiously because most research used cross-sectional data where all variables were assessed at one point in time. Such research cannot determine which variable is the cause and which variable is the outcome. For example, if a positive relation is found between off-the-job substance impairment and absenteeism, it might be that off-the-job substance impairment causes absenteeism. However, it is also possible that employees are sometimes absent so that they may engage in substance use. Moving from left to right in the model shows the expected temporal order among the variables. For example, many demographic, person, and employment variables precede and cause off-the-job substance use, off-the-job substance impairment, and absenteeism. Off-the-job substance use precedes and causes off-the-job substance impairment, which precedes and causes absenteeism. However, to determine the actual causal order among large systems of variables and to rule out common cause explanations for relations, future research should use various types of longitudinal study designs.

Moderator Variables

As shown in Figure 4.1, variables may moderate the relations between employee substance use and productivity outcomes. These moderator variables represent various pharmacological, dispositional, motivational, and situational characteristics that can influence the strength or direction (positive or negative) of a relation between two other variables. Failing to consider possible moderating processes may further account for weak and inconsistent results in prior organizational field research. In the following subsections, I summarize some characteristics that may function as important moderators of the relation between substance use and productivity outcomes, though it is not possible to consider all possible moderators. It is helpful to discuss separately the relations between substance use and substance impairment, substance impairment and productivity outcomes, and off-the-job substance impairment and on-the-job substance impairment. In terms of impairment, the focus will be on intoxication because substance withdrawal has received much less attention from researchers.

Relation Between Substance Use and Substance Intoxication

Several variables can affect the relation between substance use and intoxication. These variables affect the extent and length of bioavailability (blood concentration or level of intoxication) of a substance by affecting the processes of absorption, distribution, and metabolism and elimination. *Absorption* refers to the rate and extent to which a drug leaves its site of administration and enters general systemic circulation (Jenkins, 2007; Maisto et al., 2008; Meyer & Quenzer, 2005). A primary factor affecting absorption is the mode of administration (e.g., oral, injection, inhalation, intranasal, sublingual). For example, compared with intravenous injection, inhalation, and sublingual (under-the-tongue) administration, oral ingestion is less efficient because the presence of food in the stomach and first-pass metabolism can impede absorption. *First-pass metabolism* refers to a process by which any ingested substance may be partially metabolized in the gastrointestinal tract or during the first pass of portal blood through the liver before it reaches systemic circulation (e.g., Jenkins, 2007; Meyer & Quenzer, 2005).

Once a drug enters systemic circulation, it is distributed throughout the body. Factors affecting distribution include the biochemical properties of the drug (e.g., water or fat solubility and binding properties) and physiological factors, such as diffusibility of membranes and tissues, amount of body water, and amount of body fat (e.g., Jenkins, 2007; Maisto et al., 2008; Meyer & Quenzer, 2005). Finally, either the parent substance is excreted directly from the body or, more typically, it is first metabolized into by-products called *metabolites*, which are often psychopharmacologically inactive, and then excreted. If the metabolites are psychopharmacologically active, they either are excreted directly or are further metabolized into inactive metabolites and then excreted (e.g., Jenkins, 2007; Maisto et al., 2008; Meyer & Quenzer, 2005). The speed of metabolism and excretion will affect the bioavailability of a substance.

Because of individual differences in the factors underlying absorption, distribution, and metabolism and elimination, individuals differ in the bioavailability of a substance for a given dose (e.g., Jenkins, 2007; Maisto et al., 2008; Meyer & Quenzer, 2005). For example, as implied previously, individual differences in the typical mode of self-administering a substance lead to differences in bioavailability. On average, women have a higher bioavailability than men for many substances because of their lower weight and their proportionately higher percentage of body fat, which leads to a corresponding lower amount of body water in which to distribute the substance. Older adults may experience higher bioavailability than young adults because they have less body water and their ability to metabolize substances may become compromised. Variations in genes regulating metabolism may lead to individual differences in the bioavailability of the parent drug or its active metabolites. Finally, after repeated exposure to a substance, individuals may develop pharmacokinetic tolerance (also known as dispositional or metabolic tolerance). This means that individuals who repeatedly use a drug may begin to experience an increase in the rate of metabolization and elimination of the drug (Jenkins, 2007; Maisto et al., 2008; Meyer & Quenzer, 2005), which will lead to lower bioavailability than in individuals who have not developed pharmacokinetic tolerance.

Relation Between Substance Intoxication and Productivity Outcomes

Several processes may influence the relation between substance intoxication and employee productivity. The first process that may moderate the relation of substance intoxication to productivity outcomes is *pharmacodynamic tolerance* (also known as *chronic* or *functional tolerance*; e.g., Jenkins, 2007; Maisto et al., 2008; Meyer & Quenzer, 2005). This represents a process of physiological adaptation whereby the central nervous system becomes less sensitive to the psychopharmacological effects of a given substance after repeated exposure over time.

A second process that may influence the relation between substance intoxication and productivity is *behavioral tolerance* (also known as *learned tolerance*, *conditioned tolerance*, or *context-specific tolerance*; e.g., Maisto et al., 2008; Meyer & Quenzer, 2005; Vogel-Sprott, 1992). This represents learned compensatory strategies that reduce the impact or expression of intoxication on cognitive and behavioral task performance. For example, the effect of alcohol intoxication on cognitive and behavioral performance may decrease if a person explicitly practices a set of task behaviors or mentally rehearses the task behaviors while subject to acute intoxication (e.g., Vogel-Sprott, 1992). A number of factors or cues can enhance or impede the development or expression of behavioral tolerance. For example, when behavioral tolerance is developed in a specific environment, individuals performing a task under intoxication in a new setting will fail to show behavioral tolerance (e.g., Maisto et al., 2008). Behavioral tolerance also is more likely to be developed with increased experience using a substance and when individuals are rewarded for showing nonimpaired performance (e.g., Fillmore & Vogel-Sprott, 1996; Vogel-Sprott, 1992).

A third process that might influence the effect of substance intoxication on productivity outcomes has been labeled *resistance to impairment* (George, Raynor, & Nochajski, 1992; Nochajski, 1993). Where behavioral tolerance develops over several occasions of performing a task while intoxicated, resistance to impairment refers to motivational aids that may reduce the expression of intoxication in a single occasion. For example, past laboratory research shows that visual-motor performance decrements due to alcohol intoxication at BACs of .05% (George et al., 1992) and .10% (Nochajski, 1993) were eliminated in the first and subsequent postintoxication performance trials when individuals were instructed to "concentrate very hard" on the task at hand.

Taken together, research on tolerance and resistance to impairment suggests that the positive relation of on-the-job intoxication to job injuries and accidents, as well as to other dimensions of poor performance at work and leaving work early, may be attenuated among (a) experienced substance users compared with inexperienced users, (b) workers who work in the same environment or at the same work station compared with workers who change work environments or workstations, (c) individuals rewarded for exhibiting compensatory (i.e., nonimpaired) behavior compared with individuals who are not so rewarded, and (d) individuals who use motivational strategies that focus their attention on the task to be accomplished compared with individuals who do not use such strategies. Turning to the relation of off-the-job intoxication to tardiness or absenteeism, one might expect that behavioral tolerance would attenuate the magnitude of this relation as well. For example, experienced substance users and those who perceive an immediate cost to poor attendance (e.g., being disciplined or fired) may develop compensatory responses to residual intoxication or withdrawal (hangover) the morning after a night of heavy drinking or drug use, so that they show up for work on time, unlike inexperienced users who do not perceive an immediate cost to poor attendance.

A fourth process that might influence the relation between intoxication and productivity is polysubstance use (i.e., use of multiple substances). Drug interactions occur when the use of one drug may moderate the effect of another drug. The interaction effects can be synergistic, where the effect of one drug increases impairment for a given dose of another drug, or antagonistic, where the effect of one drug decreases impairment for a given dose of another drug (e.g., Maisto et al., 2008). For example, the impact of alcohol on cognitive or behavioral impairment may become stronger with the simultaneous use of other sedative and depressant drugs. In contrast, the impact of alcohol on cognitive or behavioral impairment may be attenuated with the simultaneous use of stimulants, such as amphetamines or cocaine (e.g., Farré et al., 1993; Kerr & Hindmarch, 1998).

A fifth process specific to the relation of on-the-job substance intoxication to job injuries and accidents is between-job differences in the latent potential for being injured or having an accident. Although most studies have failed to assess on-the-job substance intoxication, some evidence exists that injury liability due to increasing levels of intoxication may depend on the characteristics of and demands inherent in the jobs under study (e.g., Dawson, 1994; Holcom, Lehman, & Simpson, 1993). For example, although on-the-job intoxication may increase the probability of a job injury among steelworkers, it is less likely to cause a job injury among office workers.

Finally, the relation between substance intoxication and productivity outcomes may be affected by the person and employment variables shown in Figure 4.1 under "Common Causes." For example, off-the-the job substance intoxication may be more strongly related to absenteeism among individuals who have high levels of tolerance for deviance or low levels of work morale. In both cases, such individuals may not care about work attendance, and this would be exacerbated by off-the-job intoxication or withdrawal from a bout of heavy substance use. Also, on-the-job intoxication may be more strongly related to poor performance or work injuries if the person has preexisting physical or mental health limitations.

Relation Between Off-the-Job Substance Impairment and On-the-Job Substance Impairment

One way for on-the-job substance impairment to occur is when a person reports to work with residual intoxication from a bout of heavy substance use that may have occurred more than a couple of hours before reporting to work. Although no research has explored this relation and the variables that may moderate it, one potential moderator is the substance use climate at work. Individuals who become impaired off the job may be more likely to report to work impaired if the climate at work is accepting of, or at least does not actively proscribe, substance use and impairment at work. Such individuals may also report to work impaired if they have low work morale and do not feel satisfied with their job or committed to their employer.

Discussion

The integrative conceptual model outlined in Figure 4.1 and described earlier presents a detailed guide to help focus future research on the relation between employee substance use and workplace productivity. To date, little research has directly tested the various processes outlined in the model, and no research has attempted a full test of the proposed model. Nonetheless, a few studies have provided partial support for the model. Two studies found that overall (i.e., off-the-job) drug use and heavy drinking was positively related to absenteeism but were unrelated to workplace accidents (Hoffmann et al., 1997; Normand et al., 1990). Also, two studies collectively found, after controlling for many common causes, that on-the-job alcohol and illicit drug use were positively related to job injuries and several other measures of poor performance, whereas overall (i.e., off-the-job) alcohol and illicit drug use were unrelated to the productivity outcomes (Ames et al., 1997; Frone, 1998). These studies suggest that more researchers should focus on the various issues outlined previously in order to understand more fully the conditions under which substance use may affect workplace productivity.

FUTURE RESEARCH

A number of suggestions were made throughout the chapter regarding directions for future research on employee substance use and work productivity. It is clear from this review that more sophisticated research should be conducted before any general conclusions can be drawn regarding the existence and importance of causal effects involving this general relation. Although the research summarized in Chapter 3 investigated the pharmacological impact of various substances on basic dimensions of cognitive and psychomotor performance, the present chapter indicates that it will be more difficult to develop an understanding of the associations between employee substance involvement and the multifaceted workplace outcomes that are embedded in complex organizational contexts. The conceptual model presented in Figure 4.1 and the discussion of its underlying processes provide one attempt to foster a more sophisticated research agenda. Finally, until better estimates are developed of the causal effects of employee substance involvement on workplace productivity outcomes, it will be impossible to develop accurate estimates of the overall cost of employee substance use to employers.

GENERAL SUMMARY AND CONCLUSIONS

On the whole, research exploring the relations of employee substance involvement to attendance and performance outcomes suggests that these relations are weak and inconsistent. The studies that have found statistically significant relations have methodological problems that undermine any conclusions regarding causal effects. Prior estimates of the costs of employee substance involvement to employers actually estimated the costs of substance use to employees and their families. The two studies that attempted to estimate costs to employers showed that the costs are much lower than previously assumed. And because of methodological issues, the employer cost estimates may still be overestimated for the outcomes employed. The general lack of support for relations between employee substance involvement and productivity outcomes may be due to the fact that research has overlooked the complexity of these relations. Although more sophisticated research may lead to a better understanding of these relations, the overall process linking substance use to productivity is likely to be complex and the causal effects may be more circumscribed than typically assumed. Nonetheless, a better understanding may lead to more focused and more effective workplace policies.

5

WORKPLACE INTERVENTIONS I: DRUG TESTING JOB APPLICANTS AND EMPLOYEES

Within the context of employee substance involvement, workplace interventions are aimed at changing environmental, cultural, social, or personal factors in an effort (a) to keep individuals from abusing alcohol or using illicit drugs and from using alcohol or illicit drugs at work and (b) to avert adverse work outcomes and, in some instances, adverse personal outcomes resulting from alcohol and illicit drug involvement. Most workplace interventions attempt to address both of these goals, at least indirectly. For example, interventions aimed at minimizing heavy alcohol or illicit drug use usually assume that such reductions will lead to improved work productivity, even if productivity is not directly targeted or assessed. Toward these ends, workplace interventions take two general approaches: (a) workforce drug testing and (b) workplace health promotion. Although some organizations use both general approaches, with the latter approach often augmenting the former approach, I discuss them in separate chapters because they have different philosophical underpinnings.

DOI: 10.1037/13944-006
Alcohol and Illicit Drug Use in the Workforce and Workplace, by M. R. Frone
Copyright © 2013 by the American Psychological Association. All rights reserved.

Workforce drug testing, the focus of this chapter, represents the more contentious type of workplace intervention and refers to chemical analysis of various biological specimens for the presence of psychoactive drugs or their metabolites. Metabolites assessed in drug testing are chemical compounds created when a psychoactive drug is metabolized (see Chapter 4). They typically have no psychoactive properties (i.e., inactive metabolites) and, as discussed later, may be detectable for long periods of time after a substance has been used. Such testing is involuntary and focuses exclusively on the person, in that the basic purpose is to identify and exclude job applicants or to identify and sanction or terminate current employees because of their illicit drug use and, less frequently, alcohol use. Drug testing programs do not attempt to evaluate and change environmental, cultural, or social conditions, within or outside the workplace, that play a role in an individual's substance involvement.

The goal in this chapter is to cover a number of issues regarding workforce substance use testing, including a brief history and prevalence of workforce substance use testing in the United States and elsewhere; characteristics of workforce substance use testing and organizations that utilize substance use testing; and the motivations underlying and effectiveness of substance use testing. However, several issues are not covered, because they go beyond the scope of this book: court rulings and laws related to workforce drug testing and the development of a drug testing program. In the United States, a number of relevant federal and state laws must be considered. Substance use testing regulations also vary widely across countries. Therefore, developing and implementing an appropriate and legally defensible testing program can be a complex issue and should be done in consultation with an attorney (DelPo & Guerin, 2011). Model guidelines for drug testing programs have been developed and presented by the U.S. federal government and the European Workplace Drug Testing Society (EWDTS).[1]

BRIEF HISTORY OF WORKFORCE SUBSTANCE USE TESTING IN THE UNITED STATES

The testing of nonmilitary employees for illicit drug use and for alcohol use in some circumstances was largely motivated in the United States by Executive Order 12564 (1986)—Drug-Free Federal Workplace—issued by

---

[1]For more detailed information, the interested reader can see Bush (2008); Caplan and Huestis (2007); Mandatory Guidelines for Federal Workplace Drug Testing Programs (http://edocket.access.gpo.gov/2008/pdf/e8-26726.pdf); the U.S. Department of Transportation guidelines (http://www.dot.gov/ost/dapc/new_docs/part40.pdf); and the EWDTS guidelines (http://www.ewdts.org/guidelines.html).

then President Ronald Reagan. This order outlined several requirements for a workplace substance use policy; made drug testing mandatory for federal employees in safety/security-sensitive jobs; allowed for the testing of all applicants to federal jobs; and allowed for testing of all federal employees, given reasonable suspicion, after an accident or unsafe practice, and as follow-up to counseling or rehabilitation for illegal drug use (Bush, 2008). Public Law 100-71 (Section 503, 5 USC 7301 note), which took effect in 1987, directed the secretary of the U.S. Department of Health and Human Services (HHS) to develop and promulgate comprehensive standards for all aspects of laboratory testing for illicit drug use by federal employees. These detailed procedures, entitled the *Mandatory Guidelines for Federal Workplace Drug Testing Programs* (*Mandatory Guidelines* hereafter), were first published in the Federal Register on April 11, 1988. The *Mandatory Guidelines* has been updated a number of times, and the most recent version was published in the *Federal Register* on November 11, 2008, to take effect on October 1, 2010. At present, the responsibility for developing and refining the standards for drug testing resides with the Division of Workplace Programs of the Substance Abuse and Mental Health Services Administration (SAMHSA), which is a division of HHS.

Following Executive Order 12564, which applied to federal employees, the U.S. Congress passed the Drug-Free Workplace Act (DFWA) in 1988, which mandated that public and private employers who are contractors receiving contracts in excess of $25,000 or receiving grants of any amount from the federal government must have in place a policy to ensure a "drug-free workplace." The DFWA also outlined the components of such a policy. Although the DFWA did not require alcohol and illicit drug use testing, it implicitly authorized and supported testing as a means of maintaining a drug-free workplace. Since the DFWA was passed, several U.S. federal agencies have mandated alcohol and drug testing for public- and private-sector employees in various safety- and security-sensitive occupations (e.g., Department of Transportation, Department of Defense, Department of Energy, Nuclear Regulatory Agency, and National Aeronautics and Space Administration).[2]

Although these federal policies and regulations do not require most nonfederal employers to engage in workforce drug testing, they did provide strong motivation for many large companies to begin testing programs. Moreover, these federal regulations and policies fueled the development of a huge industry comprising drug test manufacturers, consulting and law firms specializing in the development of drug testing policies and procedures, and laboratories that carry out the testing. This broad industry has aggressively

[2]For additional details on the history of the development of U.S. federal drug testing policies and laws, see Bush (2008); Caplan and Huestis (2007); Walsh et al. (1992); and Walsh and Trumble (1991).

marketed workforce drug testing as a means to reduce employee substance use and as a solution to potential productivity problems in the workplace. Aggressive marketing often comes with claims that are misleading regarding the extent of a problem, the effectiveness of the proposed solution, and the extent to which the solution is being used. Data addressing these issues are reviewed in detail below.

PREVALENCE OF WORKFORCE SUBSTANCE USE TESTING IN THE UNITED STATES

The exact scope of workforce substance use testing in the United States is not well documented, although estimates of various types and quality exist. All federal agencies can conduct employee substance use testing of job applicants, randomly test employees holding positions designated as safety/security sensitive, and test for reasonable suspicion and after an accident or unsafe practice among all federal employees. Nonetheless, the exact number of federal job applicants and employees tested in any year is unclear.

In the private sector, the American Management Association (AMA) has conducted a survey of its member organizations regarding illicit drug use testing since 1987, and these survey results are often cited by researchers and others. Based on these surveys, the prevalences of organizations conducting any illicit drug testing, testing of applicants, and testing of current employees are presented in Table 5.1 (AMA, 1996, 2004). Although organizations completing the surveys represent neither the AMA membership nor all employers in the United States, the results are instructive. As shown in Table 5.1, the prevalence of illicit drug testing was low in 1987, the year after Executive Order 12564 was issued. However, the prevalence of testing increased rapidly during the next 6 to 9 years and then began to decline substantially. If these data are accurate, the prevalence of companies doing any illicit drug testing increased from 21% in 1987 to 81% in 1996 and then dropped to 62% by 2004. A similar pattern exists for the prevalence of companies testing current employees for illicit drug use, increasing from 16% in 1987 to 70% in 1996 and then dropping to 44% in 2004. The prevalence of companies testing job applicants for illicit drug use peaked even faster, increasing from 19% in 1987 to 73% in 1993 and then dropping to 55% in 2004.

The National Survey of Worksites and Employee Assistance Programs (NSWEAP), conducted in 1993 and 1995, assessed the prevalence of U.S. work organizations testing for illicit drug use (Hartwell, Steele, French, & Rodman, 1996; Hartwell, Steele, & Rodman, 1998). Although surveys were conducted in only 2 years, this study provides better prevalence estimates than the AMA surveys because it used a random sample of U.S. work organizations

TABLE 5.1
Prevalence of Companies Testing for Illicit Drugs

| Year | Testing (%) | | |
	Any	Applicant	Employee
1987	21	19	16
1988	36	28	27
1989	48	39	36
1990	51	43	38
1991	63	54	53
1992	73	64	62
1993	78	*73*	66
1994	76	69	65
1995	78	63	68
1996	*81*	68	*70*
1997	74	64	62
1998	74	62	62
1999	70	63	54
2000	66	61	47
2001	67	61	50
2004	62	55	44

Note. Data provided by the American Management Association. No survey was conducted in 2002 or 2003. Percentages in boldface italics represent peak testing year.

with at least 100 employees, rather than the convenience (self-selected) samples of a single association. Data from the NSWEAP show that the estimated prevalence of organizations doing any illicit drug testing was 62% in 1993 and 54% in 1995. The prevalence of organizations testing current employees for illicit drug use was 48% in 1993 and 34% in 1995. The prevalence of organizations testing job applicants for illicit drug use was 46% in 1995 (the 1993 survey did not ask about job applicant testing). Comparison of the NSWEAP rates to those from the AMA surveys (see Table 5.1) suggests that the convenience (nonrandom) samples used in the AMA surveys may have overestimated national prevalence rates of illicit drug use testing. Nonetheless, the NSWEAP results are consistent with the AMA results in showing that the prevalence of illicit drug use testing among U.S. employers began to decline in the mid-1990s. However, the NSWEAP data suggest that the decline may have started earlier.

The 1994, 1997, and 2002–2004 National Household Survey on Drug Abuse (NHSDA; Larson et al., 2007; Zhang, Huang, & Brittingham, 1999) and the 1993, 1997, and 1999 National Employee Survey (NES; Knudsen, Roman, & Johnson, 2003; Roman & Knudsen, 2009) collected data on the prevalence of employees reporting that their employer had some form of illicit drug use testing program. Before these data are presented, it should be noted that the studies discussed previously sampled employers and provide information on the prevalence of employers who use drug testing. The NHSDA and NES studies drew random samples of U.S. workers and therefore provide data on the prevalence of employees subject to drug testing, though not necessarily the proportion that have been drug tested. Researchers sometimes fail to understand this distinction and erroneously use the NHSDA and NES data as estimates of the prevalence of employers using drug testing.

The proportion of employees in the NHSDA reporting that their employer had some form of illicit drug use testing program was 44% in 1994, 49% in 1997, and 49% in 2002 to 2004. Results from the NES indicated that preemployment testing was reported by 33.5% of employees in 1993, 45.2% in 1997, and 49.5% in 2002; for-cause testing was reported by 33.1% of employees in 1993, 41.2% in 1997, and 47.6% in 2002; and random testing was reported by 22.4% of employees in 1993, 28.8% in 1997, and 31.6% in 2002. The patterns from these studies and overall rates (overall prevalence from the NHSDA compared with preemployment prevalence from the NES) are similar. Both studies show some increase in the prevalence of employees subject to drug testing from 1993–1994 to 1997 and little change from 1997 to 2002–2004.

Even though the results from the two employee surveys (NHSDA and NES) assess the prevalence of employees subject to drug testing and the results from the two organizational surveys (AMA and NSWEAPS) assess the prevalence of organizations that use drug testing, considering the trends in the two sets of results together is useful. The organizational surveys (AMA and NSWEAP) show that the prevalence of U.S. organizations using drug testing began to decline in the mid-1990s and continued to decline through 2004, whereas the employee surveys (NHSDA and NES) show that the prevalence of U.S. employees subject to drug testing remained the same from 1997 to 2002–2004. It is not exactly clear why the prevalence of organizations testing for employee illicit drug use has been declining and there has been no increase in the proportion of employees subject to drug testing, especially in the face of growth in the development of new types of drug tests and the marketing of drug testing products and services. However, data presented later in this chapter may offer some clues. Also, the downward trend in the proportion of employers using drug testing and the fact that many employers have never used workforce drug testing suggest that there is some disagreement among U.S. employers regarding the need for and effectiveness of testing for illicit drug use.

Few data exist about the prevalence of organizations testing for illicit drug use, and even less information exists about organizations testing for alcohol use. Although the DFWA did not address the use of alcohol, several federal agencies, as noted previously, mandated alcohol testing programs for federal and many nonfederal employees in safety and security-sensitive positions. Also, some employers voluntarily use alcohol testing. The prevalence of employers that fall under mandated versus voluntary alcohol testing is not clear. The NSWEAP study (Hartwell et al., 1998) found that in 1995, 36% of organizations reported any alcohol testing; 22% of organizations reported alcohol testing among job applicants, and 28% of organizations reported alcohol testing among current employees. Further, the 2002–2004 NHSDA found that 35% of employed adults reported being subject to alcohol testing (Larson et al., 2007). Comparison of these overall alcohol testing rates with the overall drug testing rates reported previously for the 1995 NSWEAP and the 2002–2004 NHSDA shows that fewer organizations use alcohol testing than illicit drug testing (alcohol testing, 36.0%; drug testing, 53.7%), and fewer employees are subject to alcohol testing than illicit drug testing (alcohol testing, 35.0%; drug testing, 49%). A 1991 study of Fortune 1,000 companies obtained similar findings—the proportion of companies using illicit drug testing (49%) was higher than the proportion of companies using alcohol testing (24%; Guthrie & Olian, 1991). No data exist on the long-term trends in alcohol testing among organizations or among employees.

WORKFORCE SUBSTANCE USE TESTING OUTSIDE THE UNITED STATES

Workforce substance use testing also occurs in Europe, Canada, and several other countries. However, it is important to point out that because the United States is the only country to have formally declared an ideological War on Drugs, broad-scale employee testing for illicit drugs and even for alcohol use is largely an American phenomenon. To the extent that workforce substance testing occurs in other countries, it is minimal compared to that in the United States, and its use has often been introduced or imposed by U.S. multinational companies and by rules regulating federal contractors and other employers doing business in the United States (IIDTW, 2004; Pierce, 2007). However, the use of workforce substance use testing may grow outside the United States because of continued pressure from U.S. multinational companies and because of aggressive marketing from the global drug testing industry (Brännström & Hopstadius, 1994).

Europe

Minimal formal data exist about workforce substance use testing in Europe, and the legal landscape is heterogeneous (European Monitoring Centre for Drugs and Drug Addiction, 2006; EWDTS, 2011; Pierce, 2007; Verstraete &

Pierce, 2001). Only Finland, Ireland, Italy, the Netherlands, and Norway have legislation that specifically addresses workforce drug testing (European Monitoring Centre for Drugs and Drug Addiction, 2006; EWDTS, 2011; Kazanga et al., 2012). Despite a lack of direct legislation, many other countries do allow testing under certain circumstances through general labor laws or national/organizational collective bargaining agreements, such as in safety/security-sensitive positions, but they often do not support blanket testing of applicants or employees. However, a general expectation exists that employees are not under the influence of a substance while at work.

Unlike in the United States, testing is not necessarily conducted to identify job applicant or employee illicit drug use to employers; rather, it is conducted with the broader goals of enhancing health and identifying fitness for duty. Thus, in many countries, when testing is conducted under appropriate circumstances, the proximal reason would likely be a question of an employee's fitness for duty. The exact reason a job applicant or employee is not fit for duty (substance use, physical health, or mental health) is not divulged to the employer. Finally, some countries specifically penalize unjustified testing with criminal fines, either as a breach of workers' privacy or as a breach of general privacy (European Monitoring Centre for Drugs and Drug Addiction, 2006).

Verstraete and Pierce (2001) pointed out that there is no official coordination in Europe regarding workforce drug testing. Despite the existence of the EWDTS (http://www.ewdts.org), it has no regulatory power. Nonetheless, its stated goals are (a) to ensure that workforce drug testing in Europe is performed to a defined quality standard and (b) to provide an independent forum for all aspects of workforce drug testing. As part of its first goal, the EWDTS has developed and provides detailed guidelines for workforce substance use testing. However, it is not clear how many European companies follow these guidelines, and little information exists on the quality standards being used (Verstraete & Pierce, 2001).

Very few data exist on the prevalence of organizations testing employees for illicit drugs or alcohol in specific countries or across Europe as a whole. However, workforce substance use testing is probably greatest in the United Kingdom (George, 2005). To explore the prevalence of drug testing, in the United Kingdom, the IIDTW (2004) conducted a series of studies. The Ipsos MORI Social Research Institute (MORI) survey of 200 U.K. organizations found that 4% of organizations were testing for drugs or alcohol; the Confederation of British Industry (CBI) survey reported that 30% of organizations were testing; and the Chartered Management Institute (CMI) survey found that 16% of companies were conducting random drug testing and 14% of companies were conducting preemployment drug testing. The IIDTW suggested that the higher rates of drug testing in the CMI and CBI surveys than the MORI survey were because nonresponse bias existed in the former two studies and because the organizations sampled across the studies were not comparable. Finally, the IIDTW sent a survey to all members of the Federation of Small Business and received not a single response. The IIDTW took this to mean that drug testing was not an issue of importance to small businesses in the United Kingdom.

Canada

In Canada, no federal or provincial laws mandate drug testing of employees (Holmes & Richter, 2008). Nonetheless, some private employers have drug testing policies in place. Macdonald, Csiernik, Durand, Rylett, and Wild (2006) conducted a random national survey of Canadian employers with at least 100 employees in 2003. The overall prevalence of organizations engaged in any form of employee drug testing was 10.3%. However, wide variability existed across Canadian provinces, ranging 4.6% in Ontario to 25.4% in Alberta. This study also found that U.S. companies have had an influence on the prevalence of drug testing in Canada. The prevalence of drug testing was 18.2% among Canadian organizations headquartered in the United States and only 9.2% among Canadian organizations headquartered in Canada. In the only study to assess long-term trends in drug testing in Canada, Macdonald, Csiernik, Durand, Wild, et al. (2006), reported prevalence rates for the province of Ontario. The prevalence of drug testing was 1.8% in 1989, 5.9% in 1993, and 4.6% in 2003. Finally, using a national sample of Canadian employers, Keay, Macdonald, Durand, Csiernik, and Wild (2010) asked companies with drug testing why they used it and asked companies without drug testing why they did not use it. The five most important reasons for using drug testing were (a) to reduce work accidents, (b) to deter drug use, (c) to improve employee well-being, (d) to reduce absenteeism, and (e) to be cost effective. The five most important reasons for not using drug testing were (a) no need, (b) a lack of federal/provincial legislation, (c) a lack of evidence that it reduced absenteeism, (d) a lack of evidence that it improves workplace safety, and (e) a lack of evidence that it was cost effective. Consistent with the declining use of drug testing among U.S. employers, disagreement exists among Canadian employers regarding the need for and effectiveness of workforce illicit drug use testing.

The generally low rate of workforce drug testing in Canada compared with the United States may be because the political environment is less supportive of most uses of alcohol and illicit drug use testing. The Canadian Human Rights Act prohibits discrimination on the basis of disability and perceived disability, with disability including a previous or existing dependence on alcohol or a drug. The act also prohibits discrimination based on the actual or perceived possibility that an individual may develop a drug or alcohol dependency in the future (Canadian Human Rights Commission, 2009). The Canadian Human Rights Commission stated that "drug and alcohol testing is *prima facie* discriminatory under Canadian human rights law. Nevertheless, employers can justify discriminatory practices and rules if they are a *bona fide* occupational requirement" (Canadian Human Rights Commission, 2009, p. 5). Further, a key ruling emerged from *Entrop v. Imperial Oil* (2000), with the Ontario Court of Appeals noting a critical difference between alcohol and drug tests. Alcohol tests, such as the Breathalyzer, can detect impairment at the time of the test and therefore workplace impairment when administered on the job. In contrast, drug tests cannot assess impairment at the time of the test and therefore cannot determine workplace impairment.

Based on *Entrop v. Imperial Oil* (2000) and the notion of a bona fide occupational requirement, the Canadian Human Rights Commission's (2009) policy states that if testing is part of a broader program of medical assessment, monitoring, and support, alcohol testing can be conducted (a) on a random basis for employees in safety-sensitive positions; (b) for reasonable suspicion, where an employee reports for work in an unfit state and there is evidence of substance abuse; (c) after a significant incident or accident has occurred and there is evidence that an employee's act or omission may have contributed to the incident or accident; and (d) following treatment for alcohol abuse or disclosure of a current alcohol dependency or abuse. Also, if testing is part of a broader program of medical assessment, monitoring, and support, drug testing can be done in the following situations: (a) for reasonable suspicion, where an employee reports for work in an unfit state and there is evidence of substance abuse; (b) after a significant incident or accident has occurred and there is evidence that an employee's act or omission may have contributed to the incident or accident; and (c) following treatment for drug abuse or disclosure of a current drug dependency or abuse. Nonetheless, reasonable suspicion, postaccident, and return to duty alcohol and illicit drug use testing are viewed as more acceptable among employees holding safety- and security-sensitive positions. Finally, the policy states that the following types of testing are not permitted: (a) preemployment alcohol or drug testing, (b) random drug testing, and (c) random alcohol testing of employees in non-safety-sensitive positions. Although preemployment testing for alcohol or drugs is not viewed as acceptable by the Canadian Human Rights Commission, if a preemployment alcohol or drug test is conducted and the employee fails, the policy states that an employer cannot automatically withdraw an offer of employment from the prospective employee without first addressing the issue of accommodation.[3]

---

[3]For a more detailed discussion of Canadian laws and regulations regarding workforce drug testing, see Holmes and Richter (2008) and the Canadian Human Rights Commission's policy on alcohol and drug testing (Canadian Human Rights Commission, 2009).

Other Countries

Workforce drug testing in New Zealand began in the 1990s, partly in response to U.S. multinational companies requiring their global subsidiaries to adopt workforce testing (Nolan, 2008). Testing began in safety-sensitive industries, such as forestry, fishing, mining, and aluminum manufacturing, and since 2000 most other high-risk industries (e.g., transportation and road construction) have established testing programs (Nolan, 2008). However, few data exist on the prevalence of organizations using workforce drug testing in New Zealand. Haar and Spell (2007) reported that 6% of employers with 50 or more employees tested in 1996 and that 8% of employers with 10 or more employees reported testing in 2007. Thus, little growth has been observed in the prevalence of employers engaged in drug testing in New Zealand. In contrast, Nolan (2008) reported that the number of employee urine tests conducted for illicit drugs increased from approximately 4,000 in 1998–1999 to approximately 24,000 in 2004–2005. Nonetheless, it remains unclear whether this change represents an increase in the prevalence of employers who conduct drug testing, an increase in the prevalence of employees subject to drug testing, or an increase in the number of yearly tests conducted on employees subject to testing.

Alcohol and drug testing in New Zealand are regulated in part by the Human Rights Act, Privacy Act, Bill of Rights Act, Employment Relations Act, and common law (Nolan, 2008; Thomas, 1997). A comprehensive drug-and alcohol-free workplace model has been developed and is accepted by employment courts and most unions. The model has four main components, which are (a) development of policies and procedures that "fit," (b) education and training, (c) alcohol and drug testing, and (d) rehabilitation and case management. Many steps and issues exist within each of these components. For more details on this model, see Nolan (2008).

Drug testing also occurs in Australia (Pierce, 2007). As in New Zealand, substance use testing was introduced by U.S. multinational companies, with most testing taking place in mining, transportation, and construction industries. No data exist on the prevalence of organizations conducting workforce alcohol and illicit drug use testing (Pierce, 2007). Workforce drug testing also is not common in South America (Pierce, 2007), but where workforce substance use testing does occurs, it is generally performed due to the global policies of U.S. multinational companies. Although the impact of U.S. multinational companies may extend to Asian countries, no information could be located exploring the prevalence of and regulations regarding alcohol and drug testing in this part of the world.

CHARACTERISTICS OF WORKFORCE SUBSTANCE USE TESTING

Testing Circumstances and Outcomes of Testing

Workforce substance use testing occurs under several difference circumstances (e.g., Normand et al., 1994). *Preemployment testing* occurs during the screening and selection process for job applicants. To contain costs and avoid litigation, preemployment testing in the United States typically occurs after a job offer is made that is contingent on passing a test for illicit drug use, and the applicant is informed of this at the beginning of the screening process. Whether preemployment testing takes place before or after a job offer may vary across countries. Among the current employees of an organization, *postemployment testing* occurs under several different circumstances. *Random testing* requires that a prespecified proportion of employees (e.g., 50% annually) be randomly selected to submit to a substance use test without warning. *Postaccident testing* occurs after an employee is involved in a qualifying accident or serious incident. The characteristics of the qualifying accident or incident may differ across companies, collective bargaining agreements, and countries. *Reasonable suspicion* or *probable cause testing* occurs when a trained representative of an employer (e.g., supervisor) has reasonable suspicion that an employee has used a prohibited drug or alcohol at work. The basis for reasonable suspicion may vary across companies, collective bargaining agreements, and countries, although it often requires that specific, contemporaneous, and articulable observations be documented by a trained supervisor concerning the appearance, behavior, speech, or body odor of an employee. *Return to duty and follow-up testing* occurs (a) after employees who had an alcohol or drug violation return to work to resume their duties or (b) when employees undergoing substance abuse treatment return to their job duties. The number and spacing of tests required after returning to duty may vary across companies, collective bargaining agreements, and countries.

But what happens when an employee has a positive test result in one of these circumstances? After a positive preemployment drug test in the United States, an applicant is typically not hired (e.g., Guthrie & Olian, 1991; Murphy & Thornton, 1992). However, among Fortune 1,000 companies, a person is more likely to be rejected after an initial failure of a preemployment illicit drug use test (71.7%) than an initial failure of a preemployment alcohol test (47.4%; Guthrie & Olian, 1991). Differences also exist in the outcome of a failed preemployment drug test across countries. For example, as already noted, if a preemployment alcohol or drug test is positive, the Canadian Human Rights Commission policy states that an employer cannot automatically withdraw an offer of employment from a job applicant without first addressing the issue of accommodation.

The possible outcomes of a positive postemployment test can include immediate dismissal, punishment (e.g., suspension), or mandated treatment (e.g., Knudsen, Roman, & Johnson, 2004). Each of these three outcomes can be viewed as punitive in nature. Although the employer's perspective might be that mandated treatment is rehabilitative and therefore not punitive, mandated treatment in order to avoid job termination may be viewed as punishment by an employee (e.g., Brunet, 2002), especially if the employee does not view his or her infrequent off-the-job substance use as a potential threat to performance and workplace safety (see limitations of drug testing below). The exact outcome of a postemployment drug or alcohol violation will vary across organizations, the nature of the job, government regulations, characteristics of the labor market, and collective bargaining agreements (e.g., Blum, Fields, Milne, & Spell, 1992; Knudsen et al., 2004; Murphy & Thornton, 1992). Nonetheless, in the NES (Knudsen et al., 2004), 54.2% of U.S. employees stated that the most common employer response for failing a drug test was mandated counseling; 29.9% reported dismissal, 6.6% reported punishment (e.g., suspension), and 9.3% reported some other reaction, perhaps a combination of the three just mentioned. If employees are not immediately dismissed and then fail a return to duty or follow-up test, they will likely be terminated at that point. However, the number of chances an employee may get before being terminated likely depends on the various characteristics mentioned previously (e.g., specific organization or government regulations, characteristics of the labor market, and collective bargaining agreements). No research has directly explored this issue.

Finally, what happens when a person refuses to submit to a preemployment or postemployment test for alcohol or illicit drug use? Submitting to a substance use test must be mandatory for a testing policy and program to work. Therefore, refusing to submit to a substance use test is viewed as an attempt to evade detection and invariably treated as testing positive, leading to the various sanctions mentioned above.

Types of Drugs Tested

Which substances are tested? Again, there is wide variability, though job applicants and employees who are not in security- and safety-sensitive jobs are more likely to be tested for illicit drug use than for alcohol use. In the *Mandatory Guidelines*, the U.S. federal government identified a panel of five substances that must be tested for by any of the federal government agencies or any employer that is required by federal regulation to do workforce drug testing. These five drug classes are marijuana, cocaine, opiates, amphetamine (including methamphetamine), and phencyclidine (PCP). No requirement exists to test for illicit use of other drugs, though many federal agencies impose testing for alcohol use under a variety of circumstances. Nonetheless, the *Mandatory Guidelines* states that a specimen may be tested for any Schedule I or II drugs on a case-by-case basis for reasonable suspicion, post-accident, or unsafe practice testing. But not all federal agencies make this exception. The Department of Transportation guidelines for drug testing state that specimens may not be tested for illicit drug use beyond the five classes of drugs mentioned previously, though they do allow for alcohol testing. Private-sector employers that engage in pre- or postemployment drug testing and are not required to follow federal regulations are free to test for any psychoactive substance, and many do so. Common additional drugs are barbiturates, benzodiazepines, additional opioids (methadone, propoxyphene, oxycodone, hydrocodone, and buprenorphine), and tricyclic antidepressants. One class of drugs not tested for in the workforce is inhalants.

Biological Specimens Tested and What They Tell Us

A number of biological specimens can be used to test for alcohol or illicit drug use. Table 5.2 details the major biological specimens that may be used, their strengths and weaknesses, and the detection time for the major classes of substances (cf. Bosker & Huestis, 2009; Couper & Logan, 2004; Cowan, Osselton, & Robinson, 2007; Crouch, 2005; Dolan, Rouen, & Kimber, 2004; Drummer, 2005, 2008; Dyer & Wilkinson, 2008; Huestis, 2002; IIDTW, 2004; Jaffee, Trucco, Teter, Levy, & Weiss, 2008; Jones, 2006; Kadehjian, 2005; Kapur, 1993; Lee et al., 2011; Musshoff & Madea, 2007; Pill & Verstraete, 2008; Pragst & Balivova, 2006; Tsanaclis & Wicks, 2007; Verstraete, 2004; Wolff et al., 1999). The primary biological specimen used for workforce testing of illicit drug use has been urine, and the primary specimen used for workforce testing of alcohol use has been breath. Although blood testing has been available for a long time, it is rarely used for workforce testing for the reasons presented in Table 5.2. However, other biological specimens, such as oral fluids (saliva) and hair, are being used in workforce substance use testing programs for alcohol and illicit drug use.

Although Table 5.2 outlines the major strengths and limitations of each biological specimen, some attention should be devoted to a particular issue that is related to the motivation for using drug tests (also see the discussion of motives for and effectiveness of substance use testing below). If the primary goal of workforce testing is to identify *any illicit drug use* among job applicants or employees, biological specimens with the longest window of detection will be optimal. In order of preference, one would want to use hair, urine, and then any of the other three specimens. In contrast, if the primary goal of workforce testing is to identify *substance impairment at work*, the use of biological specimens with the shortest detection times, such as blood and

TABLE 5.2

Biological Matrices Used for Workplace Drug Testing: Strengths, Weaknesses, and Typical Drug and Drug Metabolite Detection Times

Biological matrix	Strengths	Weaknesses	Detection times
Breath (alcohol only)	Concentration of alcohol in breath can be converted into blood alcohol content (BAC). A positive test indicates that a person has alcohol in their blood at the time of testing and BAC correlates reasonably well with alcohol-induced cognitive and psychomotor impairment.	Despite the fact that BAC correlates with impairment, there can be large variations in impairment to the same BAC across persons largely due to various types of tolerance	1 to 12 hours. With a BAC of .10% or less, which would be likely in the workplace, alcohol could be detected up to 5 to 6 hours depending on the weight and gender of the individual, though the level at time of assessment might not meet criteria for reportability based on company policy.
Urine	Available in sufficient quantity. Easy to collect. Drugs or metabolites are present in relatively high concentration. Easy and inexpensive to analyze.	Observed collection of urine is seen as invasive, though direct observation often is used only when attempts at adulteration might be suspected. Typically contains metabolites and little parent drug. Easily adulterated or diluted in an effort to produce a false negative result. Results cannot determine dose; frequency of use (daily vs. weekly vs. monthly); chronic or single dosing; dependence; route of administration; where the substance was used; and impairment at the time of use or testing. For alcohol, if a double-voided urine sample is collected and the time between voids is known, the BAC	Alcohol: Less than 12 hours for ethanol; up to 3 days for certain alcohol metabolites Cannabis: 1 to 3 days for single use; up to 7 days for occasional use; up to 30 days for chronic heavy use Stimulants: 1 to 3 days Depressants: 1 day to 4 weeks depending on type of depressant and the frequency of use Opiates/Opioids: 1 to 3 days Hallucinogens: 1 to 7 days for occasional use; up to 30 days for chronic use; but depends on the hallucinogen (e.g. LSD vs. PCP).

(continues)

TABLE 5.2

Biological Matrices Used for Workplace Drug Testing: Strengths, Weaknesses, and Typical Drug and Drug Metabolite Detection Times (*Continued*)

Biological matrix	Strengths	Weaknesses	Detection times
		at the time midway between the two voids can be *approximately* estimated from urine alcohol content (UAC). However, the single-void urine samples typical of workforce drug testing generally cannot be used to estimate BAC. Also, the use of UAC for the purpose of back extrapolation of BAC at an earlier time should be avoided.	Alcohol: 1 to 12 hours Cannabis: 1 to 36 hours, and up to 7 or more days in some chronic heavy users. Stimulants: 1 to 2 days Depressants: 1 to 2 days Opiates/Opioids: 1 to 24 hours Hallucinogens: 1 to 24 hours
Blood	Assessment of drug and metabolite concentrations is possible and can be compared to standards for therapeutic, toxic, and fatal levels, though it is not commonly used for workforce substance use testing.	The collection of blood is viewed as the most invasive procedure compared with other biological specimens. Collection requires trained personnel and has the potential for disease transmission. More difficult to handle and store than other biological specimens Analysis is more complex and costly. Results cannot determine dose; frequency of use (daily vs. weekly vs. monthly); chronic or single dosing; dependence; route of administration; where the substance was used; and impairment at the time of use or testing.	

Hair

Collection of head hair is easy and relatively noninvasive.
Results can determine chronicity of use. By analyzing segments of hair, a monthly history of use can be compiled. Difficult to adulterate the sample to avoid detection

If head hair is too short or not available, collection of other body hair may be more invasive. Prone to external contamination necessitating decontamination (washing). Decontamination procedures can affect outcomes, but no standardized procedure exists.
Drugs acidic in nature may not incorporate well into the hair shaft. Also, alcohol does not incorporate into hair. Therefore, hair tests for alcohol detect minor metabolites. Even with other drugs, the focus may be on the detection of specific metabolites rather than the parent drug in order to rule out passive or external contamination. Hair treatments, differences in hair color, and differences in hair structure, and the physicochemical properties of different drugs complicate interpretation of test results. Tests using hair are among the most expensive.
Results cannot determine dose; frequency of use (daily vs. weekly vs. monthly); chronic or single dosing; dependence; route of administration; where the substance was used; and impairment at the time of use or testing.

Alcohol: 1 to 3 months
Cannabis: 1 to 3 months
Stimulants: 1 to 3 months
Depressants: 1 to 3 months
Opiates/Opioids: 1 to 3 months
Hallucinogens: 1 to 3 months

(continues)

TABLE 5.2
Biological Matrices Used for Workplace Drug Testing: Strengths, Weaknesses, and Typical Drug and Drug Metabolite Detection Times (*Continued*)

Biological matrix	Strengths	Weaknesses	Detection times
Oral fluid	Collection of oral fluid is easy and noninvasive. Parent drug is more likely to be present than a metabolite. Difficult to adulterate. The possibility of estimating drug concentrations in blood from oral fluid drug concentrations. This may provide information on potential impairment at the time of testing. However, the accuracy of this estimation can be greatly affected by several factors, including oral contamination during drug use, oral fluid pH, the collection device used, time between drug test and drug use, characteristics of the drug (e.g., half-life), and large interindividual variability. Because of these issues, the correlations between oral fluid and blood drug concentration are often low, thereby only allowing for a qualitative determination of recent drug use.	Oral fluid is available in small quantities that may be inadequate for testing in some individuals. Drug concentrations may be low making analysis difficult. Oral fluid has the potential for errors in the collection process because collection devices are not standardized. Results can determine recent use, but cannot determine dose; frequency of use (daily vs. weekly vs. monthly); chronic or single dosing; dependence; route of administration; where the substance was used; and impairment at the time of use or testing is not always possible.	Alcohol: Less than 12 hours for ethanol; up to 3 days for certain alcohol metabolites Marijuana: 1 to 24 hours for THC, and up to 7 or more days in some chronic heavy users when assessing metabolites. Stimulants: 1 to 36 hours Depressants: 1 to 48 hours Opiates/Opioids: 1 to 36 hours Hallucinogens: 1 to 48 hours

Note. See Table 1.1 for a list of the specific drugs that fall into each of the broad drug classes listed in this table. Time of detection refers to the maximum time a drug can be detected after last use of the substance. Variation in estimates exists because the detection time is affected by many factors, such as the amount of the substance consumed per occasion; frequency of consumption; individual differences in metabolism; pH of urine or oral fluid; analytic cut-off values used for a positive test result; and on the parent drug or its specific metabolite being analyzed. Detection time for hair depends on the length of the hair sample, so it can be longer than 3 months.

oral fluids, would be preferable. The underlying assumption is that the use of biological specimens with short windows of detection might better identify individuals who may be working impaired. However, this assumption may be problematic. As noted in Table 5.1, with the exception of breath tests for alcohol, determination of the level of intoxication at a given point in time is not possible when using urine and hair, and it is difficult to impossible even for biological specimens with short detection times, such as oral fluids and blood (e.g., Couper & Logan, 2004; Crouch, 2005; Huestis, 2002; Kadehjian, 2005; Kapur, 1993; Wennig, 2000). Consistent with this argument, it was shown in Chapter 4 that the positivity rates for illicit drug use were not substantially higher for postaccident tests than they were for random tests, and this applied to urine, oral fluid, and breath (in the case of alcohol) tests. The lack of relation between drug test results and accidents for urine and oral fluid is most likely due to the inability of drug tests to detect impairment at the time of testing. In contrast, as noted in Chapter 4, the lack of relation for alcohol tests is more likely due to the low blood alcohol content (BAC) used for an alcohol violation and to the fact that most individuals who fail an alcohol test probably have BACs that are low (i.e., not high enough to be associated with consistent functional impairment; see Chapter 3).

Drug Testing Methods

A defensible workforce drug testing program comprises a complex set of procedures (e.g., see the *Mandatory Guidelines*) but has three basic stages. However, no data exist on how many companies follow each of these stages. The first stage is use of an initial or screening test to rule out employees who have not used a substance. Until recently, employees were usually sent to an off-site facility to have a biological specimen collected. In large companies with a medical department, the collection may have occurred on the employer's premises. Although other biological specimens are now being analyzed, as discussed previously, urine is tested most frequently for illicit drug use, because the detection of substances in urine has a long history and is well understood (e.g., Wolff et al., 1999). The *Mandatory Guidelines* still allow for only the use of urine when testing for illicit drugs. Breath is used for alcohol testing, and more recently oral fluids may be used for the initial screening test. After a specimen is collected, it is sent to a laboratory for the initial screening using some form of immunoassay test. Such screening tests are designed to be maximally sensitive in order to minimize missing a positive specimen, and this sensitivity increases the probability of false positive test results (e.g., Dolan et al., 2004).

Because of the implications of a positive screening result for job applicants or employees, in the second stage of testing all positive results should be confirmed with a qualitatively different confirmation test. The gold standard for confirmation of drug use is gas or liquid chromatography coupled with mass spectrometry (e.g., GC/MS, LC/MS; Cowan et al., 2007). A study by Stuck, English, and Chandler (1998) compared the results of laboratory immunoassay urine screening with the results of more rigorous GC/MS confirmatory tests. Their conclusion was that a GC/MS confirmation test is needed to avoid false positives. Following a positive screening test for alcohol using either oral fluid or a portable screening Breathalyzer, a confirmation test uses an evidentiary breath testing device with technology that differs from the portable Breathalyzers used for screening. Another option is to screen and confirm for alcohol using two different evidentiary breath testing devices. A confirmatory result over a prespecified BAC obtained from breath is treated as evidence that an alcohol violation has occurred. It is possible to screen and confirm for recent or any heavy alcohol using a biological specimen other than breath (e.g., urine, hair). This is uncommon, however, because the main motive for alcohol testing is to estimate the level of alcohol in blood at the time of testing.

Following a positive confirmatory test for drugs other than alcohol, a third stage is required by the *Mandatory Guidelines*, to further avoid a false positive test result, and is often used by employers not bound by federal regulations. The third stage is for a trained medical review officer (MRO) to interview the employee to see if a legitimate reason exists for the positive drug test. If not, it is reported as a positive test for illicit drug use. If there is a legitimate reason (e.g., medical prescription, consumption of certain foods), the outcome of testing is reported as negative to the employer. Some drug testing companies offer the services of a MRO for smaller companies that do not have the resources to employ their own.

Although immunoassay screening tests for illicit drugs have traditionally taken place in laboratories, a new form of immunoassay screening test exists. It is called a *point of collection test* (POCT) because it can be conducted outside a laboratory (e.g., at a worksite or at roadside; Crouch, 2007). The POCTs are growing in popularity and are being marketed because they provide immediate results, require little training, and are relatively inexpensive. For example, a POCT for illicit drugs may require (a) collecting a sample of urine, dipping a set of test strips into the urine, and using a color chart or the presence or absence of a bar to determine whether an individual fails any of the tests or (b) placing an oral fluid collection device in an employee's mouth for a specified time and then reading a color line. However, as with laboratory immunoassay screening, false positive test results are a potential problem with POCTs (e.g., Dolan et al., 2004). Therefore, the use of a confirmatory test and an MRO review are as important after a POCT screening test as after a laboratory screening test in order to minimize false positives (e.g., Pil &

Verstraete, 2008; Verstraete & Walsh, 2007). Schults (2007) pointed out that some, though not all, manufacturers and distributors of POCTs recommend the use of confirmatory tests and review of results by an MRO.

With the exception of the Department of Transportation's allowed use of certain oral fluid POCTs for initial alcohol screening, which then requires a confirmatory evidentiary Breathalyzer test, POCTs do not presently meet scientific standards required for federally regulated workforce drug testing in the United States (e.g., Baylor, Sutheimer, & Crumpton, 2007; Schults, 2007). Nonetheless, in the absence of state laws regulating the use of POCTs, private-sector employers can and do use them, and there may be no requirement or policy to follow up a positive POCT result with a confirmatory test and an MRO review involving job applicants or current employees (Schults, 2007).

Few data exist on the use of confirmatory tests or MRO review among U.S. employers, and those that exist are dated. For example, using a small convenience sample of 177 organizations (ranging between one and 5,000 employees) that were regional, national, or international in scope, Murphy and Thornton (1992) reported that 31% of organizations did not use a confirmatory test after a failed initial urine screening test. In a 1991–1992 survey of 342 medium to large (200+ employees) U.S. worksites in Georgia that were part of local, regional, national, or international organizations, 18% of the worksites did not use a confirmatory test after a failed initial urine screening test (Blum et al., 1992). The difference in the percentage of worksites or organizations not using a confirmatory test between these studies may be due to the use of nonrepresentative samples in each study. Another possibility is that the size of the organization matters. The proportion of worksites not using confirmatory tests increased as worksites got smaller in Blum et al.'s (1992) analysis. Therefore, because Murphy and Thornton's sample had many more small organizations, a higher percentage of organizations failing to use confirmatory tests would be expected. With the relatively recent introduction and use of POCTs, the proportion of companies not following up failed screening tests with confirmatory tests may have grown in the United States. The extent to which POCT screening tests, confirmatory tests, and MRO review are used outside the United States is unclear.

Finally, in most of the major countries that allow for workforce drug testing, the cutoff values for screening and confirmatory tests that determine whether a person passes or fails a drug test are set by government agencies, accrediting agencies, or professional societies. For each psychoactive substance, the cutoff values differ according to the type of biological specimen being analyzed and whether the test is for screening or confirmation. Also, the cutoff values used can differ across test manufactures, unregulated employers, and countries.

ORGANIZATIONAL CHARACTERISTICS RELATED TO VOLUNTARY ADOPTION OF WORKFORCE SUBSTANCE USE TESTING

Among U.S. private-sector employers not required by federal regulations to test for illicit drugs or alcohol, what factors predict whether organizations use drug testing? The adoption and use of various human resource management practices are influenced by an organization's internal and external environments (e.g., Jackson & Schuler, 1995; Jackson, Schuler, & Rivero, 1989; Spell & Blum, 2001).

Internal Environment

Of all organizational characteristics studied, organizational size has received the most attention. The prevalence of organizations using illicit drug and alcohol testing among job applicants and employees increases substantially as worksites or organizations get larger, in terms both of number of employees and of amount of revenue (e.g., Blum et al., 1992; Guthrie & Olian, 1991; Hartwell, Steele, French, & Rodman, 1996; Hayghe, 1991; Knudsen et al., 2003; Macdonald, Csiernik, Durand, Rylett, & Wild, 2006; National Federation of Independent Business, 2004; Roman & Knudsen, 2009; Zhang et al., 1999). Several reasons have been offered for this relation. Compared with smaller organizations, larger organizations (a) may perceive the need to rely on formal social control of large applicant pools or large workforces rather than the more informal monitoring of supervisors, (b) are more likely to have the financial resources to engage in alcohol and drug testing, (c) may be more interested in the symbolic management functions of substance testing and other methods of social control and employee surveillance, and (d) are more visible and under more perceived pressure to gain legitimacy by conceding to external normative pressures for workforce testing (Hecker & Kaplan, 1989; Jackson & Schuler, 1995; Roman & Knudsen, 2009).

Also, a study of small businesses (fewer than 250 employees) by the National Federation of Independent Business (2004) suggests that most small businesses may not use substance use testing because they do not perceive employee alcohol and drug use to be a problem. In this study, only 14% of small businesses reported that an employee was tested for alcohol or drugs during the preceding 3 years. Moreover, 78.2% of small businesses reported that employee abuse of alcohol and its consequences were neither a concern nor an unusual concern, and 82.2% of small businesses reported the same for employee use of illicit drugs and its consequences. Also, recall that in the United Kingdom, the IIDTW (2004) sent a survey on the use of drug testing to all members of the Federation of Small Business and did not receive a single response, which was interpreted to mean that drug testing was not an issue of importance to small businesses. Finally, other research has shown that the prevalence of drug testing is lower among organizations that do not perceive drug use to be a problem (Spell & Blum, 2005).

Another factor that may affect the adoption of drug testing by organizations is their internal turnover rate. Applicant and employee drug testing may be less likely when an organization is experiencing high rates of turnover because individuals may not apply to organizations that drug test, even if they do not use drugs. Some research supports this inverse relation between turnover rates and the use of preemployment drug testing (Spell & Blum, 2005). Other internal organizational characteristics that have been associated with a higher likelihood of alcohol and illicit drug use testing are having a higher proportion of safety-sensitive jobs, having a stronger rules-oriented culture, having a written alcohol and drug policy, having a union, and having an employee assistance program (e.g., Blum et al., 1992; Guthrie & Olian, 1991; Hartwell, Steele, French, Potter, et al., 1996; Knudsen et al., 2003; Spell & Blum 2005). A higher likelihood of illicit drug use testing in organizations is also related to having a higher percentage of male employees (Blum et al., 1992; Borg & Arnold, 1997). Because male employees are more likely than female employees to use illicit drugs, this relation may reflect the fact that employers are more concerned about illicit drug use as the proportion of male employees gets larger. Alternately, this relation may merely reflect the possibility that employers with more male employees have a larger proportion of safety-sensitive jobs.

External Environment

Organizations are sensitive to external contingencies that pressure or allow for drug testing. As shown in Table 5.1 and discussed previously, the prevalence of drug testing increased among organizations after the U.S. federal government declared its War on Drugs and applied pressure on organizations to assist in this effort (e.g., Spell & Blum, 2005). Also, organizations are more likely to engage in drug testing (a) as an increasing proportion of organizations in their industry begins to use drug testing (referred to as organizational mimicry or a lemming effect; Draper, 1998) and (b) as negative media attention devoted to drug use and positive media attention devoted to drug testing increase (Spell & Blum, 2005). Consistent with this seeming organizational sensitivity to the antidrug zeitgeist caused by the War on Drugs, the prevalence of organizations testing for illicit drug use is much higher than the prevalence of organizations testing for alcohol use, although the heavy use of alcohol and alcohol dependence is more prevalent than illicit drug use and dependence (see Chapter 1).

MOTIVATIONS FOR WORKFORCE SUBSTANCE USE TESTING: RATIONALES AND EFFECTIVENESS

Although a number of explicit and implicit reasons have been offered to support the use of workforce drug testing (e.g., Brunet, 2002; Keay et al., 2010; Murphy & Thornton, 1992; Walsh, 2008; Zwerling, 1993), they generally fall into two primary and two secondary motivational themes (e.g., Brunet, 2002). The first primary motive, promoted by the U.S. federal government's initiatives described previously, is to deter the use of illicit drugs in the workforce and in society and to deter alcohol use and impairment in the workplace. The second primary motive is to improve the attendance, performance, and safety of employees and the public. These two motives also underlie the promotional materials and arguments used by drug testing consultants, laboratories, and test manufacturers to sell their services or products. The research evaluating the extent to which workforce substance use testing effectively addresses substance use deterrence and productivity enhancement is summarized below.

However, before I turn to these two primary motives for drug testing, two secondary motives must be briefly discussed. One secondary motive is the use of drug testing as a form of symbolic management (a) to control employee behavior and show that management is in charge; (b) to show constituents that the organization is addressing a perceived social problem; and (c) to control the image and reputation of the organization and public trust in various industries (e.g., Brunet, 2002). With regard to control of employee behavior, research discussed below on the deterrent value of drug testing partly addresses this issue. No research has explored whether workplace drug testing has any useful impact on an organization's constituencies. With regard to using drug testing to manage an organization's image, the IIDTW (2004) stated that it is "extremely difficult to assess the impact of drug and alcohol use among employees on a company's reputation" (p. 53). No research has attempted to explore the impact of drug testing on organizational image or on public confidence in an organization or industry. Another secondary motive is to meet federal or state regulations or to obtain desired financial incentives. One might assume that organizations required to drug test do so to avoid penalties and because formal reporting requirements may exist. One also might assume that some proportion of employers use drug testing because of financial incentives (e.g., reduced insurance premiums) offered by state governments and insurance companies that are perceived to exceed the cost of the testing program. However, there is a lack of data on the proportion of companies that test because of financial incentives, and no research exists on whether such incentives exceed the cost of testing.

Deterring Employee Substance Use and Impairment

A major motivation for workforce substance use testing is to deter any illicit drug use or any on-the-job use of alcohol through the use of punishment, such as denial or termination of employment, suspension, or mandated treatment. Although the often stated goal underlying the deterrence motive is to produce a drug-free workplace, the actual goal is to create an illicit-drug-free workforce and, in the case of alcohol, an alcohol-free workplace.

With respect to illicit drug use, the basic question is whether drug testing has a deterrent effect and if so, what exactly is being deterred? Testing can deter the use of any illicit substances among the workforce; it can deter the use of only those substances for which organizations test; or it can simply deter substance-using individuals from seeking employment from employers who engage in testing. The first outcome is the primary intent of drug testing, whereas the second and third outcomes might be viewed as unintended consequences of testing. Yet, no direct and credible evidence exists showing that drug testing reduces the use of illicit drugs (e.g., Crown & Rosse, 1988; Harris & Heft, 1993; IIDTW, 2004; Macdonald et al., 2010; Walsh, Elinson, & Gostin, 1992; Zwerling, 1993). Some of the studies summarized in these reviews showed evidence that after a drug testing program was introduced, drug positivity rates decreased over time (e.g., Lange et al., 1994). However, these studies have a number of important methodological shortcomings, such as (a) not directly assessing substance use among employees subject to drug testing, (b) failing to use a no-drug-testing comparison group where employee substance use was assessed over the same period of time, and (c) failing to discuss whether other changes that could have resulted in the decline in positivity rates might have occurred simultaneously with drug testing.

Other studies in these reviews used cross-sectional data to show that, compared with drug users, nonusers are more likely to report that their employer tests for drugs (e.g., Carpenter, 2007; French, Roebuck, & Alexandre, 2004). The primary problem with these studies is that it is not possible to determine whether drug testing deters illicit drug use or deters substance users from applying to organizations that test for illicit drug use. To date, no research has been conducted (experimental or longitudinal) that can demonstrate whether workforce drug testing has a casual deterrent effect on employee drug use. Walsh et al. (1992) pointed out that, given the design flaws in past research, the deterrence effect of drug testing on drug use is a matter of conjecture. It is instructive, nonetheless, to consider several broader patterns of data indirectly addressing the potential deterrence value of workforce drug testing that were not part of previous reviews.

First, as shown in Table 5.1, the proportion of U.S. employers that tested job applicants or current employees for illicit drug use increased substantially from 21% in 1987 to 81% in 1996. Although the proportion of employers testing for illicit drug use has apparently fallen, most employers (62%) were still testing in 2004. With nearly three decades of workforce drug testing behind us, is the prevalence of illicit substance use among workers low, and has it changed considerably during the period of growth in drug testing? According to Quest Diagnostics' Drug Testing Index for the combined U.S. workforce (Quest Diagnostics Incorporated, 2011), overall positivity rates for drug use across all forms of testing (preemployment, postaccident, for cause) dropped from 13.6% in 1988 to 4.5% in 2004. On the surface, this pattern of results suggests that drug testing may have caused a decrease in illicit drug users in the workforce. However, the inverse association between these two aggregate trends cannot be used to support a causal deterrent effect of drug testing on illicit drug use in the workforce, because unmeasured changes in society (e.g., growing media attention to drug use) may have caused both an increase in testing and a decrease in positivity rates. Moreover, other data are not consistent with decreasing workforce illicit drug use. For example, Table 1.9 shows that across three national studies conducted from 2001 to 2003, the average 12-month prevalence of illicit drug use in the U.S. workforce was 15.9%. Data from Table 1.15 show that the prevalence of illicit drug use in the 2002–2003 NSWHS was 43.4% among young women and 56.7% among young men in high-risk occupations. Finally, using data from the annual NSDUH, Walsh (2008) showed that the overall prevalence of illicit drugs use in the U.S. workforce changed little between 1988 and 2004. It is not clear why drug positivity rates declined as the use of drug testing increased, yet the estimated prevalence of workforce illicit drug use remained high in some subgroups, and overall workforce prevalence rates for illicit drug use did not change during the time when the use of drug testing was increasing. Walsh (2008) concluded that "more research is needed to better understand what these laboratory drug-testing results really mean, and to determine the effectiveness of the current system of workplace drug testing programs in detecting illegal drug use by workers" (p. 122).

Although the actual meaning of these inconsistent results is unclear, the pattern is consistent with two related explanations. First, frequent, heavy, or dependent drug users are more likely to be detected through drug testing, although their actual drug use is not likely to be responsive to drug testing programs. Rather than stop using illicit drugs, such individuals may look for employment in workplaces that do not test (French et al., 2004). This means that during the time the use of drug testing was increasing, the prevalence of workforce drug use would not decrease, although drug testing positivity rates would decrease.

Second, Table 1.7 shows that 58% of employees who use illicit drugs do so three times per month or less, and most may not be heavy users. Although

Walsh (2008) showed that the overall proportion of the workforce using illicit drugs did not change from 1988 to 2004, it is possible that the frequency of use declined during this period. If this were true, testing of urine, which is the most widely used specimen, may fail to identify most infrequent casual users, because the window of detection for most drugs is about one to three days (see Table 5.2). In fact, DuPont, Griffin, Siskin, Shiraki, and Katze (1995) estimated that with a 50% annual random urine testing rate (50% of a workforce is randomly tested per year), approximately 40% of daily users would be detected, 8% of monthly users would be detected, and 1% of less than monthly users would be detected. Moving to a more costly 100% testing rate (every employee is tested randomly once during the year), the detection rate would increase to 79% for daily users, 15% for monthly users, and 2% for less than monthly users. Moving to a much more costly 300% testing rate (every employee is tested randomly three times per year), the detection rate would increase to 99% for daily users, 45% for monthly users, and 5% for less than monthly users. Even with a 300% random urine testing rate, the majority of infrequent users would not be detected. Thus, a downward shift in the frequency of illicit drug use would not result in a reduction in the overall prevalence of illicit drug use in the workforce, although drug testing positivity rates would decrease.

Both of these explanations obtain additional support from two national cross-sectional studies. Larson et al. (2007) reported that the frequency of illicit drug use was positively related to reports of being less willing to work for employers who used preemployment or random drug testing. Further, Hoffmann and Larison (1999) found that compared with nonusers, those who used marijuana or cocaine at least once per week were less likely to report working for companies that drug tested. The results also showed that, relative to nonusers, those who used marijuana or cocaine less than once per week were as likely to report working for companies that drug tested.

Finally, although no research has explicitly examined whether drug testing deters the use of only those substances for which organizations test, this outcome is unlikely. Even though every organization that tests for illicit drug use tests for marijuana, it has been and remains the most frequently used illicit drug and the mostly frequently detected illicit drug in drug testing programs.

These results do not provide convincing support for the notion that illicit drug use testing deters the overall use of illicit drugs in the workforce. Rather, the research on the deterrent effect of illicit drug use is most consistent with the conclusion that (a) drug testing redistributes frequent heavy and dependent illicit drug users among employers who do not drug test and (b) drug testing may reduce the frequency of use among some users, which reduces the likelihood of detection. Thus, infrequent illicit drug users may be as likely as nonusers to work for employers who drug test.

With regard to alcohol testing, Spicer and Miller (2005) explored the change in alcohol positivity rates for one company in the transportation industry when industry-wide alcohol testing went into effect and 5 years later. The positivity rate for random alcohol testing declined from 0.5% in 1995 to 0.1% in 2000. Likewise, data from the Federal Transit Authority (FTA; 1997, 2010) show that the overall alcohol violation rate for random testing declined from 0.25% in 1995 to 0.15% in 2008. Given the already low base rate of on-the-job alcohol use in 1995 in both of these studies, it is not surprising that random alcohol testing would be associated with a very small absolute decline in alcohol positivity rates through 2008. The low positivity rates from 1995 to 2008 are even more notable when one considers that an alcohol violation can result from a BAC as low as .04%. As with illicit drug use, random alcohol testing may be most effective at detecting a portion of the minority of workers with an alcohol dependence disorder (see Table 1.5) and may be less effective at detecting workers who infrequently work with a BAC of .04 or above. The alcohol positivity rates and the potential deterrent effect of alcohol testing in other industries are unknown.

The results discussed to this point refer largely to preemployment and random postemployment testing. Although no research has explicitly compared various drug testing circumstances, it might be expected that relative to other testing circumstances, probable-cause testing would be more likely than random testing to identify substance use or abuse among current employees. After all, a probable-cause test is initiated after a trained observer has reason to believe that a person is under the influence of a substance at work. According to Quest Diagnostics' 2010 Drug Testing Index for the general workforce (Quest Diagnostics Incorporated, 2011), the positivity rate for illicit drug testing for probable cause (26.9%) is much higher than the overall positivity rate for all testing circumstances combined (4.2%). The positivity rate for illicit drug testing for probable cause (9.7%) is also higher than the overall positivity rate for all testing circumstances combined (1.5%) in the federally mandated, safety-sensitive workforce. Likewise, 2008 data from the FTA (2010) for safety-sensitive positions show that the positivity rate for illicit drug testing for probable cause (10.9%) is much higher than the overall positivity rate for all testing circumstances combined (1.5%). With regard to alcohol, 2008 data from the FTA for safety-sensitive positions show that the positivity rate for an alcohol violation based on probable cause testing (19.7%) is much higher than the overall violation rate for all testing circumstances combined (0.3%).

Despite the higher positivity rates resulting from probable cause testing, these results show that among employees who are believed to be under the influence of an illicit drug or alcohol at work, 73% to 90% have not used an illegal drug during the past 1 to 30 days and are not under the influence of alcohol at work. In addition, probable cause tests may be of limited value in identifying employees who have used illicit drugs or alcohol at work because the proportion of such tests conducted and proportion of identified positives from such testing are likely to be small. This, of course, would reduce the deterrent value of probable cause testing. Although Quest Diagnostics' Drug Testing Index does not provide the proportion of tests conducted under various circumstances, the FTA data show that of all 207,342 illicit drug tests conducted in 2008, only 0.3% were conducted for probable cause, and of all 3,063 positive test results, only 2.0% were the result of probable cause testing. Further, of all 74,556 alcohol tests conducted in 2008, only 0.7% were conducted for probable cause. However, in contrast to the data for illicit drugs, of all 207 alcohol violations detected, 51.2% were the result of probable cause testing.

These results suggest that relative to preemployment and random testing, probable cause testing leads to higher positivity rates. Nonetheless, probable cause testing for illicit drugs is unlikely to have much of a deterrent effect, because very few probable cause tests are conducted and only a small percent of positive results for illicit drug use comes from such testing. Probable cause alcohol testing might have a slightly stronger deterrent effect. As much as 50% of positive alcohol violations may come from probable cause testing. Nonetheless, few such tests are conducted. It is not clear why the proportion of alcohol positives coming from probable cause testing is much higher than that found for illicit drugs. One possibility is that the smell of alcohol is more likely to trigger a probable cause alcohol test, whereas a probable cause illicit drug test is triggered by behaviors (fatigue, argument, poor performance) that can be caused by many other factors (e.g., depression, personality, family problems, financial problems, poor work conditions).

Productivity Enhancement

Employers have an obligation to maintain a safe workplace, and they have a direct interest in maximizing employee attendance and performance and reducing dysfunctional workplace behavior (e.g., theft, aggression) at work. Therefore, another primary motivation for illicit drug use testing is to achieve these outcomes, and a primary sales pitch in the drug testing industry is that drug testing will lead to these outcomes. So what does research have to say about the causal impact of drug testing on improving employee productivity?

Before looking at the research evaluating drug testing's effects on improving productivity, one needs to consider the key assumptions underlying the use of illicit drug testing to improve employee productivity. The first assumption is that drug testing can identify most individuals who use drugs. As discussed in the previous section on deterrence, it may be difficult to identify most infrequent users, and this would be true for most biological specimens that are tested. A second assumption is that a positive drug test can detect individuals who are likely to be impaired at work. But it has been noted throughout this chapter that a positive drug test merely indicates that an illicit drug has been used in the recent past (oral fluid or urine testing) or distant past (hair testing). A positive drug test provides no information on when an illicit substance was used, how often or how much is typically used, or if the person was or has ever been impaired at work. The third assumption is that any illicit drug use has a causal effect on employee productivity. This issue has been discussed in detail in Chapters 3 and 4, which show that the relation of employee substance use to cognitive and psychomotor performance and productivity outcomes is not strong and may be more complex than typically acknowledged.

Because research generally fails to support the three main assumptions underlying the use of drug testing to improve employee productivity, one might anticipate that research will provide little support for a meaningful effect of drug testing on improving worker productivity. Prior research on the relation of drug testing programs to employee productivity supports several conclusions (Beach et al., 2006; Cashman, Ruotsalainen, Greiner, Beirne, & Verbeek, 2009; Dell & Berkout, 1998; IIDTW, 2004; Kitterlin & Moreo, 2012; Kraus, 2001; Lockwood, Klaas, Logan, & Sandberg, 2000; Macdonald et al., 2010; Macdonald, Wells, & Fry, 1993; Morantz, 2008; Normand et al., 1994; Ozminkowski et al., 2003; Snowden, Miller, Waehrer, & Spicer, 2007; Swena & Gaines, 1999).[4] First, little research has directly tested the effect of alcohol and illicit drug testing programs on employee productivity outcomes. Second, this area of research has focused almost entirely on injury or accident outcomes, with virtually no research on attendance or turnover (for one exception, see Kitterlin & Moreo, 2012) and no research on job performance or other dysfunctional work behaviors. Third, many studies have employed data from companies that used more than one type of drug testing (e.g., preemployment, random, for cause, postaccident), and their separate effects could not be evaluated. Fourth, most studies have focused on illicit drug testing, with little attention paid to alcohol testing. Fifth, the available research provides no convincing evidence that workforce alcohol or

---

[4]Studies by Normand et al. (1990) and Zwerling et al. (1990) have been described as testing the effectiveness of preemployment drug testing. However, these studies did not actually test the effects of preemployment drug testing on workplace productivity outcomes. To do so, a study would have to compare organizations or organizational units that did and did not utilize testing. In contrast, these two studies used preemployment drug tests to identify individuals who did and did not engage in recent illicit drug use and then estimated the relation of employee substance use to various productivity outcomes. For this reason, these studies have been cited in Chapter 4 and are not mentioned in this chapter.

drug testing programs improve employee productivity outcomes, and when statistically significant relations are reported, they tend to be small and of limited practical utility. Sixth, failure to attend to unanticipated results of drug testing may affect conclusions regarding their effectiveness. For example, Morantz (2008) provided some evidence that decreases in injury rates following the implementation of a drug testing program may be partly due to underreporting of injuries. To the extent that few employees want to undergo substance use testing—even those who do not use illicit drugs at all and do not use alcohol at work—injured employees may be motivated not to report their injury. Unless the injury is very serious, if some medical attention is required, employees may hide the injury, obtain medical treatment later, and report it as occurring off the job. Higher levels of underreporting of injuries among individuals subject to drug testing than among those not subject to testing would artificially inflate or create a spurious negative relation between drug testing and job injuries.

Most important, this general body of research suffers from many methodological problems and most studies have more than one limitation, which prevents us from drawing any causal conclusions with confidence. Some examples of methodological problems include (a) no experimental research designs with random assignment of employees or work units to drug testing and no drug testing conditions; (b) among the nonexperimental studies, failure to use an appropriate random or matched comparison group; (c) failure to assess and control for environmental changes or other relevant organizational programs that occurred along with or preceded the implementation of drug testing, such as improvements in technology, implementation of policies and organizational cultures enforcing safety and sanctioning dysfunctional behavior of various sorts, and implementation of substance use policies and education programs; (d) failure to assess and control for organizational characteristics and individual differences that might be related to illicit drug use and performance outcomes, such as work stressors, dysfunctional management styles, personality, and comorbid mental health problems; (e) low response rates and small and/or nonrandom samples, which jeopardize generalizing the results beyond the self-selected sample of study participants; and (f) use of aggregate or ecological data across companies and/or time, which limits conclusions regarding the effect of drug testing on individual workers.

FUTURE RESEARCH

The research conducted to date does not provide an evidence base supporting the use of workforce substance use testing. Nonetheless, because of methodological problems outlined in this chapter, more sophisticated field research, both experimental and observational, should be designed to better evaluate whether substance use testing has a practically important causal deterrent effect on employee illicit drug use or alcohol use. Such research must differentiate between the various types of testing circumstances, assess changes in the overall prevalence of use, and assess changes in patterns (frequency and quantity) and contexts (off the job and on the job) of use. Researchers also need to explore whether workforce substance use testing has a practically important causal effect on employee productivity. Because a positive test for illicit drug use generally reflects off-the-job use, the research and model presented in Chapter 4 can inform this research. It might be anticipated that the process linking drug testing to employee productivity is more complex and the relation more circumscribed than typically assumed. Regardless of the outcome, additional studies are needed so that substance use testing policies can be informed by more rigorous scientific evidence rather than ideology or the marketing strategies of a large drug testing industry wanting to promote its products and services. Finally, this research must include estimates of the potential savings due to workforce substance use testing as well as the cost of testing. Estimating the potential savings due to testing cannot be done until reasonable estimates of the size of any causal effects can be made. It is not useful to pretend or assume that some noncausal association provides a reasonable estimate of the causal effect of workforce substance use testing on productivity, especially if most studies do not support a relation.

GENERAL SUMMARY AND CONCLUSIONS

Motivated by federal initiatives (Executive Order 12564 of 1986 and the Drug-Free Workplace Act of 1988), workforce illicit drug use testing and workplace alcohol testing in U.S. organizations increased substantially from the late 1980s to the mid-1990s. Although the proportion of organizations testing employees for alcohol and illicit drug use has been on a decline, a large proportion of organizations still test. Pre- and postemployment testing are more prevalent for illicit drugs than for alcohol use. Workforce substance use testing is largely a U.S. phenomenon. Although less is known about alcohol and drug testing in other countries, the available evidence suggests that it is much less prevalent and has often been introduced by U.S. multinational companies. Also, other countries are generally less accepting of illicit drug use testing, because it cannot determine use or impairment during the workday.

A defensible workforce testing program includes an initial screening test to rule out individuals who have not used a substance or set of substances;

confirmatory testing to exclude false positives based on initial screening tests; and, for illicit drugs, a final review by a medical review officer to further minimize false positive results. Among employers who are not regulated by U.S. federal or state policies, a large proportion may not go beyond an initial screening test, and this may become more common with the introduction and increased use of point of collection testing.

Two primary motives exist for alcohol and illicit drug use testing. The first is to deter any employee use of illicit drugs and alcohol use during the workday. The second is to improve workplace productivity. In the research that exists, little support exists for a deterrent effect of workforce substance use testing on illicit drug use or workplace alcohol use. The data are more consistent with the conclusion that illicit drug use testing deters dependent or very frequent drug users from applying to organizations that use testing and may have no effect on their drug use per se. For other drug users, drug testing may reduce the frequency of use but not use per se. Infrequent drug users may be less likely to be detected through most types of drug testing (e.g., urine) and may be as likely as nonusers to work for organizations that employ workforce substance use testing. In terms of improving workplace productivity, little evidence exists to support the main assumptions underlying the use of testing for this purpose. It is no surprise that research evaluating workforce substance use testing does not support a relation to improved employee productivity.

The lack of support for the deterrent and enhanced productivity effects of workforce substance use testing calls into question the usefulness of testing employees. Nonetheless, the common use of drug testing for safety- and security-sensitive positions is a reasonable exception. Many large employers may continue testing non-safety- and non-security-sensitive employees, because they are unaware of the issues reviewed in this chapter or because they use workforce substance use testing for its symbolic social control function.

6

WORKPLACE INTERVENTIONS II: WORKPLACE HEALTH PROMOTION

Workplace health promotion (WHP) has the broad goal of providing preventive and rehabilitative interventions to address all manner of problems among workers: health (behavioral, mental, physical), personal (social, family, financial, legal, gambling), and workplace (stress, coworkers, manager). Although WHP is broad in scope, the focus of this chapter is on the use and effectiveness of WHP for addressing employee substance involvement and improving productivity affected by substance involvement. Because approximately 75% of illicit drug users and heavy alcohol users are employed, the workplace is viewed as a convenient place to identify substance use problems early and motivate employees with substance abuse or dependence problems to seek treatment, especially those whose productivity has begun to suffer (Roman & Blum, 2002). The workplace also is viewed as a convenient context in which to provide basic information to a large proportion of the general population on the acute and chronic effects of alcohol and illicit drug use and

DOI: 10.1037/13944-007
Alcohol and Illicit Drug Use in the Workforce and Workplace, by M. R. Frone

the signs of substance abuse and dependence, with the goal of preventing or ameliorating abusive substance use and potential productivity problems.

In theory, WHP interventions can target both the employee and the work environment. With regard to employee substance involvement, such interventions can focus on building employee resilience, offering substance abuse education and treatment to employees, and facilitating changes in workplace environmental factors that may cause substance involvement and impaired productivity. In practice, though, WHP interventions generally target the employee. For example, the focus of most WHP interventions is on development of the resilience and coping skills of employees or on treatment interventions that target employee substance use and performance rather than on redesign of the work environment.

In contrast to workforce substance use testing, which is aimed at identifying substance users and either excluding the user from the workplace or eliminating the use through largely punitive methods, WHP represents a more holistic and nonpunitive approach to employee health and productivity. Today, almost all interventions aimed at minimizing employee illness, maximizing employee health and well-being, and sustaining or improving employee productivity fall under the general rubric of WHP. However, a historical and substantive distinction exists between employee assistance programs (EAPs) and workplace wellness programs (WWPs). Therefore, each is discussed separately. In particular, EAPs and WWPs are described briefly, and their effectiveness for addressing employee substance involvement and substance-related performance problems is reviewed.

EAPS

Brief History and Description

The phrase *employee assistance program* emerged in the United States during the 1970s (Steele, 1989). EAPs are an extension of earlier *occupational alcoholism programs* (OAPs; also called *industrial* or *job-based alcoholism programs*).[1] OAPs began to form in the 1940s and 1950s as an attempt to deal with growing recognition and concern over the negative workplace effects of heavy drinking and alcohol dependence among workers. Concern about employee alcohol abuse and dependence grew during World War II, when

---

[1]Although a detailed historical review of the earlier OAP movement and its transition into EAPs is beyond the scope of this chapter, a cumulative history of such programs and their underlying philosophy from 1900 into the 1990s was collectively provided by Steele (1989, 1995); Trice and Schonbrunn (1981); and Weiss (2005).

employers had to rely on marginal workers because of labor shortages and, after the war, because of readjustment problems of millions of returning soldiers (Trice & Schonbrunn, 1981). OAPs focused on employees who were alcohol dependent or alcoholic, and they were based on the increasingly promoted and accepted philosophy that alcohol dependence represented a treatable health condition rather than a moral weakness (Steele, 1995; Trice, Beyer, & Hunt, 1978; Walsh, 1982).

The main motivation underlying OAPs (and to some extent modern EAPs) was what Roman and Blum (2002) broadly referred to as "human resource conservation" (p. 49) rather than corporate humanitarianism. For example, in their research on the early development of OAPs, Trice and Schonbrunn (1981) pointed out that many corporate alcoholism programs evolved from necessity rather than benevolence. Holder and Cunningham (1992) highlighted two main reasons why employers might engage in human resource conservation. First, tight labor markets or collective-bargaining agreements with labor unions might limit the ability of employers to terminate employees with substance abuse or dependence problems. Second, because many employees with substance abuse or dependence problems are highly skilled, their termination might represent a substantial loss. Despite occasional relapses, rehabilitation may be a less costly alternative to hiring and training a replacement.

OAPs basically consisted of a written policy statement introducing the OAP and its philosophy. They emphasized the role of supervisors through performance monitoring and constructive confrontation; were operated internally, thereby minimizing the need for outside treatment, although referrals to Alcoholics Anonymous (AA) were often made; and allowed for posttreatment follow-up (Steele, 1995). These programs were usually linked to organizational medical departments and staffed by individuals knowledgeable about alcohol dependence (e.g., recovering members of AA). The backbone of OAPs was constructive confrontation by supervisors of employees having performance problems (e.g., Roman & Baker, 2002). In constructive confrontation, the role of the supervisor was not to diagnose, criticize, or directly address an employee's personal problems. Instead, the supervisor met with the employee to deal directly with documented performance problems. During this meeting, the supervisor confronted the employee with documented evidence of performance problems. The employee was told what needed to be done to bring performance back to acceptable levels. It was also explained that disciplinary steps could be avoided if performance was improved, and use of the OAP was emphasized to help deal with any problems that might be causing the poor performance. However, the employee also was told that continued poor performance might lead to progressive discipline and possible dismissal. Thus, the meeting combined a constructive element by temporarily suspending discipline and offering help through the OAP and a confrontational element by emphasizing future discipline and possible dismissal if performance did not improve (e.g., Roman & Baker, 2002).

The use by OAPs of poor work performance as the defining characteristic of a problem employee made it apparent that many personal problems in addition to alcohol were implicated in poor performance by employees (Walsh, 1982). Thus, to address fully an organization's interest in reducing impaired work performance, OAPs developed into broader EAPs. Although many definitions and descriptions of EAPs exist, the Employee Assistance Society of North America (EASNA) described EAPs as follows:

> EAPs are employer-sponsored programs designed to alleviate and assist in eliminating a variety of workplace problems. EAPs typically provide screening, assessments, brief interventions, referrals to other services and case management with longitudinal follow-up for mental health concerns and substance abuse problems. The source of these employee problems can be either personal or work-related. Those who work for EAPs come from many different professions including social workers, psychologists, counselors, substance abuse specialists, occupational nurses, and others. Many types of EAPs are available today and there are thus some differences on the definition of what is an EAP. Regardless of the specific definition, what ultimately distinguishes the EAP profession from other forms of mental health counseling, coaching, and occupational health services, is that it emphasizes *employee work performance* as a central theme guiding all program practices and services to the organization. (EASNA, 2009, p. 12)

Two general themes come from this definition. First, EAPs benefit both the employee and the employer (Weiss, 2005). In fact, Weiss (2005) suggested that employers stand to gain more than employees; therefore, *employee* assistance programs should be called *employer* assistance programs. Second, no standard structure or model exists for an EAP. Masi et al. (2004; see for more details) reviewed a number of dimensions on which EAPs may vary, such as the range of EAP services available (basic model or add-on service model), relationship between the EAP and treatment providers (stand-alone model or integrated mode), EAP location (on-site model, off-site model, virtual or web-based model, or a mixed-site model), EAP service provider (internal staff model, external staff model, blended model of internal and external staff, peer model, or affiliate model), EAP eligibility (employee and family assistance program, member assistance program, or labor assistance program), and sponsor or payer of EAP services (management model, professional organization model, consortium model, joint labor–management model, or union model). Variation across all of these dimensions produces many variants of EAPs that may affect their absolute and relative utilization and effectiveness.[2]

Roman and Baker (2002) suggested that to deal effectively with substance use problems, EAPs must incorporate a minimum of five components. First, the EAP's policy and philosophy should be based on addressing job performance first and foremost. Second, the EAP must be appropriately staffed to provide substance abuse services or appropriate referrals. Third, the EAP is directly and readily accessible to supervisors and employees. Fourth, supervisors, employees, and union representatives need to be aware of and to support the use of constructive confrontation. Fifth, staff specialists are able to link employees with appropriate resources for assistance, engage in case management through treatment, and implement long-term follow-up in the workplace. Although not mentioned directly by Roman and Baker, a sixth component applicable to all EAPs, regardless of their overall focus, is that they must engender in employees absolute trust in an EAP's policy of confidentiality regarding the services provided.

Prevalence of EAP Availability and Utilization for Substance Involvement

As with drug testing, EAPs were developed in the United States, and their use expanded quickly. Several national studies have estimated the prevalence of employers providing EAPs and the prevalence of employees having access to an EAP. The National Survey of Worksites and Employee Assistance Programs (NSWEAP) found that 33% of organizations offered EAP services in 1993 and 36% of organizations did so in 1995 (Hartwell, Steele, French, & Rodman, 1996; Hartwell, Steele, & Rodman 1998). On the basis of several sources, Attridge et al. (2009) estimated that the prevalence of organizations offering EAPs was 31% in 1985, 33% in 1995, 70% in 2004, and 75% in 2008. The 2008 Global Wellness Survey reported that 95% of U.S. employers offered an EAP (Buck Consultants, 2008). With regard to the prevalence of employees having access to an EAP, the NSWEAP found that 55% of employees had access in 1993 (Hartwell, Steele, French, Potter, et al., 1996). The National Employee Survey (NES) showed that 47% of employees had access to an

---

[2]The term *employee assistance programs* (EAPs) typically refers to programs provided by employers. Another variation of assistance programs is *member assistance programs* (MAPS; also known as *peer assistance programs*, or PAPs) provided by unions to their members. MAPs are not covered in this chapter for two reasons. First, a relatively small proportion of wage-and-salary workers have access to them. The Bureau of Labor Statistics (2012) reported that only 12% of U.S. wage-and-salary workers belong to a union, and not all unions provide MAPs. Further, Golan, Bacharach, and Bamberger (2010) crudely estimated that MAPs represent "some 11% of employee assistance service frameworks in existence among American enterprises" (p. 173). Second, very little research exists on the prevalence or effectiveness of MAPs. For more information on MAPs, the interested reader can consult Bacharach, Bamberger, and Sonnenstuhl (1996) and Golan et al. (2010).

EAP in 1993 and 58% of employees had access to an EAP in 1995 (Knudsen et al., 2003; Roman, 2002). Finally, the 2002–2004 National Survey on Drug Use and Health (NSDUH) suggested that 58% of employed adults reported access to an EAP (Larson et al., 2007).

EAP availability has also grown outside the United States, both independently of and along with multinational companies and global EAP providers (e.g., Buon & Taylor, 2007; Kirk, 2006). Kirk and Brown (2003) showed that the history of Australian EAPs followed a developmental trajectory similar to that in the United States but lagged in time, beginning in the 1970s with an exclusive focus on alcohol and drug problems. This focus eventually broadened to dealing with all types of personal problems. In terms of the prevalence of EAPs outside the United States, Macdonald, Csiernik, Durand, Wild, et al. (2006) reported that the proportion of employers in Ontario, Canada, providing access to EAPs was 28% in 1989, 52% in 1993, and 67% in 2003. The Alberta Alcohol and Drug Abuse Commission (2003) found that the prevalence of employers in Alberta, Canada providing an EAP was 9% in 1992 and 28% in 2002, and the proportion of Albertan employees reporting access to an EAP was 58% in 2002. The 2008 Global Wellness Survey reported that 94% of Canadian employers offered an EAP (Buck Consultants, 2008). The prevalence of U.K. employees having access to an EAP grew from 6% in 1994 to 10% in 2005 (Arthur, 2000; Buon & Taylor, 2007). Approximately 25% of Danish workers have access to an EAP (Buon & Taylor, 2007). The 2008 Global Wellness Survey reported that overall, 62% of European employers offered an EAP (Buck Consultants, 2008). Harper (1999) found that among South Africa's 100 largest companies, 45% provided access to an EAP in at least one of their operations. The 2008 Global Wellness Survey estimated that 77% of employers in Africa offered an EAP (Buck Consultants, 2008). Finally, the 2008 Global Wellness Survey reported that 55% of employers in Asia offered an EAP (Buck Consultants, 2008). Although EAPs have expanded to many individual countries around the world, detailed prevalence data at this level are not readily available.

The major predictor of whether an organization offers an EAP and whether an employee has access to an EAP is the size of the organization (e.g., Alberta Alcohol and Drug Abuse Commission, 2003; Attridge et al., 2009; Hartwell, Steele, French, Potter, et al., 1996; Harwood & Reichman, 2000; Knudsen et al., 2003; Macdonald, Csiernik, Durand, Rylett, & Wild, 2006; Steele, 1998). For example, Attridge et al. (2009) reported that in 2008, EAPs were provided by 52% of small employers (1–99 employees), 76% of medium employers (100–499 employees), and 89% of large employers (500 or more employees). Similarly, the prevalence of employees having access to an EAP in 1997 ranged from 27% among those working for an employer with 1 to 24 employees to 75% among those working for an employer with 500 or more employees (Harwood & Reichman, 2000). An employer's beliefs about the usefulness of EAPs also affect whether or not such programs are made available to employees. In a study using a national sample of Canadian employers with 100 or more employees, Keay et al. (2010) found that the five most important reasons for providing an EAP were (a) to improve employee well-being, (b) to improve morale, (c) to reduce absenteeism, (d) to improve relations with employees, and (e) to be cost effective. The five most important reasons for not providing an EAP were (a) little evidence that it reduces absenteeism, (b) no need, (c) little evidence regarding cost effectiveness, (d) costs too much, and (e) little evidence that it improves workplace safety. As with workforce substance use testing, it appears that disagreement exists among employers regarding the need for and effectiveness of EAPs.

Compared with earlier OAPs, current EAPs are broader in terms of the presenting problems they address, and they differ in several other important ways. The goal of OAPs was to address alcohol dependence and its effect on productivity. They were primarily internal programs, in which problem employees were motivated to contact the program through supervisor-initiated constructive confrontation, and there was posttreatment follow-up. However, organizations are currently more likely to use the services of an external EAP provider that resides off company premises (Hartwell, Steele, French, Potter, et al., 1996; Macdonald, Csiernik, Durand, Rylett, & Wild, 2006; Macdonald, Csiernik, Durand, Wild, et al., 2006; Steele, 1998), which results in less use of constructive confrontation techniques and less posttreatment follow-up (Steele, 1998). For example, even as far back as 1995, 81% of organizations used an external EAP, 16% of organizations used an internal EAP, and 4% of organizations used a combination of the two. The role of constructive confrontation has declined, because its use is much less prevalent among external EAPs (26%) than internal EAPs (61%; Steele, 1998). And posttreatment follow-up through supervisors is much less prevalent among external EAPs (33%) than internal EAPs (65%; Steele, 1998). In comparison with that for earlier OAPs, contact with an EAP is much more likely due to self-referrals than to supervisor referrals (Jacobson, Jones, & Bowers, 2011; Macdonald, Csiernik, Durand, Wild, et al., 2006; Prottas, Diamante, & Sandys, 2011; Roman, 2002). For example, in an analysis of more than 90,000 EAP cases from 1999 to 2010, Prottas et al. (2011) reported that only 4% of referrals were directly attributed to managers. Although an employee's self-referral may have been partly due to informal pressure from others (e.g., supervisor or spouse), no current data exist on this issue.

Finally, OAPs dealt exclusively with heavy drinking and alcohol dependence. But what proportion of cases seen in current EAPs is related to employee substance use problems? On the basis of an examination of more than 90,000 EAP contacts from 1999 to 2010, Prottas et al. (2011) reported that the presenting problem was drug use for 3% of cases and alcohol use for 3% of cases. They also noted that the proportions of manager-referred cases for drug problems (17%) and alcohol problems (18%) were substantially higher than those for self-referred cases for drug problems (3%) and alcohol problems (3%). However, as noted previously, only 4% of referrals in this study were attributed to managers. Highley-Marchington and Cooper's (1998) survey of British organizations showed that of presenting EAP problems, 4% were due to alcohol and 1% were due to drugs. Spetch, Howland, and Lowman (2011) reported that among the EAP cases seen over 3 years from a large national Canadian retail corporation, 8% were for alcohol or drug dependency. These studies using different methods and data from different employers in different countries reported similar results, which suggests that only 5% to 8% of EAP contacts or cases have a presenting problem due primarily to alcohol or drugs. Because EAPs are now addressing a host of employee problems that individually and combined are much more prevalent than problem substance use, the relatively small proportion of EAP contacts and cases related to substance use is not surprising. The lower rate also may result if employees believe that alcohol and drug problems are more likely than other life problems to lead to stigmatization.

Effectiveness of EAPs Regarding Substance Involvement

Although information on the prevalence of individuals contacting EAPs for substance problems is useful for organizations, more important is the extent to which such programs are effective in resolving such problems. Research on the effectiveness of earlier OAPs reported high rates of alcohol treatment success—favorable outcomes in 60% or more of their cases—though most claims were based on anecdotal data or weak research designs, thereby calling into question the actual effectiveness of the programs (Kurtz, Googins, & Howard, 1984; Shain & Groeneveld, 1980). In their review of research on the effectiveness of OAPs, Kurtz et al. (1984) considered several broad outcomes: (a) changes in drinking behavior (e.g., abstinence, recovery, rehabilitation), (b) changes in performance (e.g., absenteeism, accidents, work efficacy), (c) cost reduction, and (d) penetration rate (i.e., proportion of all problem drinkers in a workforce who are identified and referred to treatment). In general, Kurtz et al. concluded that the research findings were unclear regarding OAP effectiveness, and they pointed to a number of problems with the body of research. The types of alcohol use outcomes, such as recovery or reduction in drinking, were often poorly defined, and the magnitude of change required to support a claim of success was not always clear. Results for performance outcomes were mixed, with studies that met minimum quality standards (i.e., using a control group) either showing weaker associations or failing to support an association of OAPs to job performance. Cost reduction studies had design flaws and were seen as failing to provide convincing evidence that OAPs actually reduced employer costs. Studies of penetration rates failed because estimates of the prevalence of problem drinkers in a specific workforce did not exist, forcing the use of guesses that ranged widely. Also, it was not clear how to define a successful penetration rate.

Kurtz et al. (1984) highlighted a number of other impediments to research evaluating the success of OAPs. First, managers often saw no reason for formal evaluation, because they were assured by alcoholism treatment professionals that the programs worked. Second, researchers experienced difficulty gaining access to OAPs for evaluation. Most of the research was conducted by internal program staff who may have had little research expertise or had a vested interest in the success of the program. Finally, basic flaws in research methodology existed in all studies, making their interpretation difficult. Major problems included self-selected samples of participants; small samples; lack of random control groups; use of matched control groups that may have differed in important and unknown ways from the OAP group; short follow-up periods; and the use of self-reports of alcohol use and many productivity outcomes that may have inflated the putative effect of OAPs. These various problems mean that it is difficult to say whether or not OAP participation caused changes in drinking behavior, productivity, or employer costs.

Because present-day EAPs are broad-based programs, the typical focus is on whether overall utilization of an EAP results in improved employee productivity, lower employer health care costs, and an overall cost savings for the employer that exceeds the cost of the EAP (i.e., positive return on investment). However, the lack of attention to the specific problems being addressed means that little recent research exists on the extent to which EAP utilization (a) reduces substance use problems and (b) subsequently increases productivity and reduces employer costs. In a discussion of employee alcohol problems, Gill (1994) stated that "while in theory the benefits of a workplace EAP are boundless, a considerable amount of available evidence presents a more enigmatic picture" (p. 239).

There have been several reviews of the EAP evaluation literature covering the 1970s, 1980, and 1990s (Blum & Roman, 1995; Colantonio, 1989; Csiernik, 1995, 2005; French, Zarkin, & Bray, 1995; Gill, 1994; Kirk & Brown, 2003; Walsh, 1982). As with the OAP evaluation research described previously, almost all of the studies of EAP effectiveness showed that EAP use is associated with statistically significant and sometimes practically important improvements in one or more measures of productivity (e.g., fewer attendance problems, lower absenteeism, higher job performance, fewer accidents/injuries, lower rates of dismissal) and reduced employer costs (lower health care and workers' compensation costs). Despite these positive findings, the prior reviews were unanimously critical of the study designs. They suggested that no definitive evaluations exist and that no definitive conclusions could be drawn regarding the effectiveness of EAPs for treating alcohol use, other drug use, or any other problems that bring individuals in contact with an EAP. For example, commenting on positive EAP evaluation results, Walsh (1982) stated,

> Provocative though they are, these assessments lack adequate controls to permit valid causal inferences and leave unresolved the researcher's nightmare of selection bias and the effects of secular events. What would have happened, for instance, to the treated employees with the passage of time had they been left to their own devices? "Spontaneous remission" is a clearly documented phenomenon in the alcohol-treatment field. (p. 510)

In his review of EAP evaluation research conducted during the 1990s, Csiernik (2005) commented,

> Thirty-nine studies in ten years, less than four per year, a third of which were primarily descriptive in nature and several others of which would not withstand the scrutiny of an undergraduate research methodology course. The 1990s did not provide an extensive EAP evaluation legacy. (p. 32)

These reviews demonstrate that the methodological limitations undermining the interpretation and utility of most EAP evaluation studies are nearly identical to those described previously for OAPs.

Additional EAP evaluations have been conducted since the above reviews were published, but few have focused on employee substance use. The few EAP evaluations exploring substance use continue to suffer from major methodological problems that make interpretation difficult and undermine their utility (e.g., Hargrave, Hiatt, Alexander, & Shaffer, 2008; Osilla et al., 2010; Osilla, Zellmer, Larimer, Neighbors, & Marlatt, 2008; Sieck & Heirich, 2010). For example, an evaluation study by Hargrave et al. (2008) failed to assess employee outcomes (e.g., absenteeism and work performance) prior to using the EAP, did not use a random or matched control group, and had a low response rate (13%) and a resultant small sample ($N = 133$). Any one of these limitations jeopardizes the study's interpretability and usefulness, but when all of them are combined, no credible conclusions can be derived from such a study. In addition, although a study by Osilla et al. (2010) used a randomized control group design, which is a major improvement over most prior studies, there was a large amount of nonparticipation and employee dropout during the study. Of the employees using one of five external EAPs, 365 screened positive for at-risk drinking and were eligible for the study.

Of these 365 eligible employees, 321 employees (a) were excluded from the study or declined to participate ($n = 261$), (b) dropped out of the study after treatment ($n = 32$), or (c) did not provide answers to all questions ($n = 28$). Therefore, the study's results were based on 44 employees, representing only 12% of the original eligible sample. This limitation undermines the generalizability and credibility of the study's findings and conclusions.

WWPS

Brief History and Description

A WWP can be defined as "an organized, employer-sponsored program that is designed to support employees (and sometimes their families) as they adopt and sustain behaviors that reduce health risks, improve quality of life, enhance personal effectiveness, and benefit the organization's bottom line" (Berry, Mirabito, & Baun, 2010, p. 4). Thus, one goal of WWPs is improving employee physical and mental well-being. This is partly accomplished by helping people avoid a number of physical health (heart disease, diabetes, obesity, cancer), mental health (depression, anxiety), and behavioral health (alcohol dependence, illicit drug dependence) conditions and disorders by targeting specific risk factors, such as poor nutrition, physical inactivity, stress, and substance use. A second goal is improving employee productivity and reducing employer costs. WWP interventions can include preventive screening, immunizations, health risk appraisals, lifestyle classes, behavioral coaching or brief interventions, health education, and physical fitness.

With regard to employee substance involvement, WWPs differ from EAPs in a number of ways. First, WWPs are typically aimed at all employees, not just those having performance problems. Second, WWPs generally target reducing moderate and heavy substance use that has not developed into clinical levels of substance abuse or dependence. Third, WWPs can be either preventive or rehabilitative, although focus is greater on the former. Some interventions might be viewed as serving both roles, such as when an intervention is aimed at reducing heavy alcohol use in an effort to prevent future health and workplace performance problems. Also, because WWPs target all employees, a single intervention (e.g., alcohol education) may both prevent heavy alcohol use among some employees and reduce heavy alcohol use among other employees. Despite these differences, WWPs share some similarities with EAPs. First, WWPs are broad programs that vary widely in terms of their structure and the types of preventative interventions offered. Second, WWPs focus on a wide variety of employee problems. Third, WWPs benefit both employees and employers. Finally, WWPs can operate independently or be integrated into a broad EAP.

Prevalence of WWP Availability and Utilization for Substance Involvement

WWPs began in many companies in the 1970s and 1980s, and their use has expanded globally. In early reviews, Fielding (1984) and Shain (1990) showed that across several studies conducted in the United States and Canada from the late 1970s to the late 1980s, the proportion of employers offering some form of WWP ranged from 8% to 98%. The variation in prevalence rates depended largely on the type of WWP offered (e.g., smoking cessation classes or gym facilities) and the size of the organization. As with EAPs, large organizations were much more likely to provide some form of WWP. Among the largest employers, 91% had a WWP, with an average of nine component programs, whereas among the smaller employers, 35% had a WWP, with an average of six component programs (Shain, 1990).

In the United States, the first National Survey of Worksite Health Promotion Activities, conducted in the mid-1980s, found that 65% of employers with 50 or more employees offered one wellness activity (Fielding & Piserchia, 1989). The proportion of employers in this study offering a WWP ranged from 55% among those with 55 to 99 employees to 88% among those with 750 or more employees. In the 1999 National Worksite Health Promotion Survey, 95% of employers with 50 or more employees offered one wellness activity (U.S. Department of Health and Human Services, 2000). One goal of the U.S. federal government's Healthy People 2010 initiative, rather than to focus on the provision of one or more unintegrated wellness activities, was to increase the prevalence of employers who provide a comprehensive WWP to 75% by 2010 (U.S. Department of Health and Human Services, 2000). A comprehensive WWP has five elements: (a) health education, (b) supportive social and physical environment, (c) integration among components programs, (d) linkage to related programs, and (e) worksite screening. However, the 2004 National Worksite Health Promotion Survey found that only 7% of employers provide a comprehensive WWP, with the prevalence ranging from 5% of employers with 50 to 99 employees to 24% of employers with 750 or more employees (Linnan et al., 2008).

Finally, the 2010 Global Wellness Survey collected data from 1,248 employers based in 47 countries with more than 13 million employees (Buck Consultants, 2010). This study found that globally, 66% of employers provided a WWP. The prevalence rates varied somewhat across regions: 74% in North America, 45% in Middle/South America, 49% in Europe, 41% in Africa/Middle East, 47% in Asia, and 47% in Australia/New Zealand.

Among multinational employers, 54% provided a WWP. However, only 21% of employers had a comprehensive WWP. Although the overall prevalence of having a comprehensive WWP found in the 2010 Global Wellness Survey (21%) is larger than the overall prevalence reported in the 2004 National Worksite Health Promotion Survey (7%), the former study had more large companies and did not use the more stringent definition outlined in Healthy People 2010. Among employers with no plans for a WWP, the 2008 Global Wellness Survey found, the main reasons were lack of budget (47%), lack of knowledge on how to get started (29%), perceived lack of a business case to support implementation (24%), insufficient internal ownership (18%), insufficient management support (18%), preference for incremental programs (12%), a company culture incompatible with the wellness message (12%), and the belief that managing employee health is not the role of the organization (12%). For those companies providing access to at least one wellness activity, the menu of intervention options is large, and many employers offer several options. Although some information exists on the prevalence of various broad wellness program components (e.g., Buck Consultants, 2008, 2010), no information exists on the prevalence of wellness programs and interventions specifically addressing employee substance use.

Effectiveness of WWPs Regarding Substance Involvement

Most large-scale evaluation studies and reviews of the effectiveness of WWPs focus almost exclusively on the overall association of WWPs with reductions in cumulative risk across many risk factors, overall performance outcomes, and overall costs (e.g., Goetzel, Juday, & Ozminkowski, 1999; Goetzel & Ozminkowski, 2008; Harden, Peersman, Oliver, Mauthner, & Oakley, 1999; Kuoppala, Lamminpää, & Husman, 2008; Parks & Steelman, 2008). When these broad evaluation studies and reviews do address specific health conditions and risk factors, alcohol and illicit drug use often are not considered. This means that little detailed information exists from large-scale evaluation studies and recent reviews on the extent to which WWP interventions (a) reduce employee substance use and (b) subsequently increase productivity or reduce employer costs. Nonetheless, two reviews and a number of smaller studies have presented and evaluated substance-related WWPs that could be used by employers.

Reviews of WWP Effectiveness for Substance Involvement

Webb, Shakeshaft, Sanson-Fisher, and Havard (2009) undertook a systematic review of 10 intervention studies focused on alcohol involvement that were conducted from January 1995 to February 2007. Bennett, Reynolds, and Lehman (2003) provided a review of 11 intervention studies focusing on either alcohol use or illicit drug use, which were all published from 1991 to 2003. The two reviews had only two intervention studies in common. The studies encompassed a variety of interventions, which included psychosocial skills training, screening with brief intervention, and alcohol education. With regard to effectiveness, Webb et al. concluded that the results were mixed. Although only one study failed to report any statistically significant associations, the pattern of results in the remaining studies showed little consistency regarding which interventions might be most effective and which dimensions of alcohol involvement were more likely to be affected. Although the relations between interventions and alcohol outcomes were evaluated in terms of statistical significance, Webb et al. made no attempt to evaluate the size and practical importance of the associations. Bennett et al.'s review suggested that all studies found at least one statistically significant relation between the interventions and some measure of substance use, although the effects were classified as generally weak. With regard to methodological issues, Webb et al. (2009) found that none of the studies were methodologically sound and concluded, "These methodological weaknesses have grave implications for the credibility of the study results" (p. 374). Among the main methodological problems were selection bias due to self-selected, nonrandom samples; low response and participation rates; high dropout rates; low integrity of intervention implementation; issues regarding data analysis, such as no attempt to adjust analyses for the impact of participant dropout; and short follow-up periods. Bennett et al. did not provide a detailed analysis of study limitations, although they warned appropriately that the observed effects might overestimate true intervention effects because studies that fail to find statistically significant relations are not likely to be submitted to journals or to be published if submitted.

Additional WWP Evaluation Studies

A number of additional intervention studies evaluating the relation of WPPs to employee substance use exist but were not included in either of the two prior reviews. These studies are briefly summarized next, with a focus on intervention studies that used some type of control group. Even studies that use control groups may have methodological problems that undermine their utility. Nonetheless, under the best of methodological circumstances, intervention studies without control groups simply cannot provide credible evidence regarding causal effects. The intervention studies are grouped into two categories: (a) educational and psychosocial skills training and (b) screening and brief intervention.

Educational and psychosocial skills training. Lapham, Gregory, and McMillan (2003) examined the effect of an educational intervention on several measures of alcohol involvement. Of two worksites, one ($N = 3,442$ employees) served as the intervention group, and the other ($N = 2,032$) served as the control group. Of these populations, 576 employees from the intervention worksite (17% response rate) and 381 employees from the control worksite (19% response rate) participated in the study, but employees were not randomly assigned to conditions. The goal of the intervention was to reduce binge drinking (5 or more drinks) days during the course of a month. The intervention lasted 24 months and included information flyers covering eight topics about hazardous alcohol use, an alcohol awareness month, and the availability of literature and videotapes. At the end of the intervention period, 450 videos, 16,000 flyers, and 450 workbooks had been distributed. Data were collected multiple times from participants during the 8 months before the intervention and during the 24 months in which the intervention took place. The results indicated that the intervention had no statistically significant effect on the number of monthly binge drinking days.

Cook and colleagues conducted four evaluation studies. In the first study (Cook, Hersch, Back, & McPherson, 2004), 374 construction workers from four worksites voluntarily completed a preintervention questionnaire, with response rates ranging from 53% to 95%. Of the original 374 participants, 201 workers completed both the pre- and postintervention questionnaires (46% dropout rate). Employees were randomly assigned to the intervention and control groups. The intervention consisted of seven educational sessions using printed materials and video segments. Four sessions were devoted to healthy lifestyle issues, such as stress management, anger management, and goal setting, and three sessions were devoted to alcohol and drug abuse. The intervention group received all seven sessions, and the non-substance-abuse training control group (Control Group 1) received the four sessions that did not involve substance abuse training. During the study, a nonrandomly assigned, no-treatment control group of 30 individuals (Control Group 2) was added. Outcome data were collected on alcohol and illicit drug use via self-reports, and illicit drug use was assessed with urine and hair tests from a consenting subsample of individuals. The results indicated that there was no statistically significant difference between the groups in relation to three measures of alcohol use during the past month: number of drinking days, number of drinks per drinking day, and number of binge drinking (5 or more drinks) days. The intervention also had no statistically significant effect on illicit drug use (both self-reported and drug tests).

In the second study (Deitz, Cook, & Hersch, 2005), 376 office workers from two offices of an insurance company voluntarily participated (approximately 32% total response and follow-up rate). Employees from one office served as the control group, and those from another office served as the experimental group. Individual employees were not randomly assigned to experimental and control conditions, nor were individuals in the control group matched to those in the intervention group on possible confounding variables. Individuals in the control group received information on health promotion, such as stress management and healthy eating. Individuals in the intervention group received the same information and additional information on substance abuse. Outcome data on the proportion of the sample reporting binge drinking (drinking 5 or more drinks on a single occasion in the past month) and heavy drinking (5 or more days of heavy drinking in the past month) were collected before the intervention and 12 months after the intervention. The results indicate that the intervention had no statistically significant relation to binge drinking or heavy drinking.

In the third study (Billings, Cook, Hendrickson, & Dove, 2008), 309 employees of a technology company were recruited from a corporate health promotion listserv and from a health fair, and 245 workers completed both the pre- and postintervention questionnaires (21% dropout rate). Volunteers were randomly assigned to an intervention or a no-treatment control condition. The intervention consisted of access for 3 months to a web-based program on mood and stress management. Outcome data on binge drinking and four dimensions of self-reported productivity were collected before and immediately following the 3-month intervention period. The binge drinking measure contained information on drinking 5 or more drinks in the past month and in the past 6 months and on intentions to stop if the person reported binge drinking. A statistically significant effect of the intervention on binge drinking was observed. However, the change in the intervention group was small—an average change of 0.4 points on a 6-point scale. The intervention had no statistically significant effect on any of the four job performance measures.

In the fourth and final study (Deitz, Cook, & Hendrickson, 2011), 362 female hospital employees voluntarily participated (24% response rate). Of these volunteers, 346 workers completed both the pre- and postintervention questionnaires (4% dropout rate). Employees were randomly assigned to an intervention or a no-treatment control condition. The intervention consisted of 4 weeks' access to a web-based program that provided information on safe administration of prescription psychoactive drugs (analgesics, sedatives, antidepressants, and tranquilizers) and information on alternatives to psychoactive drug use for managing health. Five drug use outcomes were assessed pre- and postintervention. The intervention had no statistically significant effect on reports of illicitly using analgesics, sedatives, antidepressants, or tranquilizers. The fifth outcome was a screening measure for problematic psychoactive drug use. The results indicated that after the intervention, the mean score for the intervention group (.49) was statistically significantly smaller than the mean score for the control group (.86). However, scores on this screening measure could range from 0 to 4, with a score of 0 indicating nonrisky drug use, a score of 1 indicating risky use, a score of 2 indicating a current problem, and a score of 3 or more indicating possible dependence. Thus, the difference between the groups represented a small change in largely nonrisky prescription drug use and is not likely of practical importance.

Snow, Swan, and Wilton (2003) described two studies using the same intervention. The goal in both studies was to reduce substance use through stress management training. The intervention consisted of 15 sessions (Study 1) or 16 sessions (Study 2), each lasting 1.5 hours. Sessions 1 to 4 and 6 to 9 focused on teaching employees ways to eliminate or modify stressors in their lives. Sessions 10 to 11 taught techniques to modify appraisals of stressors to reduce distress without modifying the stressors themselves. Sessions 5 and 12 to 15 taught stress management techniques, such as deep breathing and progressive relaxation. Session 16, in Study 2, summarized and integrated all of the material from the prior 15 sessions, as well as helped individuals formulate personal stress management plans. In Study 1, the participants were 239 female secretaries who volunteered from four worksites; they were randomly assigned to either an intervention or a no-treatment control group. The number of drinks consumed per month was assessed at preintervention, postintervention, 6-month follow-up, and 22-month follow-up. Comparisons of changes in the alcohol outcome between the control group and the intervention group were made for preintervention versus postintervention and preintervention versus 6-month follow-up. No comparisons were provided for the 22-month follow-up measure. Of these two comparisons, one statistically significant intervention effect was found. No statistically significant intervention effect was found for the preintervention to postintervention comparison, but the intervention effect was statistically significantly related to the preintervention to 6-month comparison. Nonetheless, this intervention effect was small. The net difference in change between the two groups was 4 drinks per month—or a reduction of about one drink per week. Also, although no data were reported regarding daily and weekly alcohol consumption, the reported number of drinks per month at each time point for both the intervention group and the control group was likely within U.S., Canadian, and Australian safe drinking guidelines for women (Australian Institute of Health and Welfare, 2011; Butt et al., 2011; Dawson, 2000).

In Snow et al.'s (2003) second study, 468 men and women at three worksites volunteered to participate and were randomly assigned to one of three conditions: the experimental condition (all 16 sessions), the attention control condition (eight sessions of information but no skills training), or the no-treatment control condition. Of these participants, 340 employees completed the pre- and posttest measures (27% dropout rate). Three alcohol outcomes were assessed: an alcohol composite score, an alcohol use disorders test, and the number of drinks during the prior month. The assessments were made at preintervention, postintervention, 6-month follow-up, and 12-month follow-up. Comparisons of changes in alcohol scores between the control group and the intervention groups were made for preintervention to postintervention. No comparisons were reported for the 6- and 12-month follow-up measures. Compared with the attention control condition and the no-treatment control condition, the intervention was statistically significantly and negatively related to only one of the three alcohol outcomes—the alcohol composite score—although the intervention effect was weak. The analyses were then repeated in a subsample of heavy alcohol users. Compared with those for the attention control condition and the no-treatment control condition, the intervention effect in this subgroup was statistically significant and negatively related to the alcohol composite score and the number of drinks in the past month. However, the intervention effects in this subgroup were weak. For example, relative to the no-treatment control, the intervention led to a net reduction of 5 drinks in the past month. This amounted to a reduction of slightly more than one drink per week. Although no data were reported regarding daily and weekly alcohol consumption, the number of drinks per month at each time point for the intervention and control groups were likely within U.S., Canadian, and Australian safe drinking guidelines for men and women (Australian Institute of Health and Welfare, 2011; Butt et al., 2011; Dawson, 2000).

Bennett and colleagues conducted three evaluation studies. Two studies evaluated the effect of a program called Team Awareness on reducing alcohol use. This program consists of five components conducted across two 4-hour sessions separated by 2 weeks. The focus of the training is on work teams rather than individual workers. The five components cover (a) relevance of team training, (b) team ownership of workplace policies, (c) understanding stress and coping, (d) understanding tolerance for coworker substance use and poor performance, and (e) supporting and encouraging coworkers to get help for substance use problems (for a detailed description of this program, see Bennett, Lehman, & Reynolds, 2000). In the first study (Bennett, Patterson, Reynolds, Wiitala, & Lehman, 2004), participants were recruited from safety-sensitive departments of a municipal employer. A total of 587 employees volunteered for the intervention study, which represented a 73% response rate. Intact work groups, not individual employees, were randomly assigned to one of three conditions: no-treatment control group (194 employees), Team Awareness intervention (201 employees), or an intervention called enhanced information training (192 employees). The second intervention provided information on workplace policies and the negative effects of various psychoactive substances. Of the 587 employees who completed a preintervention questionnaire, 346 employees completed a postintervention questionnaire (41% dropout rate) and 265 employees completed a 6-month follow-up questionnaire (55% dropout rate). The questionnaires assessed four dimensions of alcohol use during the preceding 6 months: experiencing any of seven alcohol-related problems (e.g., drinking in the morning), drinking more than 1 day per week, getting drunk at least 1 day per month, and experiencing a job-related hangover. The enhanced information intervention had no statistically significant effect on any of the four alcohol outcomes. Also, the Team Awareness intervention had no statistically significant effect on two of the four outcomes—drinking more than 1 day per week and getting drunk at least once per month. However, compared with the control group and the enhanced information intervention, the Team Awareness intervention was related to a statistically significant reduction in experiencing an alcohol-related problem and experiencing a job-related hangover. The Team Awareness intervention led to a reduction in the proportion of employees reporting an alcohol problem in the past 6 months, from 20% at preintervention to 11% at follow-up, and to a reduction in the proportion of employees reporting a job-related hangover in the past 6 months, from 16% at preintervention to 6% at follow-up. Although these changes appear to be practically important, information on the frequency of experiencing these outcomes would have been helpful to the interpretation of these findings. Also, information on changes in job performance would have been useful, given that the results summarized in Chapter 3 provide no evidence that alcohol hangovers affect cognitive performance, psychomotor performance, or performance in a variety of workplace simulations.

In the second evaluation of Team Awareness training (Patterson, Bennett, & Wiitala, 2005), 539 participants were recruited from small businesses (fewer than 500 employees) in industries identified as being high risk for alcohol or drug abuse. No information on response rates was provided. Businesses, not employees, were randomly assigned to one of three conditions: no-treatment control group (212 employees), a short (4-hour rather than 8-hour) version of the Team Awareness intervention described previously (202 employees), and a 4-hour intervention called Choices in Health Promotion (125 employees). This second intervention provided information on the benefits of decreasing substance use and on healthy alternatives to substance use (e.g., stress management, healthy eating, an active lifestyle) and covered time management and spiritual health. Participants completed a questionnaire pre- and postintervention. Of the 539 employees who completed a preintervention questionnaire, 394 employees completed a postintervention test questionnaire (27% dropout rate). The questionnaires assessed five dimensions of alcohol and drug use: use of alcohol to unwind, use of over-the-counter drugs to unwind, use of other drugs to unwind, problem alcohol use, and experience of any of seven alcohol-related problems during the preceding 6 months (e.g., alcohol use before or during work hours). Results indicated that there were no statistically significant intervention effects for any of the five substance use outcomes.

In the third study, Broome and Bennett (2011) evaluated a program called Team Resilience, which was a version of the Team Awareness program modified for young workers. The 235 young workers (ages 16 to 35) were recruited from 28 restaurant sites from a national casual dining chain. No information on response rates was provided. Restaurant sites, not employees, were randomly assigned to one of two conditions: no-treatment control group (110 employees) or Team Resilience training (125 employees). The Team Resilience intervention consisted of nine modules covered in three 2-hour sessions that took place on three consecutive days. The focus of the training was on work teams rather than individual workers. The nine modules covered a broad array of team and psychosocial skills building (for a detailed description of the program, see Bennett, Aden, Broome, Mitchell, & Rigdon, 2010). Participants completed a questionnaire at preintervention and at 6 months and 12 months postintervention. Of the 235 employees who completed a pretest questionnaire, 190 employees completed a 6-month questionnaire (19% dropout rate) and 147 employees completed a 12-month questionnaire (37% dropout rate). The questionnaires assessed binge drinking (any day when 5 or more drinks were consumed on the same occasion) during the past month, heavy drinking (5 or more days of heavy drinking) during the past month, and the number of four work-related alcohol problems experienced during the past 6 months (e.g., going to work with a hangover).

The effect of the Team Resilience intervention on each of the three alcohol outcomes was assessed in relation to (a) change from preintervention to 6-month follow-up and (b) change from 6-month follow-up to 12-month follow-up. No comparison was made between the preintervention and 12-month follow-up scores. Neither of the two comparisons showed an intervention effect for binge drinking. There was a statistically significant difference between the control and intervention groups for one of the two comparisons involving heavy drinking—change from preintervention to 6-month follow-up. However, looking at the proportion of heavy drinkers, this effect was due to an increase in heavy drinking in the control group (preintervention, 36% heavy drinkers; 6-month follow-up, 43% heavy drinkers) and no change in heavy drinking in the intervention group (preintervention, 35% heavy drinkers; 6-month follow-up, 34% heavy drinkers). The intervention also was statistically significantly related to one of the two comparisons for work-related alcohol problems—change from 6-month follow-up to 12-month follow-up. The average number of work-related problems experienced during the preceding 6 months decreased in the intervention group (6-month follow-up, 1.1 problems; 12-month follow-up, 0.6 problems) and remained the same in the control group (6-month follow-up, 0.8 problem; 12-month follow-up, 0.8 problem). Not only was this change small, the statistically significant decrease in the intervention group from 6-month to 12-month follow-up may have been the result of an initial slight increase in work-related alcohol problems in the intervention group (preintervention, 0.9 problem; 6-month follow-up, 1.1 problems). Had the intervention been tested in relation to a change in work-related alcohol problems from preintervention to the 12-month follow-up, it is possible that no intervention effect would have been found.

Finally, Matano et al. (2007) compared the effects of two web-based interventions. The limited individualized intervention provided general information on alcohol use and its effects and individualized feedback on participants' stress levels and coping strategies. The full individualized intervention provided individualized feedback on participants' use of alcohol, stress levels, and coping strategies. Participants had access to the appropriate CopingMatters website for 90 days. It was anticipated that the full individualized intervention would have a stronger effect than the limited individualized intervention on alcohol use. Of the 8,567 employees, 145 employees participated in one of the interventions and provided data preintervention and at 3-month follow-up, which represents a 1.7% total participation rate. Ten alcohol outcomes were assessed: drinking frequency in the past 3 months, usual number of beers, usual number of glasses of wine, usual number of shots of liquor, largest number of beers consumed, largest number of glasses of wine consumed, largest number of shots of liquor consumed, frequency of beer binges, frequency of wine binges, and frequency of liquor binges. Binge drinking was defined as having 4 or more drinks of a specific beverage on a single occasion for women and 5 or more drinks of a specific beverage on a single occasion for men.

The intervention effects were examined separately for the 31 employees classified as moderate-risk drinkers and the 114 employees classified as low-risk drinkers. Among the moderate-risk drinkers, the intervention was statistically significantly related to only one of the 10 alcohol outcomes. The frequency of beer binges in the fully individualized intervention group changed from 1.4 days in the past 3 months preintervention to 0.7 day in the past 3 months at the 3-month follow-up, whereas the change for the limited individualized intervention group was from 1.0 day to 1.1 days. Among the low-risk drinkers, the intervention was statistically significantly related to only two of the 10 alcohol outcomes. The frequency of beer binges in the fully individualized intervention group changed from 1.0 day in the past 3 months preintervention to 0.6 day in the past 3 months at the 3-month follow-up, whereas the change for the limited individualized intervention group was from 1.3 days to 1.2 days. The frequency of liquor binges in the fully individualized intervention group changed from 1.0 day in the past 3 months preintervention to 0.6 day in the past 3 months at the 3-month follow-up, whereas the change for the limited individualized intervention group was from 1.0 day to 0.8 day. Not only was the number of statistically significant effects small (three out of 20 comparisons), but the size of the effects in the fully individualized intervention group was small and of limited importance.

Screening and brief intervention. This category of intervention consists of three studies that provided an initial assessment (screening) of an employee's alcohol use, followed by some form of individualized feedback or brief counseling. Anderson and Larimer (2002) developed and tested a preventive brief intervention in the workplace with the goal of decreasing negative consequences associated with alcohol use and promoting moderate alcohol use. Participants were recruited from a food and retail services company with 1,396 employees. Of all 1,396 employees, 129 chose not to participate in the study and 62 were no longer with the company. Of the remaining 1,205 employees, 458 employees were randomly selected to participate in the study. From these 458 employees, 155 employees completed the preintervention questionnaires (a 34% response rate) and 120 employees completed the postintervention questionnaire (23% dropout rate). The participants were randomly assigned either to a no-treatment control condition or to the intervention condition. The intervention involved a single 30- to 60-minute meeting with one of two trained feedback providers who provided personal feedback on the initial reports of alcohol use, alcohol education, and alcohol-related skills training. Questionnaires were completed preintervention and 6 months later, during which time individuals in the intervention group received feedback and brief intervention. Four alcohol outcomes were assessed. Alcohol problems were assessed by asking about the frequency of experiencing any of 50 alcohol-related problems during the past 3 months. Answers to several alcohol questions were used to estimate peak blood alcohol count (BAC) on any single occasion during the past month and typical BAC during the past 3 months. Finally, average number of drinking days per week during the past month was assessed.

The intervention effect was first examined among the subgroup of employees who reported experiencing at least one alcohol problem. The results showed that the intervention was statistically significantly related to lower alcohol problem scores for women, but the intervention did not affect alcohol problem scores for men. Among the women in the intervention group, alcohol problem scores changed from 7.7 at baseline to 2.0 at follow-up, whereas the change for the control group was from 5.0 to 4.8. Despite the apparent large change in the intervention group, the scores were low compared with the possible maximum score of 150 and may not have been indicative of problem drinking even at preintervention. It is not clear if the problems actually experienced were mild or severe. The intervention effect on the other three alcohol outcomes in this subgroup of employees was not tested. The intervention effect was next examined among the subgroup of individuals who reported consuming at least one drink during the month prior to baseline assessment. The results showed that the intervention was statistically significantly related to fewer drinking days per week, but the intervention was not related to peak BAC or typical BAC. The intervention effect on alcohol problems was not tested in this subgroup. Regarding the number of drinking days per week, the intervention group showed a change from 2.4 days preintervention to 1.9 days at 6-month follow-up, whereas the change for the control group was from 2.2 days to 2.3 days. The change in the intervention group was very small, and the number of drinking days per week, even before the intervention, was within U.S., Canadian, and Australian safe drinking guidelines (Australian Institute of Health and Welfare, 2011; Butt et al., 2011; Dawson, 2000), especially given the low typical BACs reported.

Doumas and Hannah (2008) compared the effects of two web-based interventions with each other and with a no-treatment control group using a sample of young workers (ages 18–24). One intervention consisted of a brief web-based program that provided personalized normative feedback on the participants' alcohol use designed to reduce high-risk drinking. The second intervention consisted of the brief web-based program plus a 15-minute, in-person motivational interviewing session with a trained counselor. Participants were recruited from five companies with high numbers of young workers. Of the 423 eligible employees, 196 participated in the study (46% response rate). Participants were randomly assigned to one of the three conditions. Of the 196 participants, 124 provided data at baseline and the 3-month follow-up (37% dropout rate). Three measures of alcohol use during the past month were assessed: average number of drinks on weekends (Friday and Saturday), frequency of intoxication, and peak number of drinks on a single occasion. The results revealed that the effects of the two interventions did not differ, suggesting that there were no differences in effectiveness between the web-based only and web-based plus brief in-person interview interventions. Therefore, the main analyses compared the pooled intervention groups with the control group. For the analyses, participants were classified as low-risk drinkers (no binge drinking during the past month) or high-risk drinkers (any binge drinking during the past month). Among the 134 low-risk drinkers, no statistically significant intervention effect was observed for any of the three alcohol outcomes. In contrast, among the 65 high-risk drinkers, there was a statistically significant intervention effect for all three outcomes. The average number of drinks on weekends in the pooled intervention group changed from 5.1 drinks preintervention to 3.4 drinks at follow-up, whereas the change for the control group was from 2.7 drinks to 2.8 drinks. The frequency of intoxication score in the pooled intervention group changed from 4.0 at preintervention to 2.3 at follow-up, whereas the change for the control group was from 2.9 to 2.6. The peak number of drinks consumed on a given occasion in the pooled intervention group changed from 10.0 drinks at baseline to 7.1 drinks at follow-up, whereas the control group reported 9.2 drinks at both preintervention and follow-up.

Thus, the practical importance of these effects is mixed. The average number of drinks consumed on weekends (Fridays and Saturdays combined) is generally within safe drinking guidelines, although information on the number of drinks consumed for each of the weekend days for each gender would help interpretation. The change in the frequency of intoxication was likely to be practically important. However, it should be pointed out that the changes in the treatment group for these two outcomes occurred because this group had higher alcohol scores at baseline than those observed in the control group. Therefore, despite random assignment to conditions, the groups were not comparable at baseline, perhaps due to different dropout rates. Finally, although the peak number of drinks was high in the control group at both assessments and in the intervention group at preintervention, the peak number of drinks at follow-up in the intervention group (7.1 drinks) was still indicative of occasional risky drinking. Thus, the intervention did not reduce peak consumption to nonrisky levels.

Hermansson, Helander, Brandt, Huss, and Ronnberg (2010) compared the effects of two interventions with each other and with that of a no-treatment control group among employees of a large Swedish organization in the transportation sector. The brief intervention provided a 15-minute session with individualized feedback on employees' alcohol use, as well as written advice on how to avoid hazardous alcohol use and minimize the risk of developing alcohol dependence. The comprehensive intervention involved three sessions. The first session was the same as that provided in the brief intervention. The second session consisted of a systematic recall of alcohol use during the preceding 2 weeks. In the third session, participants were offered the opportunity to keep a daily drinking diary for 4 weeks. Of all eligible employees, 990 volunteered for the initial alcohol screen (15% of all 6,500 employees). However, not all of employees were offered screening, and no response rate was reported. Nonetheless, the study participants represent a small proportion of all employees in this organization. Of the 990 employees who volunteered for alcohol screening, 194 employees tested positive for risky drinking based on a self-reported screening test (AUDIT; $n = 85$), an alcohol biomarker based on a blood test (carbohydrate-deficient transferrin, CDT; $n = 92$), or both ($n = 17$). These 194 employees were randomly assigned to one of the two intervention groups or the control group, and 158 of them provided data at the 12-month follow-up (19% dropout rate). The two alcohol outcomes represented scoring positive on the AUDIT or the CDT screening test. The results indicated that there was no statistically significant effect of either intervention on the two alcohol outcomes.

Discussion

Two reviews of the effect of WWPs on employee substance involvement suggested that any effects were small and that their credibility was undermined by a variety of methodological problems. Two types of additional WPP interventions were reviewed. Eleven studies were categorized as implementing educational and/or psychosocial skills training, and three studies were classified as implementing screening and brief intervention aimed at reducing employee substance use. Across these 14 studies, the number of statistically significant effects was small relative to the number of comparisons tested, and in almost all cases, the size of the statistically significant effects were small and of little practical importance. The statistically significant changes in substance use occurred among groups that were, on average, not using alcohol or illicit drugs at risky levels even at the preintervention period. Another goal of preventing risky substance use through WWPs is to have a positive impact on employee productivity; yet, only one study assessed employee productivity, and it failed to find a statistically significant effect for the intervention. Finally, this set of 14 studies suffered from all of the methodological problems identified in the two literature reviews described previously.

Dusenbury (1999) stated that WWPs aimed at employee substance use are in their infancy and that it is premature to say that the field has identified the elements of program effectiveness. The research reviewed above strongly supports this sentiment. Yet, the lack of support for many workplace wellness interventions summarized above may not be surprising. One set of studies employed educational and/or psychosocial skill development. Prior reviews of research on substance abuse education in other contexts, such as mass media and schools, suggest that such efforts are ineffective (e.g., Faupel et al., 2004; Maisto et al., 2008). Maisto et al. (2008) pointed out that "increased knowledge about alcohol and other drugs does not necessarily translate into modification in their use" (p. 413). The present results support this contention. General research on resistance skills training may show a little more promise than educational interventions (Maisto et al., 2008). However, workplace research to date fails to support such interventions, which include the stress management training used in several of the intervention studies. As noted in Chapter 2, work stressors and other stressors outside work (e.g., Cooper et al., 1992) are not likely to be a consistent cause of substance involvement for most individuals. Instead, work and life stressors may be a cause of substance involvement for certain, as yet not well-defined, vulnerable subgroups of employees. If this is true, stress-resistance training applied to general samples of employees will not likely show strong effects, if any effects at all.

The final group of studies used a combination of alcohol screening and some form of brief intervention. This group of studies showed a little more evidence for statistically significant intervention effects, although the size of the effects was small and of limited practical importance. But this is consistent with other research on brief interventions. Prior meta-analytic reviews of brief intervention research in other settings (e.g., primary care) among individuals who were not seeking help for substance use support statistically significant reductions in alcohol and illicit drug use (e.g., Bertholet, Daeppen, Wietlisbach, Fleming, & Burnand, 2005; Kaner et al., 2009; Lundahl & Burke, 2009; Moyer, Finney, Swearingen, & Vergun, 2002). Nonetheless, the reviews have generally found that the size of brief intervention effects tends to be small. For example, two meta-analyses showed that brief interventions reduced alcohol intake, on average, by roughly 38 grams per week (Bertholet et al., 2005; Kaner et al., 2009). To better gauge the size of this effect, it is helpful to convert the results into standard drinks, which are used to define safe drinking guidelines. However, variability exists across countries in the number of grams of alcohol used to define a standard drink. The International Center for Alcohol Policies (1998) reported that across 18 countries, the number of grams in a standard drink ranged from 6 in Austria to 19.75 in Japan, with most in the 10-gram to 14-gram range. In North America (United States and Canada), a standard drink contains roughly 14 grams of alcohol, and taking the mean across the 18 countries leads to 11.5 grams per standard drink. Thus, a reduction of 38 grams of alcohol per week is about 2.7 drinks per week based on North American standards and 3.3 drinks per week based on the average across countries.

FUTURE RESEARCH

To the extent that EAPs and WWPs have not been successful in reducing problem alcohol or drug use among employees, researchers need to reconsider the theoretical underpinning of their interventions. Equally important, the methodological problems highlighted above have persisted for several decades and should be addressed. A number of researchers have discussed the measurement, analytic, and program and study design issues that must be considered when evaluating any intervention program, including EAPs and WWPs (e.g., Bennett & Beaudin, 2000; Bray, Schlenger, Zarkin, & Galvin, 2008; Colantonio, 1989; Csiernik, 1995; French, Zarkin, & Bray, 1995; Kurtz et al., 1984; Lahtinen, Koskinen-Ollonqvist, Rouvinen-Wilenius, Tuominen, & Mittelmark, 2005; Leukefeld & Bukowski, 1991; Macdonald, Lothian, &

Wells, 1997; Nielsen, Randall, Holten, & Gonzalez, 2010; Ozminkowski & Goetzel, 2001). Although no single study can address every methodological problem, a growing body of better designed studies may provide more credible support for such programs, as well as important information on program and intervention design to best address specific problems and specific populations of workers.

EAP and WWP researchers also need to assess on-the-job substance impairment and productivity outcomes. Changes in heavy off-the-job substance may reduce absenteeism and tardiness to some extent. However, as pointed out in Chapters 3 and 4, only workplace interventions that have an impact on substance impairment at work are likely to reduce most substance-related productivity problems. Workplace interventionists also need to move beyond reporting whether or not comparisons across experimental and control groups are statistically significant. Attention should be devoted to determining whether or not such differences have any practical or clinical importance. As discussed above, many, if not most, statistically significant effects were small and of limited utility for employers who might use such programs to reduce problem substance involvement and improve resulting productivity problems.

GENERAL SUMMARY AND CONCLUSIONS

EAPs and WWPs focus on a wide range of potential employee problems and have expanded worldwide. The overall prevalence of organizations offering and employees having access to both types of programs is high. Nonetheless, the prevalence of providing and having access to these programs increases with the size of the organization. Because of the broad focus of EAPs, a small proportion (5% to 8%) of contacts and cases involve alcohol or illicit drug use, and no information exists on the extent to which available WWPs specifically target employee substance involvement. Although EAPs and WWPs have potential for reducing or preventing problematic substance use in the workforce and workplace and subsequently increasing employee performance and reducing employer costs, past research does not provide a strong evidence base supporting the effectiveness of current EAPs and WWPs in reducing employee substance involvement. The use of EAPs and WWPs to address employee substance involvement issues will require much more development before these programs will be of general use to employers.

7

GENERAL IMPLICATIONS FOR WORKPLACE POLICY AND ISSUES FOR FUTURE RESEARCH

The research reviewed in this book provides detailed information on what is and is not known about the prevalence, causes, and productivity outcomes of employee substance involvement; the use and effectiveness of drug testing and workplace health promotion programs in reducing employee substance involvement and increasing subsequent productivity; and the putative costs to employers of lost productivity due to employee substance involvement. In this final chapter, I first briefly discuss the general implications of the reviewed research for workplace substance use policy. I then discuss several often recurring findings that have general implications for future research.

IMPLICATIONS FOR WORKPLACE SUBSTANCE USE POLICY

The U.S. Department of Labor (1990) outlined five components that make up a comprehensive workplace substance use program. The first component is a written substance use policy. The actual policy statement must be

DOI: 10.1037/13944-008
Alcohol and Illicit Drug Use in the Workforce and Workplace, by M. R. Frone

customized for each organization because its focus can be affected by the types of occupations found in an organization (e.g., safety and security sensitive vs. nonsensitive), relevant federal and state laws, and whether specific collective bargaining agreements must be considered.[1] With regard to the timing of employee substance use, research summarized in Chapters 3 and 4 suggests that a policy statement should focus primarily on substance use and impairment on the job, because workplace impairment is more likely than use off the job to affect most productivity outcomes (job performance, dysfunctional behaviors at work, and workplace accidents and injuries). Also, despite federal initiatives, research in Chapters 1, 3, and 4 suggests that alcohol should be given greater attention in workplace policies than illicit drug use. Heavy drinking, alcohol abuse, and alcohol dependence are more prevalent and occur more frequently than illicit drug use. Also, although the relation between employee substance use and employee productivity is not as clear cut as typically assumed, misuse of alcohol is more likely than the use of illicit drugs to present a problem.

The second component of a workplace substance use program is supervisor training. This training should include information on specific drugs, the employer's written substance use policy, and potential workplace performance and behavioral problems associated with substance use and impairment at work and frequent impairment outside of work. Nonetheless, the key role of supervisors should be to observe, document, and address specific performance problems and proscribed workplace behaviors. Supervisors should not attempt to diagnose or treat perceived substance use problems. The inability of supervisors to successfully differentiate performance and behavioral problems due to potential substance involvement versus other potential causes at work and outside work is demonstrated in Chapter 5. Of all probable-cause substance use tests, approximately 73% to 90% are negative. This means that most individuals suspected of being under the influence of a substance at work have not used an illegal drug during the past 1 to 30 days and are not under the influence of alcohol at work. The variation in the proportion of tests that are negative is due to the substance use test (breath tests for alcohol vs. urine tests for illicit drugs) and workforce (general vs. safety sensitive) under consideration.

The third component of a workplace substance use program is employee education. Employees should be provided the same type of information mentioned for supervisors. They need to be aware of all workplace policies

---

[1]The U.S. Department of Labor has an online drug-free workplace advisor that summarizes the five components of a workplace substance use policy and will help develop a customized written substance use policy statement that addresses each of 13 key issues (http://www.dol.gov/elaws/asp/drugfree/drugs/screen1.asp). However, a written policy statement and some other elements of a workplace substance use program, such as a drug testing program, should be reviewed by a labor attorney to avoid potential legal problems (e.g., DelPo & Guerin, 2011).

and how these policies might affect them. The provision of information about psychoactive substances and their potential effects can be done inexpensively. However, research in Chapter 6 fails to demonstrate that increasing employees' knowledge about alcohol and illicit drugs will translate into modification of employees' use of these substances.

The fourth component of a workplace substance use program is providing employee assistance through employee assistance programs (EAPs) or workplace wellness programs (WWPs), which are discussed in detail in Chapter 6. Although originally developed to assist alcohol-dependent employees, EAPs have evolved into broad programs that address any potential life problem. However, because of the breadth of these programs, only a small proportion of those accessing EAPs (fewer than 10%) directly seek help for alcohol or drug use problems. Moreover, little sound research has examined and demonstrated the effectiveness of modern EAPs in reducing employee substance use problems or substance-related performance problems. WWPs are programs that address a broad spectrum of health and lifestyle issues in an effort to improve employee health (physical, mental, and behavioral) and improve performance. However, little information exists on the extent to which WWPs address alcohol and illicit drug use issues compared with other health-related issues (e.g., smoking cessation, obesity, diabetes, depression). As with EAPs, little research has examined and demonstrated the effectiveness of WWPs in reducing employee substance use problems or substance-related performance problems. Nonetheless, research continues to focus on the development of more effective workplace substance use interventions. Employers interested in such interventions need to keep abreast of future developments and to critically evaluate claims regarding their effectiveness.

The last component of a workplace substance use program is drug testing, which is discussed in detail in Chapter 5. Although all federal agencies and many private-sector employers are required by federal regulations to develop a testing program for illicit drug use and sometimes for workplace alcohol use, most private-sector employers are not required to test their workforce. Among those employers who are not required to do so, the development of a drug testing program should be given serious consideration. It is a contentious issue, and the development of a fair (to minimize false positive results) and legally defensible program is a complex issue that should occur within the context of the first four components. Employers should fully understand an important distinction between illicit drug use testing and alcohol use testing. Whereas alcohol testing can identify on-the-job alcohol use and impairment, illicit drug use testing cannot identify on-the-job use or impairment. In general, illicit drug use testing of the workforce can detect use of a specific drug in the recent or distant past, but it cannot determine level of impairment or where and when any impairment might have occurred.

The primary reasons for workforce substance use testing are (a) to deter any illicit drug use and on-the-job alcohol impairment and (b) to improve productivity (e.g., improve attendance and performance and reduce injuries). However, the research summarized in Chapter 5 fails to support the effectiveness of workforce substance use testing for these reasons. Employers should, therefore, closely examine their motives for testing. If workforce substance use testing is desired, the circumstances under which testing might occur and the outcomes of a positive test should be considered and conveyed to employees. The Canadian Human Rights Commission's (2009) recommendations concerning the circumstances under which testing for alcohol and illicit drug use is allowable or not allowable provide a policy that is most consistent with past research findings on this issue. These recommendations are provided in Chapter 5.

ISSUES FOR FUTURE RESEARCH

Lack of Important Distinctions

Two important distinctions often are overlooked when studying and discussing employee substance involvement. Those interested in this issue need to differentiate between (a) workforce (off-the-job) and workplace (on-the-job) substance involvement and (b) general patterns of substance use and acute impairment. These distinctions were shown to be important when estimating the prevalence and when studying the putative causes and outcomes of employee substance involvement. Although not considered to date, these differences also may be relevant when evaluating the effectiveness of EAPs and workplace health promotion programs (WHPs). Failure to consider these distinctions impairs our ability to develop a sound understanding of employee substance involvement.

Illicit Drugs Versus Alcohol

The media, organizations, and policymakers have paid undue attention to the use of and testing for illicit drugs, given that past research suggests employee alcohol involvement may be a more salient concern for employers. Heavy use, impairment, abuse, and dependence are more prevalent for alcohol than for illicit drugs. Also, if substance involvement causally affects employee productivity, at least in certain subgroups of employees, alcohol is likely to be more important than illicit drugs. These observations further suggest that more resources should be devoted to providing, developing, and evaluating workplace interventions for alcohol than for illicit drugs.

Lack of Research Addressing Causality

Over the past 20 to 30 years, a fair amount has been learned about the correlates of workforce substance involvement, although less progress has been made concerning workplace substance involvement. These correlates include person characteristics, workplace environmental characteristics, various types of employee productivity, and drug testing and WHP programs. However, we do not have a good understanding of which variables cause employee substance involvement, which productivity outcomes are caused by employee substance involvement, and the types of workplace interventions that cause a reduction in employee substance involvement and subsequent increase in productivity. There are three reasons for this lack of knowledge regarding causal processes.

First, as shown for the putative causes and productivity outcomes of employee substance involvement (see Figures 2.1 and 4.1), the underlying causal processes are likely to be much more complex than assumed in prior research. More sophisticated research is needed to understand how multiple person and environmental characteristics combine to cause workforce/off-the-job and workplace/on-the-job substance involvement. Also, more advanced research is needed to explore the causal processes linking substance involvement to employee productivity. Prior research suggests that overall patterns of alcohol and illicit drug use are not likely to cause productivity problems. Instead, poor productivity may be an outcome of the joint effects of acute impairment (intoxication and withdrawal), the context of substance impairment (off-the-job vs. on-the-job), and the type of productivity outcome. Moreover, these relations may be affected by a number of other variables, such as tolerance to the effects of a substance and the work environment.

Second, the research designs used in the majority of past research studies did not allow for the estimation of causal effects. Instead, this research provided information on associations between employee substance involvement and other variables. Foster (2010) pointed out that causal inference is of central importance to science but that much observational research involves implausible causal inference. When possible, such as when evaluating the effect of workplace interventions on employee substance involvement and productivity, the use of experimental designs with participants randomly assigned to experimental conditions provides the strongest evidence of causal effects. However, the study of many relations involving employee substance involvement is possible only with observational field research. Although drawing sound causal inference from observational research in real-world settings is not easy, there are ways to strengthen researchers' ability to infer causation (e.g., Antonakis, Bendahan, Jacquart, & Lalive, 2010; Foster, 2010). Properly designed observational studies that provide the strongest inference regarding causality are costly in terms of time, effort, and money, but there may be more important costs to poorly designed research. As noted by Foster (2010), "Bad causal inference can indeed do real harm" (p. 1456). One type of harm is social and occurs when a noncausal association is incorrectly interpreted as causal, leading to individuals being inappropriately sanctioned and/or stigmatized. Another type of harm is economic and occurs when financial resources are devoted to developing and implementing workplace policies and interventions that are based on noncausal rather than causal relations between a presumed cause and outcome. Such interventions and policies may not have the intended outcome of reducing substance involvement in the workforce and workplace or improving employee productivity.

Third, many studies are based on simplistic models and have inadequate designs because they are unfunded or underfunded and run into resistance from work organizations. Thus, financial support through governments, private foundations, and employers is essential. High-quality research is costly. Also important to this endeavor is partnering between work organizations and researchers. Employers are often reluctant to participate in research, especially when it involves the study of undesirable behaviors, because of concerns about monetary costs, potential workplace disruption, and public impressions if negative results are associated with their organization. However, research can be designed to minimize costs and workplace disruptions to some extent, and the reporting of findings in scientific publications can be done in such a way that the identities of participating employees and organizations are not made public. If employers are truly interested in the causes and outcomes of employee substance involvement, effective workplace interventions and policies, and potential costs to their organizations, they will have to partner with researchers and accept some of the cost and inconvenience that come with conducting high-quality research.

REFERENCES

Adams, I. B., & Martin, B. (1996). Cannabis: Pharmacology and toxicology in animals and humans. *Addiction, 91,* 1585–1614. doi:10.1111/j.1360-0443.1996. tb02264.x

Agrawal, A., Balasubramanian, S., Smith, E. K., Madden, P. A. F., Bucholz, K., Heath, A. C., & Lynskey, M. T. (2010). Peer substance involvement modifies genetic influence on regular substance involvement in young women. *Addiction, 105,* 1844–1853. doi:10.1111/j.1360-0443.2010.02993.x

Agrawal, A., & Lynskey, M. T. (2006). The genetic epidemiology of cannabis use, abuse, and dependence. *Addiction, 101,* 801–812. doi:10.1111/j.1360-0443.2006.01399.x

Agrawal, A., & Lynskey, M. T. (2008). Are there genetic influences on addiction: Evidence from family, adoption, and twin studies. *Addiction, 103,* 1069–1081. doi:10.1111/j.1360-0443.2008.02213.x

Agrawal, A., Lynskey, M. T., Bucholz, K. K., Martin, N. G., Madden, P. A. F., & Heath, A. C. (2007). Contrasting models of genetic co-morbidity for cannabis and other illicit drugs in adult Australian twins. *Psychological Medicine, 37,* 49–60. doi:10.1017/S0033291706009287

Akobundu, E., Ju, J., Blatt, L., & Mullins, C. D. (2006). Cost-of-illness studies: A review of current methods. *PharmacoEconomics, 24,* 869–890. doi:10.2165/ 00019053-200624090-00005

Alaska Oil Spill Commission. (1990). *Spill: The wreck of the* Exxon Valdez. Anchorage, AK: Oil Spill Public Information Center.

Alberta Alcohol and Drug Abuse Commission. (2003). *Substance use and gambling in the Alberta workplace, 2002: A replication study: technical report.* Edmonton, Alberta, Canada: Author.

American Management Association. (1996). *1996 AMA survey: Workplace drug testing and drug abuse policies.* New York, NY: Author.

American Management Association. (2004). *AMA 2004 workplace testing survey: Medical testing.* New York, NY: Author.

American Psychiatric Association. (2000). *Diagnostic and statistical manual of mental disorders* (4th ed., text revision). Washington, DC: Author.

Ames, G. M. (1989). Alcohol-related movements and their effects on drinking policies in the American workplace: An historical review. *Journal of Drug Issues, 19,* 489–510.

Ames, G. M. (1993). Research and strategies for the primary prevention of workplace alcohol problems. *Alcohol Health & Research World, 17,* 19–27.

Ames, G. M., & Grube, J. W. (1999). Alcohol availability and workplace drinking: Mixed method analyses. *Journal of Studies on Alcohol, 60,* 383–393.

Ames, G. M., Grube, J. W., & Moore, R. S. (1997). The relationship of drinking and hangovers to workplace problems: An empirical study. *Journal of Studies on Alcohol, 58,* 37–47.

Ames, G. M., Grube, J. W., & Moore, R. S. (2000). Social control and workplace drinking norms: A comparison of two organizational cultures. *Journal of Studies on Alcohol, 61*, 203–219.

Ames, G. M., & Janes, C. R. (1992). A cultural approach to conceptualizing alcohol and the workplace. *Alcohol Health & Research World, 16*, 112–119.

Anderson, B. K., & Larimer, M. E. (2002). Problem drinking and the workplace: An individualized approach to prevention. *Psychology of Addictive Behaviors, 16*, 243–251. doi:10.1037/0893-164X.16.3.243

Anglin, M. D., Caulkins, J. P., & Hser, Y.-I. (1993). Prevalence estimation, policy needs, current status, and future potential. *Journal of Drug Issues, 23*, 345–360.

Anthony, J. C., & Arria, A. M. (1999). Epidemiology of substance abuse in adulthood. In P. J. Ott, R. E. Tarter, & R. T. Ammerman (Eds.), *Sourcebook on substance abuse: Etiology, epidemiology, assessment, and treatment* (pp. 32–49). Boston, MA: Allyn & Bacon.

Anthony, J. C., Eaton, W. W., Mandell, W., & Garrison, R. (1992). Psychoactive drug dependence and abuse: More common in some occupations than in others? *Journal of Employee Assistance Research, 1*, 148–186.

Antonakis, J., Bendahan, S., Jacquart, P., & Lalive, R. (2010). On making causal claims: A review and recommendations. *Leadership Quarterly, 21*, 1086–1120. doi:10.1016/j.leaqua.2010.10.010

Arthur, A. R. (2000). Employee assistance programmes: The emperor's new clothes of stress management? *British Journal of Guidance & Counselling, 28*, 549–559. doi:10.1080/03069880020004749

Attridge, M., Amaral, T., Bjornson, T., Goplerud, E., Herlihy, P., McPherson, T., . . . Teems, L. (2009). History and growth of the EAP field. *EASNA Research Notes, 1*(1), 1–4.

Australian Institute of Health and Welfare. (2011). *Measuring alcohol risk in the 2010 National Drug Strategy Household Survey: Implementation of the 2009 alcohol guidelines* (Drug Statistics Series No. 26). Canberra, Australia: Author.

Axelsson, R. (1998). Towards an evidence based health care management. *International Journal of Health Planning and Management, 13*, 307–317. doi:10.1002/(SICI)1099-1751(199810/12)13:4<307::AID-HPM525>3.0.CO;2-V

Bacharach, S. B., Bamberger, P., & Biron, M. (2010). Alcohol consumption and workplace absenteeism: The moderating effect of social support. *Journal of Applied Psychology, 95*, 334–348. doi:10.1037/a0018018

Bacharach, S. B., Bamberger, P., & McKinney, V. M. (2007). Harassing under the influence: The prevalence of male heavy drinking, the embeddedness of permissive drinking norms, and the gender harassment of female coworkers. *Journal of Occupational Health Psychology, 12*, 232–250. doi:10.1037/1076-8998.12.3.232

Bacharach, S. B., Bamberger, P. A., & Sonnenstuhl, W. J. (1996). MAPs: Labor-based peer assistance in the workplace. *Industrial Relations, 35*, 261–275. doi:10.1111/j.1468-232X.1996.tb00406.x

Bacharach, S. B., Bamberger, P. A., & Sonnenstuhl, W. J. (2002). Driven to drink: Managerial control, work-related risk factors, and employee problem drinking. *Academy of Management Journal, 45*, 637–658. doi:10.2307/3069302

Baker, C. (2004). *Behavioral genetics: An introduction to how genes and environments interact through development to shape differences in mood, personality, and intelligence.* Washington, DC: American Association for the Advancement of Science.

Baldwin, W. (2000). Information no one else knows: The value of self-report. In A. A. Stone, J. S. Turkkan, C. A. Bachrach, J. B. Jobe, H. S. Kurtzman, & V. S. Cain (Eds.), *The science of self-report: Implications for research and practice* (pp. 3–7). Mahwah, NJ: Erlbaum.

Balster, R. L. (1998). Neural basis of inhalant abuse. *Drug and Alcohol Dependence, 51,* 207–214. doi:10.1016/S0376-8716(98)00078-7

Bamberger, P., & Bacharach, S. B. (2006). Abusive management and subordinate problem drinking: Taking resistance, stress, and subordinate personality into account. *Human Relations, 59,* 723–752. doi:10.1177/0018726706066852

Bamberger, P., & Biron, M. (2006). The prevalence and distribution of employee substance-related problems and programs in the Israeli workplace. *Journal of Drug Issues, 36,* 755–786. doi:10.1177/002204260603600401

Bandura, A. (1977). *Social learning theory.* Englewood Cliffs, NJ: Prentice-Hall.

Barbee, J. G. (1993). Memory, benzodiazepines, and anxiety: Integration of theoretical and clinical perspectives. *Journal of Clinical Psychiatry, 54*(Suppl. 10), 86–97.

Barker, M. J., Greenwood, K. M., Jackson, M., & Crowe, S. F. (2004). Cognitive effects of long-term benzodiazepine use. *CNS Drugs, 18,* 37–48. doi:10.2165/00023210-200418010-00004

Barling, J., & Frone, M. R. (Eds.). (2004). *The psychology of workplace safety.* Washington, DC: American Psychological Association. doi:10.1037/10662-007

Barling, J., Kelloway, E. K., & Frone, M. R. (Eds.). (2005). *Handbook of work stress.* Thousand Oaks, CA: Sage.

Bass, A. R., Bharucha-Reid, R., Delaplane-Harris, K., Schork, M. A., Kaufmann, R., McCann, D., . . . Cook, S. (1996). Employee drug use, demographic characteristics, work reactions, and absenteeism. *Journal of Occupational Health Psychology, 1,* 92–99. doi:10.1037/1076-8998.1.1.92

Baumberg, B. (2006). The global economic burden of alcohol: A review and some suggestions. *Drug and Alcohol Review, 25,* 537–551. doi:10.1080/09595230600944479

Baylor, M. R., Sutheimer, C. A., & Crumpton, S. D. (2007). Regulatory concerns for point of collection testing in the workplace. In S. B. Karch (Ed.), *Drug abuse handbook* (pp. 917–926). New York, NY: CRC Press.

Bazargan-Hejazi, S., Gaines, T., Duan, N., & Cherpitel, C. J. (2007). Correlates of injury among ED visits: Effects of alcohol, risk perception, impulsivity, and sensation seeking behaviors. *American Journal of Drug and Alcohol Abuse, 33,* 101–108. doi:10.1080/00952990601087455

Beach, J., Ford, G., & Cherry, N. (2006). *A literature review of the role of alcohol and drugs in contributing to work-related injury.* Edmonton, Alberta, Canada: University of Alberta.

Becker, W. C., Sullivan, L. E., Tetrault, J. M., Desai, R. A., & Fiellin, D. A. (2008). Non-medical use, abuse, and dependence on prescription opioids among

U.S. adults: Psychiatric, medical, and substance use correlates. *Drug and Alcohol Dependence, 94*, 38–47. doi:10.1016/j.drugalcdep.2007.09.018

Belsky, J., & Pluess, M. (2009). Beyond diathesis stress: Differential susceptibility to environmental influences. *Psychological Bulletin, 135*, 885–908. doi:10.1037/a0017376

Bennett, J. B., Aden, C. A., Broome, K., Mitchell, K., & Rigdon, W. D. (2010). Team resilience for young restaurant workers: Research-to-practice adaptation and assessment. *Journal of Occupational Health Psychology, 15*, 223–236. doi:10.1037/a0019379

Bennett, J. B., & Beaudin, C. L. (2000). Collaboration for preventing substance abuse in the workplace: Modeling research partnerships in prevention. *Journal for Healthcare Quality, 22*, 24–30. doi:10.1111/j.1945-1474.2000.tb00136.x

Bennett, J. B., & Lehman, W. E. K. (1998). Workplace drinking climate, stress, and problem indicators: Assessing the influence of teamwork (group cohesion). *Journal of Studies on Alcohol, 59*, 608–618.

Bennett, J. B., Lehman, W. E. K., & Reynolds, G. S. (2000). Team awareness for workplace substance prevention: The empirical and conceptual development of a training program. *Prevention Science, 1*, 157–172. doi:10.1023/A:1010025306547

Bennett, J. B., Patterson, C. R., Reynolds, S., Wiitala, W. L., & Lehman, W. E. K. (2004). Team awareness, problem drinking, and drinking climate: Workplace social health promotion in a policy context. *American Journal of Health Promotion, 19*, 103–113. doi:10.4278/0890-1171-19.2.103

Bennett, J. B., Reynolds, G. S., & Lehman, W. E. K. (2003). Understanding employee alcohol and other drug use: Toward a multilevel approach. In J. B. Bennett & W. E. K. Lehman (Eds.), *Preventing workplace substance abuse: Beyond drug testing to wellness* (pp. 29–56). Washington, DC: American Psychological Association. doi:10.1037/10476-001

Berry, J. G., Pidd, K., Roche, A. M., & Harrison, J. E. (2007). Prevalence and patterns of alcohol use in the Australian workforce: Findings from the 2001 National Drug Strategy Household Survey. *Addiction, 102*, 1399–1410. doi:10.1111/j.1360-0443.2007.01893.x

Berry, L. L., Mirabito, A. M., & Baun, W. B. (2010). What's the hard return on employee wellness programs? *Harvard Business Review, 88*(12), 2–9.

Bertholet, N., Daeppen, J.-B., Wietlisbach, V., Fleming, M., & Burnand, B. (2005). Reduction of alcohol consumption by brief alcohol invention in primary care. *Archives of Internal Medicine, 165*, 986–995. doi:10.1001/archinte.165.9.986

Billings, D. W., Cook, R. F., Hendrickson, A., & Dove, D. C. (2008). A web-based approach to managing stress and mood disorders in the workforce. *Journal of Occupational and Environmental Medicine, 50*, 960–968. doi:10.1097/JOM.0b013e31816c435b

Blum, T. C., Fields, D. L., Milne, S. H., & Spell, C. S. (1992). Workplace drug testing programs: A review of research and a survey of worksites. *Journal of Employee Assistance Research, 1*, 315–349.

Blum, T. C., & Roman, P. M. (1995). *Cost-effectiveness and preventive implications of employee assistance programs* (DHHS Publication No. SMA 95-3053). Rockville, MD: Substance Abuse and Mental Health Services Administration.

Blum, T. C., Roman, P. M., & Martin, J. K. (1993). Alcohol consumption and work performance. *Journal of Studies on Alcohol, 54,* 61–70.

Boles, M., Pelletier, B., & Lynch, W. (2004). The relationship between health risks and work productivity. *Journal of Occupational and Environmental Medicine, 46,* 737–745. doi:10.1097/01.jom.0000131830.45744.97

Borg, M. J., & Arnold, W. P., III. (1997). Social monitoring as social control: The case of drug testing in a medical workplace. *Sociological Forum, 12,* 441–460. doi:10.1023/A:1024629311818

Borges, G., Cherpitel, C., & Mittleman, M. (2004). Risk of injury after alcohol consumption: A case-crossover study in the emergency department. *Social Science & Medicine, 58,* 1191–1200. doi:10.1016/S0277-9536(03)00290-9

Bosker, W. M., & Huestis, M. A. (2009). Oral fluid testing for drugs of abuse. *Clinical Chemistry, 55,* 1910–1931. doi:10.1373/clinchem.2008.108670

Bouchard, T. J., Jr. (2004). Genetic influence on human psychological traits. *Current Directions in Psychological Science, 13,* 148–151. doi:10.1111/j.0963-7214.2004.00295.x

Bouchery, E. E., Harwood, H. J., Sacks, J. J., Simon, C. J., & Brewer, R. D. (2011). Economic costs of excessive alcohol consumption in the U.S., 2006. *American Journal of Preventive Medicine, 41,* 516–524. doi:10.1016/j.amepre.2011.06.045

Brännström, G., & Hopstadius, B. (1994). A comparative study between the ILO's guiding principles and drug testing at workplaces in Stockholm, Sweden. *Journal of Workplace Learning, 6,* 4–6. doi:10.1108/13665629410795826

Bray, J. W., Schlenger, W. E., Zarkin, G. A., & Galvin, D. (2008). *Analyzing data from nonrandomized group studies.* Triangle Park, NC: RTI Press. doi:10.3768/rtipress.2008.mr.0008.0811

Bromet, E. J., Dew, M. A., & Parkinson, D. K. (1990). Spillover between work and family: A study of blue-collar working women. In J. Eckenrode & S. Gore (Eds.), *Stress between work and family* (pp. 133–151). New York, NY: Plenum Press.

Broome, K. M., & Bennett, J. B. (2011). Reducing heavy alcohol consumption in young restaurant workers. *Journal of Studies on Alcohol and Drugs, 72,* 117–124.

Brownson, R. C., Chriqui, J. F., & Stamatakis, K. A. (2009). Understanding evidence-based public health policy. *American Journal of Public Health, 99,* 1576–1583. doi:10.2105/AJPH.2008.156224

Brunet, J. R. (2002). Employee drug testing as social control: A typology of normative justification. *Review of Public Personnel Administration, 22,* 193–215. doi:10.1177/0734371X0202200302

Buck Consultants. (2008). *Working well: A global survey of health promotion and workplace wellness strategies.* San Francisco, CA: Author.

Buck Consultants. (2010). *Working well: A global survey of health promotion and workplace wellness strategies.* San Francisco, CA: Author.

Buckland, P. R. (2001). Genetic association studies of alcoholism: Problems with the candidate gene approach. *Alcohol and Alcoholism, 36*, 99–103. doi:10.1093/alcalc/36.2.99

Buon, T., & Taylor, J. (2007). *A review of the employee assistance programme (EAP) market in the UK and Europe.* Aberdeen, Scotland: Robert Gordon University.

Bureau of Economic Analysis. (2000). National estimates: Selected NIPA tables. *Survey of Current Business Online, 79*(12). Retrieved from http://www.bea.gov/scb/toc/1200cont.htm

Bureau of Labor Statistics. (2012). *Union members—2011* [Press release]. Retrieved from http://www.bls.gov/news.release/pdf/union2.pdf

Burmeister, M., McInnis, M. G., & Zöllner, S. (2008). Psychiatric genetics: Progress amid controversy. *Nature Reviews Genetics, 9*, 527–540. doi:10.1038/nrg2381

Burton, W. N., Chen, C.-Y., Conti, D. J., Schultz, A. B., Pransky, G., & Edington, D. W. (2005). The association of health risks with on-the-job productivity. *Journal of Occupational and Environmental Medicine, 47*, 769–777.

Bush, D. M. (2008). The U.S. mandatory guidelines for federal workplace drug testing programs: Current status and future considerations. *Forensic Science International, 174*, 111–119. doi:10.1016/j.forsciint.2007.03.008

Butt, P., Beirness, D., Cesa, F., Gliksman, L., Paradis, C., & Stockwell, T. (2011). *Alcohol and health in Canada: A summary of evidence and guidelines for low-risk drinking.* Ottawa, Ontario, Canada: Canadian Centre on Substance Abuse.

Bywood, P., Pidd, K., & Roche, A. (2006). *Illicit drugs in the Australian workforce: Prevalence and patterns of use.* Canberra, Australia: National Centre for Education and Training on Addiction.

Caetano, R., Clark, C. L., & Greenfield, T. K. (1998). Prevalence, trends, and incidence of alcohol withdrawal symptoms: Analysis of general population and clinical samples. *Alcohol Health & Research World, 22*, 73–79.

Canadian Human Rights Commission. (2009). *Canadian Human Rights Commission's policy on alcohol and drug testing.* Ottawa, Ontario, Canada: Author.

Caplan, Y. H., & Huestis, M. A. (Eds.). (2007). Workplace testing. In S. B. Karch (Ed.), *Drug abuse handbook* (pp. 727–893). New York, NY: CRC Press.

Carey, G. (2003). *Human genetics for the social sciences.* Thousand Oaks, CA: Sage.

Carlson-Berne, E. (Ed.). (2007). *Cocaine.* New York, NY: Greenhaven Press.

Carpenter, C. S. (2007). Workplace drug testing and worker drug use. *Health Services Research, 42*, 795–810. doi:10.1111/j.1475-6773.2006.00632.x

Cascio, W., & Boudreau, J. (2008). *Investing in people: Financial impact of human resource initiatives.* Upper Saddle River, NJ: FT Press.

Cashman, C. M., Ruotsalainen, J. H., Greiner, B. A., Beirne, P. V., & Verbeek, J. H. (2009). Alcohol and drug screening of occupational drivers for preventing injury. *Cochrane Database of Systematic Reviews, 2009*(2). doi:10.1002/14651858.CD006566.pub2

Caulkins, J. P., Reuter, P., & Coulson, C. (2011). Basing drug scheduling decisions on scientific ranking of harmfulness: False promise from false premises. *Addiction, 106*, 1886–1890. doi:10.1111/j.1360-0443.2011.03461.x

Chait, L. D., & Perry, J. L. (1994). Acute and residual effects of alcohol and marijuana, alone and in combination, on mood and performance. *Psychopharmacology, 115*, 340–349. doi:10.1007/BF02245075

Chen, M.-J., & Cunradi, C. (2008). Job stress, burnout and substance use among urban transit operators: The potential mediating role of coping behavior. *Work & Stress, 22*, 327–340. doi:10.1080/02678370802573992

Cherpitel, C. J. (2007). Alcohol and injuries: A review of international emergency room studies since 1995. *Drug and Alcohol Review, 26*, 201–214. doi:10.1080/09595230601146686

Cherpitel, C. J., Giesbrecht, N., & Macdonald, S. (1999). Alcohol and injury: A comparison of emergency room populations in two Canadian provinces. *American Journal of Drug and Alcohol Abuse, 25*, 743–759. doi:10.1081/ADA-100101890

Christiansen, B. A., & Goldman, M. S. (1983). Alcohol related expectancies vs. demographic/background variables in the prediction of adolescent drinking. *Journal of Consulting and Clinical Psychology, 51*, 249–257. doi:10.1037/0022-006X.51.2.249

Cialdini, R. B., & Trost, M. R. (1998). Social influence: Social norms, conformity, and compliance. In D. T. Gilbert, S. T. Fiske, & G. Lindzey (Eds.), *The handbook of social psychology* (4th ed., Vol. 2, pp. 151–192). New York, NY: McGraw-Hill.

Coggans, N., Dalgarno, P., Johnson, L., & Shewan, D. (2004). Long-term heavy cannabis use: Implications for health education. *Drugs: Education, Prevention, and Policy, 11*, 299–313. doi:10.1080/09687630410001687860

Coghlan, M., & Macdonald, S. (2010). The role of substance use and psychosocial characteristics in explaining unintentional injuries. *Accident Analysis & Prevention, 42*, 476–479. doi:10.1016/j.aap.2009.09.010

Cohen, M. A. (1999). Alcohol, drugs and crime: Is "crime" really one-third of the problem? *Addiction, 94*, 644–647.

Colantonio, A. (1989). Assessing the effects of employee assistance programs: A review of employee assistance program evaluations. *Yale Journal of Biology and Medicine, 62*, 13–22.

Colder, C. R., & Chassin, L. (1997). Affectivity and impulsivity: Temperament risk for adolescent alcohol involvement. *Psychology of Addictive Behaviors, 11*, 83–97. doi:10.1037/0893-164X.11.2.83

Collins, D. J., & Lapsley, H. M. (2002). *Counting the cost: Estimates of the social costs of drug abuse in Australia in 1998–9*. Canberra, Australia: Commonwealth Department of Health and Ageing.

Conger, J. J. (1956). Reinforcement theory and the dynamics of alcoholism. *Quarterly Journal of Studies on Alcohol, 17*, 296–305.

Connors, G. J., & Maisto, S. A. (2003). Drinking reports from collateral individuals. *Addiction, 98*(Suppl. 2), 21–29. doi:10.1046/j.1359-6357.2003.00585.x

Controlled Substances Act, 21 U.S.C § 812 (1970).

Cook, R. F., Hersch, R. K., Back, A. S., & McPherson, T. L. (2004). The prevention of substance abuse among construction workers: A field test of a social-cognitive program. *Journal of Primary Prevention, 25,* 337–357. doi:10.1023/B:JOPP.0000048025.11036.32

Cooper, M. L., Frone, M. R., Russell, M., & Mudar, P. (1995). Drinking to regulate positive and negative emotions: A motivational model of alcohol use. *Journal of Personality and Social Psychology, 69,* 990–1005. doi:10.1037/0022-3514.69.5.990

Cooper, M. L., Russell, M., & Frone, M. R. (1990). Work stress and alcohol effects: A test of stress-induced drinking. *Journal of Health and Social Behavior, 31,* 260–276. doi:10.2307/2136891

Cooper, M. L., Russell, M., Skinner, J. B., Frone, M. R., & Mudar, P. (1992). Stress and alcohol use: The moderating effect of gender, coping and alcohol expectancies. *Journal of Abnormal Psychology, 101,* 139–152. doi:10.1037/0021-843X.101.1.139

Couper, F. J., & Logan, B. K. (2004). *Drugs and human performance fact sheets* (DOT HS 809 725). Washington, DC: U.S. Department of Transportation.

Cowan, D., Osselton, D., & Robinson, S. (2007). Drug testing. In D. Nutt, T. W. Robbins, G. V. Stimson, M. Ince, & A. Jackson (Eds.), *Drugs and the future: Brain science, addiction and society* (pp. 315–336). New York, NY: Academic Press.

Crouch, D. J. (2005). Oral fluid collection: The neglected variable in oral fluid testing. *Forensic Science International, 150,* 165–173. doi:10.1016/j.forsciint.2005.02.028

Crouch, D. J. (Ed.). (2007). Point of collection drug tests. In S. B. Karch (Ed.), *Drug abuse handbook* (pp. 895–959). New York, NY: CRC Press.

Crown, D. F., & Rosse, J. G. (1988). A critical review of the assumptions underlying drug testing. *Journal of Business and Psychology, 3,* 22–41. doi:10.1007/BF01016746

Cruickshank, C. C., & Dyer, K. R. (2009). A review of the clinical pharmacology of methamphetamine. *Addiction, 104,* 1085–1099. doi:10.1111/j.1360-0443.2009.02564.x

Crum, R. M., Muntaner, C., Eaton, W. W., & Anthony, J. C. (1995). Occupational stress and the risk of alcohol abuse and dependence. *Alcoholism: Clinical and Experimental Research, 19,* 647–655. doi:10.1111/j.1530-0277.1995.tb01562.x

Csiernik, R. (1995). A review of research methods used to examine employee assistance program delivery options. *Evaluation and Program Planning, 18,* 25–36. doi:10.1016/0149-7189(94)00043-W

Csiernik, R. (2005). A review of EAP evaluation in the 1990s. *Employee Assistance Quarterly, 19,* 21–37. doi:10.1300/J022v19n04_02

Cunradi, C. B., Greiner, B. A., Ragland, D. R., & Fisher, J. (2005). Alcohol, stress-related factors, and short-term absenteeism among urban transit operators. *Journal of Urban Health, 82,* 43–57. doi:10.1093/jurban/jti007

Dar-Nimrod, I., & Heine, S. J. (2011). Genetic essentialism: On the deceptive determinism of DNA. *Psychological Bulletin, 137,* 800–818. doi:10.1037/a0021860

Dawson, D. A. (1994). Heavy drinking and the risk of occupational injury. *Accident Analysis and Prevention, 26*, 655–665. doi:10.1016/0001-4575(94)90027-2

Dawson, D. A. (2000). U.S. low-risk drinking guidelines: An examination of four alternatives. *Alcoholism: Clinical and Experimental Research, 24*, 1820–1829. doi:10.1111/j.1530-0277.2000.tb01986.x

Deitz, D. K., Cook, R. F., & Hendrickson, A. (2011). Preventing prescription drug misuse: Field test of the SmartRx web program. *Substance Use & Misuse, 46*, 678–686. doi:10.3109/10826084.2010.528124

Deitz, D., Cook, R., & Hersch, R. K. (2005). Workplace health promotion and utilization of health services: Follow-up data findings. *Journal of Behavioral Health Services & Research, 32*, 306–319. doi:10.1007/BF02291830

Dell, T., & Berkout, J. (1998). Injuries at a metal foundry as a function of job classification, length of employment, and drug screening. *Journal of Safety Research, 29*, 9–14. doi:10.1016/S0022-4375(97)00024-8

DelPo, A., & Guerin, L. (2011). *Dealing with problem employees: A legal guide* (6th ed.). Berkeley, CA: Nolo.

Dick, D. M., & Agrawal, A. (2008). The genetics of alcohol and other drug dependence. *Alcohol Research & Health, 31*, 111–118.

Dick, D. M., Agrawal, A., Schuckit, M. A., Bierut, L., Hinrichs, A., Fox, L., . . . Begleiter, H. (2006). Marital status, alcohol dependence, and GABRA2: Evidence for gene–environment correlation and interaction. *Journal of Studies on Alcohol, 67*, 185–194.

Dimich-Ward, H., Gallagher, R. P., Spinelli, J. J., Threlfall, W. J., & Band, P. R. (1988). Occupational mortality among bartenders and waiters. *Canadian Journal of Public Health, 79*, 194–197.

Dindo, L., McDade-Montez, E., Sharma, L., Watson, D., & Clark, L. A. (2009). Development and initial validation of the Disinhibition Inventory: A multifaceted measure of disinhibition. *Assessment, 16*, 274–291. doi:10.1177/1073191108328890

Dolan, K., Rouen, D., & Kimber, J. (2004). An overview of the use of urine, hair, sweat, and saliva to detect drug use. *Drug and Alcohol Review, 23*, 213–217. doi:10.1080/09595230410001704208

Dorafshar, A. H., O'Boyle, D. J., & McCloy, R. F. (2002). Effects of a moderate dose of alcohol on simulated laproscopic surgical performance. *Surgical Endoscopy, 16*, 1753–1758. doi:10.1007/s00464-001-9052-3

Doumas, D. M., & Hannah, E. (2008). Preventing high-risk drinking in youth in the workplace: A web-based normative feedback program. *Journal of Substance Abuse Treatment, 34*, 263–271. doi:10.1016/j.jsat.2007.04.006

Draper, E. (1998). Drug testing in the workplace: The allure of management technologies. *International Journal of Sociology and Social Policy, 18*, 62–103. doi:10.1108/01443339810788380

Drug-Free Workplace Act, 41 U.S.C. § 701 (1988).

Drummer, O. H. (2005). Review: Pharmacokinetics of illicit drugs in oral fluid. *Forensic Science International, 150*, 133–142. doi:10.1016/j.forsciint.2004.11.022

Drummer, O. H. (2008). Introduction and review of collection techniques and applications of drug testing of oral fluid. *Therapeutic Drug Monitoring, 30*, 203–206.

Ducci, F., & Goldman, D. (2008). Genetic approaches to addiction: Genes and alcohol. *Addiction, 103*, 1414–1428. doi:10.1111/j.1360-0443.2008.02203.x

Dumont, G. J. H., & Verkes, R. J. (2006). A review of acute effects of 3,4-methylenedioxymethamphetamine in health volunteers. *Journal of Psychopharmacology, 20*, 176–187. doi:10.1177/0269881106063271

DuPont, R. L., Griffin, D. W., Siskin, B. R., Shiraki, S., & Katze, E. (1995). Random drug tests at work: The probability of identifying frequent and infrequent users of illicit drugs. *Journal of Addictive Diseases, 14*, 1–17. doi:10.1300/J069v14n03_01

Dusenbury, L. (1999). Workplace drug abuse prevention initiatives: A review. *Journal of Primary Prevention, 20*, 145–156. doi:10.1023/A:1021442016197

Dyer, K. R., & Wilkinson, C. (2008). The detection of illicit drugs in oral fluids: Another potential strategy to reduce illicit drug-related harm. *Drug and Alcohol Review, 27*, 99–107. doi:10.1080/09595230701727583

Earleywine, M. (2002). *Understanding marijuana: A new look at the scientific evidence.* New York, NY: Oxford University Press.

El-Bassel, N., Schilling, R. F., Schinke, S., Orlandi, M., Sun, W.-H., & Back, S. (1997). Assessing the utility of the Drug Abuse Screening Test in the workplace. *Research on Social Work Practice, 7*, 99–114.

Eliyahu, U., Berlin, S., Hadad, E., Heled, Y., & Moran, D. S. (2007). Psychostimulants and military operations. *Military Medicine, 172*, 383–387.

Elkins, I. J., King, S. M., McGue, M., & Iacono, W. G. (2006). Personality traits and the development of nicotine, alcohol, and illicit drug disorders: Prospective links from adolescence to young adulthood. *Journal of Abnormal Psychology, 115*, 26–39. doi:10.1037/0021-843X.115.1.26

Employee Assistance Society of North America. (2009). *Selecting and strengthening employee assistance programs: A purchaser's guide.* Arlington, VA: Author.

Enoch, M.-A., & Goldman, D. (2002). Molecular and cellular genetics of alcohol addiction. In K. L. Davis, D. Charney, J. T. Coyle, & C. Nemeroff (Eds.), *Neuropsychopharmacology: The fifth generation of progress* (pp. 1413–1423). Philadelphia, PA: Lippincott Williams & Wilkins.

Entrop v. Imperial Oil, 50 O.R. (3rd) 18 (C.A. 2000).

European Monitoring Centre for Drugs and Drug Addiction. (2006). *Legal status of drug testing in the workplace.* Lisbon, Portugal: Author.

European Workplace Drug Testing Society. (2011). *Workplace drug testing in Europe.* Retrieved from http://www.ewdts.org/euwdt.html

Evidence-Based Medicine Working Group. (1992). Evidence-based medicine: A new approach to teaching the practice of medicine. *JAMA, 268*, 2420–2425. doi:10.1001/jama.1992.03490170092032

Executive Order No. 12564, 51 Fed. Reg. 32889, 3 C.F.R. 224 (1986).

Falk, D., Yi, H.-Y., & Hiller-Sturmhofel, S. (2008). An epidemiologic analysis of co-occurring alcohol and drug use and disorders. *Alcohol Research & Health*, *31*, 100–110.

Farid, B. T., Lucas, G., & Williams, R. (1994). Occupational risk factors in patients with alcoholic or non-alcoholic liver disease. *Alcohol and Alcoholism*, *29*, 459–463.

Farré, M., de la Torre, R., Llorente, M., Lamas, X., Ugena, B., Segura, J., & Camí, J. (1993). Alcohol and cocaine interactions in humans. *Journal of Pharmacology and Experimental Therapeutics*, *266*, 1364–1373.

Faupel, C. E., Horowitz, A. M., & Weaver, G. S. (2004). *The sociology of American drug use*. New York, NY: McGraw-Hill.

Fava, M. (1996). Traditional and alternative research designs and methods in clinical pediatric psychopharmacology. *Journal of the American Academy of Child & Adolescent Psychiatry*, *35*, 1292–1303. doi:10.1097/00004583-199610000-00016

Federal Transit Authority. (1997). *Drug and alcohol testing results: 1996 annual report* (FTA Publication No. FTA-MA-18X018-98-1). Washington, DC: Author.

Federal Transit Authority. (2008). *Drug and alcohol testing results: 2006 annual report* (FTA Publication No. FTA-MA-26-5562-08-1). Washington, DC: Author.

Federal Transit Authority. (2009). *Drug and alcohol testing results: 2007 annual report* (FTA Publication No. FTA-MA-26-5562-09-1). Washington, DC: Author.

Federal Transit Authority. (2010). *Drug and alcohol testing results: 2008 annual report* (FTA Publication No. FTA-MA-26-5566-10-1). Washington, DC: Author.

Fein, G., Torres, J., Price, L. J., & Di Sciafani, V. (2006). Cognitive performance in long-term abstinent alcoholics. *Alcoholism: Clinical and Experimental Research*, *30*, 1538–1544. doi:10.1111/j.1530-0277.2006.00185.x

Feinauer, D. M. (1990). The relationship between workplace accident rates and drug and alcohol abuse: The unproven hypothesis. *Labor Studies Journal*, *15*, 3–15.

Fenoglio, P., Parel, V., & Kopp, P. (2003). The social cost of alcohol, tobacco, and illicit drugs in France, 1997. *European Addiction Research*, *9*, 18–28. doi:10.1159/000067730

Fielding, J. E. (1984). Health promotion and disease prevention at the worksite. *Annual Review of Public Health*, *5*, 237–265. doi:10.1146/annurev.pu.05.050184.001321

Fielding, J. E., & Piserchia, P. V. (1989). Frequency of worksite health promotion activities. *American Journal of Public Health*, *79*, 16–20. doi:10.2105/AJPH.79.1.16

Fillmore, K. M. (1984). Research as a handmaiden of policy: An appraisal of estimates of alcoholism and its costs in the workplace. *Journal of Public Health Policy*, *5*, 40–64. doi:10.2307/3342383

Fillmore, M. T., & Vogel-Sprott, M. (1996). Social drinking history, behavioral tolerance and the expectation of alcohol. *Psychopharmacology*, *127*, 359–364.

Finnigan, F., Hammersley, R., & Cooper, T. (1998). An examination of next-day hangover effects after a 100 mg/ml dose of alcohol in heavy social drinkers. *Addiction*, *93*, 1829–1838. doi:10.1046/j.1360-0443.1998.931218298.x

Finnigan, F., Schulze, D., Smallwood, J., & Helander, A. (2005). The effects of self-administered alcohol induced "hangover" in a naturalistic setting on psychomotor and cognitive performance and subjective state. *Addiction, 100,* 1680–1689. doi:10.1111/j.1360-0443.2005.01142.x

Firebaugh, G. (1997). *Analyzing repeated surveys.* Thousand Oaks, CA: Sage.

Fishbain, D. A., Cutler, B., Rosomoff, H. L., & Rosomoff, R. S. (2003). Are opioid-dependent/tolerant patients impaired in driving-related skills? A structured evidence-based review. *Journal of Pain and Symptom Management, 25,* 559–577. doi:10.1016/S0885-3924(03)00176-3

Fisk, J. E., Montgomery, C., Wareing, M., & Murphy, P. N. (2006). The effects of concurrent cannabis use among ecstasy users: Neuroprotective or neurotoxic? *Human Psychopharmacology: Clinical and Experimental, 21,* 355–366. doi:10.1002/hup.777

Foltin, R. W., & Evans, S. M. (1993). Performance effects of drugs of abuse: A methodological survey. *Human Psychopharmacology: Clinical and Experimental, 8,* 9–19. doi:10.1002/hup.470080104

Ford, M. T., Cerasoli, C. P., Higgins, J. A., & Decesare, A. L. (2011). Relationships between psychological, physical, and behavioural health and work performance: A review and meta-analysis. *Work & Stress, 25,* 185–204. doi:10.1080/02678373.2011.609035

Foroud, T., Edenberg, H. J., & Crabbe, J. C. (2010). Genetic research: Who is at risk for alcoholism? *Alcohol Research & Health, 33,* 64–75.

Foster, E. M. (2010). Causal inference and developmental psychology. *Developmental Psychology, 46,* 1454–1480. doi:10.1037/a0020204

Foster, W. H., & Vaughan, R. D. (2005). Absenteeism and business costs: Does substance abuse matter? *Journal of Substance Abuse Treatment, 28,* 27–33. doi:10.1016/j.jsat.2004.10.003

Franken, I. H. A., & Muris, P. (2006). BIS/BAS personality characteristics and college students' substance use. *Personality and Individual Differences, 40,* 1497–1503. doi:10.1016/j.paid.2005.12.005

French, M. T., Rachal, J. V., & Hubbard, R. L. (1991). Conceptual framework for estimating the social cost of drug abuse. *Journal of Health & Social Policy, 2,* 1–22. doi:10.1300/J045v02n03_01

French, M. T., Roebuck, C., & Alexandre, P. K. (2004). To test or not to test: Do workplace drug testing programs discourage employee drug use? *Social Science Research, 33,* 45–63. doi:10.1016/S0049-089X(03)00038-3

French, M. T., Zarkin, G. A., & Bray, J. W. (1995). A methodology for evaluating the costs and benefits of employee assistance programs. *Journal of Drug Issues, 25,* 451–470.

French, M. T., Zarkin, G. A., & Dunlap, L. J. (1998). Illicit drug use, absenteeism, and earnings at six U.S. worksites. *Contemporary Economic Policy, 16,* 334–346. doi:10.1111/j.1465-7287.1998.tb00523.x

French, M. T., Zarkin, G. A., Hartwell, T. D., & Bray, J. W. (1995). Prevalence and consequences of smoking, alcohol use, and illicit drug use at five worksites. *Public Health Reports, 110,* 593–599.

Friedman, A. S., Granick, S., Utada, A., & Tomko, L. A. (1992). Drug use/abuse and supermarket workers' job performance. *Employee Assistance Quarterly, 7,* 17–34. doi:10.1300/J022v07n04_02

Frone, M. R. (1998). Predictors of work injuries among employed adolescents. *Journal of Applied Psychology, 83,* 565–576. doi:10.1037/0021-9010.83.4.565

Frone, M. R. (1999). Work stress and alcohol use. *Alcohol Research & Health, 23,* 284–291.

Frone, M. R. (2000). Work–family conflict and employee psychiatric disorders: The National Comorbidity Survey. *Journal of Applied Psychology, 85,* 888–895. doi:10.1037/0021-9010.85.6.888

Frone, M. R. (2003). Predictors of overall and on-the-job substance use among young workers. *Journal of Occupational Health Psychology, 8,* 39–54. doi:10.1037/1076-8998.8.1.39

Frone, M. R. (2004). Alcohol, drugs, and workplace safety outcomes: A view from a general model of employee substance use and productivity. In J. Barling & M. R. Frone (Eds.), *The psychology of workplace safety* (pp. 127–156). Washington, DC: American Psychological Association. doi:10.1037/10662-007

Frone, M. R. (2006a). Prevalence and distribution of alcohol use and impairment in the workplace: A U.S. national survey. *Journal of Studies on Alcohol, 67,* 147–156.

Frone, M. R. (2006b). Prevalence and distribution of illicit drug use in the workforce and in the workplace: Findings and implications from a U.S. national survey. *Journal of Applied Psychology, 91,* 856–869. doi:10.1037/0021-9010.91.4.856

Frone, M. R. (2008). Are work stressors related to employee substance use? The importance of temporal context in assessments of alcohol and illicit drug use. *Journal of Applied Psychology, 93,* 199–206. doi:10.1037/0021-9010.93.1.199

Frone, M. R., & Brown, A. L. (2010). Workplace substance-use norms as predictors of employee substance use and impairment: A survey of U.S. workers. *Journal of Studies on Alcohol and Drugs, 71,* 526–534.

Frone, M. R., Russell, M., & Barnes, G. M. (1996). Work–family conflict, gender, and health-related outcomes: A study of employed parents in two community samples. *Journal of Occupational Health Psychology, 1,* 57–69. doi:10.1037/1076-8998.1.1.57

Frone, M. R., Russell, M., & Cooper, M. L. (1993). Relationship of work–family conflict, gender, and alcohol expectancies to alcohol use/abuse. *Journal of Organizational Behavior, 14,* 545–558. doi:10.1002/job.4030140604

Frone, M. R., Russell, M., & Cooper, M. L. (1995). Job stressors, job involvement, and employee health: A test of identity theory. *Journal of Occupational and Organizational Psychology, 68,* 1–11. doi:10.1111/j.2044-8325.1995.tb00684.x

Frone, M. R., Russell, M., & Cooper, M. L. (1997). Relation of work–family conflict to health outcomes: A four-year longitudinal study of employed parents. *Journal of Occupational and Organizational Psychology, 70,* 325–335. doi:10.1111/j.2044-8325.1997.tb00652.x

Frone, M. R., & Trinidad, J. R. (2011). *Workplace physical availability of substances as a risk factor for employee substance use and impairment*. Unpublished manuscript, Research Institute on Addictions, State University of New York at Buffalo.

Frone, M. R., & Trinidad, J. R. (2012). Relation of supervisor social control to employee substance use: Considering the dimensionality of social control, temporal context of substance use, and substance legality. *Journal of Studies on Alcohol and Drugs, 73,* 303–310.

García-Altés, A., Ollé, J. M., Antoñanzas, F., & Colom, J. (2002). The social cost of illegal drug consumption in Spain. *Addiction, 97,* 1145–1153. doi:10.1046/j.1360-0443.2002.00170.x

George, S. (2005). A snapshot of workplace drug testing in the UK. *Occupational Medicine, 55,* 69–71. doi:10.1093/occmed/kqi017

George, W. H., Frone, M. R., Cooper, M. L., Russell, M., Skinner, J. B., & Windle, M. (1995). A revised Alcohol Expectancy Questionnaire: Factor structure confirmation and invariance in a general population sample. *Journal of Studies on Alcohol, 56,* 177–185.

George, W. H., Raynor, J. O., & Nochajski, T. H. (1992). Resistance to alcohol impairment of visual-motor performance. *Journal of Studies on Alcohol, 53,* 507–513.

Ghoneim, M. M., & Medwaldt, S. P. (1990). Benzodiazepines and human memory: A review. *Anesthesiology, 72,* 926–938.

Gigerenzer, G., Gaissmaier, W., Kurz-Milke, E., Schwartz, L. M., & Woloshin, S. (2008). Helping doctors and patients make sense of health statistics. *Psychological Science in the Public Interest, 8,* 53–96.

Gill, J. (1994). Alcohol problems in employment: Epidemiology and responses. *Alcohol and Alcoholism, 29,* 233–248.

Gimeno, D., Amick, B. C., Barrientos-Gutiérrez, T., & Mangione, T. W. (2009). Work organization and drinking: An epidemiological comparison of two psychosocial work exposure models. *International Archives of Occupational and Environmental Health, 82,* 305–317. doi:10.1007/s00420-008-0335-z

Gjerde, H., Christophersen, A. S., Moan, I. S., Yttredal, B., Walsh, J. M., Normann, P. T., & Morland, J. (2010). Use of alcohol and drugs by Norwegian employees: A pilot study using questionnaires and analysis of oral fluid. *Journal of Occupational Medicine and Toxicology, 5,* Article 13. doi:10.1186/1745-6673-5-13

Glencross, D. J. (1990). Alcohol and human performance. *Drug and Alcohol Review, 9,* 111–118. doi:10.1080/09595239000185161

Goetzel, R. Z., Juday, T. R., & Ozminkowski, R. J. (1999). What's the ROI? A systematic review on return-on-investment studies of corporate health and productivity management initiatives. *AWHP's Worksite Health, 6,* 12–21.

Goetzel, R. Z., & Ozminkowski, R. J. (2008). The health and cost benefits of work site health-promotion programs. *Annual Review of Public Health, 29,* 303–323. doi:10.1146/annurev.publhealth.29.020907.090930

Golan, M., Bacharach, Y., & Bamberger, P. (2010). Peer assistance programs in the workplace. In J. Houdmont & S. Leka (Eds.), *Contemporary occupational health psychology: Global perspectives on research and practice* (Vol. 1, pp. 169–187). New York, NY: Wiley. doi:10.1002/9780470661550.ch9

Gold, M. S., Melker, R. J., Dennis, D. M., Morey, T. E., Bajpai, L. K., Pomm, R., & Frost-Pineda, K. (2006). Fentanyl abuse and dependence: Further evidence for second hand exposure hypothesis. *Journal of Addictive Diseases, 25*, 15–21. doi:10.1300/J069v25n01_04

Golding, J. F., Groome, D. H., Rycroft, N., & Denton, Z. (2007). Cognitive performance in light current users and ex-users of ecstasy (MDMA) and controls. *American Journal of Drug and Alcohol Abuse, 33*, 301–307. doi:10.1080/00952990601175052

Goldman, D., Oroszi, G., & Ducci, F. (2005). The genetics of addictions: Uncovering the genes. *Nature Reviews Genetics, 6*, 521–532. doi:10.1038/nrg1635

Goldman, M. S., Brown, S. A., & Christiansen, B. A. (1987). Expectancy theory: Thinking about drinking. In H. T. Blane & K. E. Leonard (Eds.), *Psychological theories of drinking and alcoholism* (pp. 181–226). New York, NY: Guilford Press.

Grant, B. F., & Dawson, D. A. (2006). Introduction to the National Epidemiologic Survey on Alcohol and Related Conditions. *Alcohol Research & Health, 29*, 74–78.

Grant, J. D., Agrawal, A., Bucholz, K. K., Madden, P. A., Pergadia, M. L., Nelson, E. C., . . . Heath, A. C. (2009). Alcohol consumption indices of genetic risk for alcohol dependence. *Biological Psychiatry, 66*, 795–800. doi:10.1016/j.biopsych.2009.05.018

Grant, S., & Langan-Fox, J. (2007). Personality and the occupational stressor–strain relationship: The role of the Big Five. *Journal of Occupational Health Psychology, 12*, 20–33. doi:10.1037/1076-8998.12.1.20

Gray, J. A. (1987). *The psychology of fear and stress*. Cambridge, England: Cambridge University Press.

Greenberg, E. S., & Grunberg, L. (1995). Work alienation and problem alcohol behavior. *Journal of Health and Social Behavior, 36*, 83–102. doi:10.2307/2137289

Greenberg, L., & Barling, J. (1999). Predicting employee aggression against coworkers, subordinates and supervisors: The roles of person behaviors and perceived workplace factors. *Journal of Organizational Behavior, 20*, 897–913. doi:10.1002/(SICI)1099-1379(199911)20:6<897::AID-JOB975>3.0.CO;2-Z

Grube, J. W., & Agostinelli, G. E. (1999). Perceived consequences and adolescent drinking: Nonlinear and interactive models of alcohol expectancies. *Psychology of Addictive Behaviors, 13*, 303–312. doi:10.1037/0893-164X.13.4.303

Grube, J. W., Ames, G. M., & Delaney, W. (1994). Alcohol expectancies and workplace drinking. *Journal of Applied Social Psychology, 24*, 646–660. doi:10.1111/j.1559-1816.1994.tb00605.x

Grunberg, L., Moore, S., Anderson-Connolly, R., & Greenberg, E. S. (1999). Work stress and self-reported alcohol use: The moderating role of escapist reasons for drinking. *Journal of Occupational Health Psychology, 4*, 29–36. doi:10.1037/1076-8998.4.1.29

Grunberg, L., Moore, S., & Greenberg, E. S. (1998). Work stress and problem alcohol behavior: A test of the spillover model. *Journal of Organizational Behavior, 19,* 487–502. doi:10.1002/(SICI)1099-1379 (199809)19:5<487::AID-JOB852>3.0.CO;2-Z

Guthrie, J. P., & Olian, J. D. (1991). Drug and alcohol testing programs: Do firms consider their operating environment? *Human Resource Planning, 14,* 221–232.

Haar, J. M., & Spell, C. S. (2007). Factors affecting employer adoption of drug testing in New Zealand. *Asia Pacific Journal of Human Resources, 45,* 200–217. doi:10.1177/1038411107079116

Halkitis, P. N. (2009). *Methamphetamine addiction: Biological foundations, psychological factors, and social consequences.* Washington, DC: American Psychological Association. doi:10.1037/11883-000

Hall, W., & Babor, T. F. (2000). Cannabis use and public health: Assessing the burden. *Addiction, 95,* 485–490. doi:10.1046/j.1360-0443.2000.9544851.x

Hansell, N. K., Agrawal, A., Whitfield, J. B., Morley, K. I., Zhu, G., Lind, P. A., . . . Martin, N. G. (2008). Long-term stability and heritability of telephone interview measures of alcohol consumption and dependence. *Twin Research and Human Genetics, 11,* 287–305. doi:10.1375/twin.11.3.287

Harden, A., Peersman, G., Oliver, S., Mauthner, M., & Oakley, A. (1999). A systematic review of the effectiveness of health promotion interventions in the workplace. *Occupational Medicine, 49,* 540–548. doi:10.1093/occmed/49.8.540

Harden, K. P., Hill, J. E., Turkheimer, E., & Emery, R. E. (2008). Gene–environment correlation and interaction in peer effects on adolescent alcohol and tobacco use. *Behavior Genetics, 38,* 339–347. doi:10.1007/s10519-008-9202-7

Harford, T. C., & Brooks, S. D. (1992). Cirrhosis mortality and occupation. *Journal of Studies on Alcohol, 53,* 463–468.

Hargrave, G. E., Hiatt, D., Alexander, R., & Shaffer, I. A. (2008). EAP treatment impact on presenteeism and absenteeism: Implications for return on investment. *Journal of Workplace Behavioral Health, 23,* 283–293. doi:10.1080/15555240802242999

Harper, T. (1999). Employee assistance programming and professional developments in South Africa. *Employee Assistance Quarterly, 14,* 1–18. doi:10.1300/J022v14n03_01

Harris, M., & Heft, L. L. (1992). Alcohol and drug use in the workplace: Issues, controversies, and directions for future research. *Journal of Management, 18,* 239–266. doi:10.1177/014920639201800203

Harris, M. M., & Heft, L. L. (1993). Preemployment urinalysis drug testing: A critical review of psychometric and legal issues and effects on applicants. *Human Resource Management Review, 3,* 271–291. doi:10.1016/1053-4822(93)90002-L

Harris, N. (Ed.). (2005). *Opiates.* New York, NY: Greenhaven Press.

Hart, C. L., Haney, M., Nasser, J., & Foltin, R. W. (2005). Combined effects of methamphetamine and zolpidem on performance and mood during simulated night shift work. *Pharmacology Biochemistry and Behavior, 81,* 559–568. doi:10.1016/j.pbb.2005.04.008

Hart, C. L., Marvin, C. B., Silver, R., & Smith, E. E. (2012). Is cognitive functioning impaired in methamphetamine users? A critical review. *Neuropsychopharmacology, 37,* 586–608. doi:10.1038/npp.2011.276

Hart, C. L., van Gorp, W., Haney, M., Foltin, R. W., & Fishman, M. W. (2001). Effects of acute smoked marijuana on complex cognitive performance. *Neuropsychopharmacology, 25,* 757–765. doi:10.1016/S0893-133X(01)00273-1

Hart, C. L., Ward, A. S., Haney, M., & Foltin, R. W. (2003). Zolpidem-related effects on performance and mood during simulated night-shift work. *Experimental and Clinical Psychopharmacology, 11,* 259–268. doi:10.1037/1064-1297.11.4.259

Hart, C. L., Ward, A. S., Haney, M., Nasser, J., & Foltin, R. W. (2003). Methamphetamine attenuates disruptions in performance and mood during simulated night-shift work. *Psychopharmacology, 169,* 42–51. doi:10.1007/s00213-003-1464-4

Hartman, S. J., & Crow, S. M. (1993). Drugs in the workplace: Setting Harris straight. *Journal of Drug Issues, 23,* 733–738.

Hartwell, T. D., Steele, P., French, M. T., Potter, F. J., Rodman, N. F., & Zarkin, G. A. (1996). Aiding troubled employees: The prevalence, cost, and characteristics of employee assistance programs in the United States. *American Journal of Public Health, 86,* 804–808. doi:10.2105/AJPH.86.6.804

Hartwell, T. D., Steele, P. D., French, M. T., & Rodman, N. F. (1996). Prevalence of drug testing in the workplace. *Monthly Labor Review, 119,* 35–42.

Hartwell, T. D., Steele, P. D., & Rodman, N. F. (1998). Workplace alcohol-testing programs: Prevalence and trends. *Monthly Labor Review, 121,* 27–34.

Harwood, H. (2000). *Updating estimates of the economic cost of alcohol abuse: Estimates, updating methods, and data.* Retrieved from http://pubs.niaaa.nih.gov/publications/economic-2000

Harwood, H., Fountain, D., & Livermore, G. (1998). *The economic costs of alcohol and drug abuse in the United States—1992.* Retrieved from http://archives.drugabuse.gov/EconomicCosts/Index.html

Harwood, H. J., & Reichman, M. B. (2000). The cost to employers of employee alcohol abuse: A review of the literature in the United States of America. *Bulletin on Narcotics, 52,* 39–51.

Hasin, D. S., & Katz, H. (2010). Genetic and environmental factors in substance use, abuse, and dependence. In L. M. Scheier (Ed.), *Handbook of drug use etiology: Theory, methods, and empirical findings* (pp. 247–267). Washington, DC: American Psychological Association.

Hayaki, J., Hagerty, C. E., Herman, D. S., de Dios, M. A., Anderson, B. J., & Stein, M. D. (2010). Expectancies and marijuana use frequency and severity among young females. *Addictive Behaviors, 35,* 995–1000. doi:10.1016/j.addbeh.2010.06.017

Hayghe, H. V. (1991). Antidrug programs in the workplace: Are they here to stay? *Monthly Labor Review, 114,* 26–29.

Head, J., Stansfeld, S. A., & Siegrist, J. (2004). The psychosocial work environment and alcohol dependence: A prospective study. *Occupational and Environmental Medicine, 61*, 219–224. doi:10.1136/oem.2002.005256

Heath, A. C., Madden, P. A. F., Bucholz, K. K., Dinwiddie, S. H., Slutske, W. S., Bierut, L. J., . . . Martin, N. G. (1999). Genetic differences in alcohol sensitivity and the inheritance of alcoholism risk. *Psychological Medicine, 29*, 1069–1081. doi:10.1017/S0033291799008909

Hecker, S., & Kaplan, M. S. (1989). Workplace drug testing as social control. *International Journal of Health Services, 19*, 693–707. doi:10.2190/CTDA-5W30-XP4V-AM6E

Heien, D. M., & Pittman, D. J. (1989). The economic costs of alcohol abuse: An assessment of current methods and estimates. *Journal of Studies on Alcohol, 50*, 567–579.

Heishman, S. J. (1998). Effects of abused drugs on human performance: Laboratory assessment. In S. B. Karch (Ed.), *Drug abuse handbook* (pp. 206–235). New York, NY: CRC Press.

Heishman, S. J., Kleykamp, B. A., & Singleton, E. G. (2010). Meta-analysis of the acute effects of nicotine and smoking on human performance. *Psychopharmacology, 210*, 453–469. doi:10.1007/s00213-010-1848-1

Heishman, S. J., & Meyers, C. S. (2007). Effects of abused drugs on human performance: Laboratory assessment. In S. B. Karch (Ed.), *Drug abuse handbook* (2nd ed., pp. 209–238). New York, NY: CRC Press.

Hemmingsson, T., & Lundberg, I. (1998). Work control, work demands, and work social support in relation to alcoholism among young men. *Alcoholism: Clinical and Experimental Research, 22*, 921–927. doi:10.1111/j.1530-0277.1998.tb03890.x

Hermansson, U., Helander, A., Brandt, L., Huss, A., & Ronnberg, S. (2010). Screening and brief intervention for risky alcohol consumption in the workplace: Results of a 1-year randomized control study. *Alcohol and Alcoholism, 45*, 252–257. doi:10.1093/alcalc/agq021

Hertz, R. P., & Baker, C. L. (2002). *The impact of mental disorders on work*. Groton, CT: Pfizer Pharmaceuticals.

Hesse, M., & Tutenges, S. (2010). Predictors of hangover during a week of heavy drinking on holiday. *Addiction, 105*, 476–483. doi:10.1111/j.1360-0443.2009.02816.x

Highley-Marchington, J. C., & Cooper, C. L. (1998). *An assessment of employee assistance and workplace counselling programmes in British organizations* (Research Report 198). London, England: Health and Safety Executive.

Hodgins, D. C., Williams, R., & Munro, G. (2009). Workplace responsibility, stress, alcohol availability and norms as predictors of alcohol consumption-related problems among employed workers. *Substance Use & Misuse, 44*, 2062–2069. doi:10.3109/10826080902855173

Hoffmann, J. P., Brittingham, A., & Larison, C. (1996). *Drug use among U.S. workers: Prevalence and trends by occupation and industry categories* (DHHS Publication No. SMA 96–3089). Washington, DC: U.S. Government Printing Office.

Hoffmann, J. P., & Larison, C. L. (1999). Worker drug use and workplace drug-testing programs: Results from the 1994 National Household Survey on Drug Abuse. *Contemporary Drug Problems, 26,* 331–354.

Hoffmann, J. P., Larison, C., & Sanderson, A. (1997). *An analysis of worker drug use and workplace policies and programs* (DHHS Publication No. SMA 97-3142). Washington, DC: U.S. Government Printing Office.

Holcom, M. L., Lehman, W. E. K., & Simpson, D. D. (1993). Employee accidents: Influences of personal characteristics, job characteristics, and substance use in jobs differing in accident potential. *Journal of Safety Research, 24,* 205–221. doi:10.1016/0022-4375(93)80002-S

Holder, H. D., & Cunningham, D. W. (1992). Alcoholism treatment for employees and family members. *Alcohol Health & Research World, 16,* 149–153.

Holmes, N., & Richter, K. (2008). *Drug testing in the workplace.* Ottawa, Ontario, Canada: Library of Parliament.

Howard, L. W., & Cordes, C. L. (2010). Flight from unfairness: Effects of perceived injustice on emotional exhaustion and employee withdrawal. *Journal of Business and Psychology, 25,* 409–428. doi:10.1007/s10869-010-9158-5

Howland, J., Rohsenow, D. J., Allensworth-Davies, D., Greece, J., Almeida, A., Minsky, S. J., . . . Hermos, J. (2008). The incidence and severity of hangover the morning after moderate drinking. *Addiction, 103,* 758–765. doi:10.1111/j.1360-0443.2008.02181.x

Howland, J., Rohsenow, D. J., Bliss, C. A., Almeida, A. B., Calise, T. V., Heeren, T., & Winter, M. (2010). Hangover predicts residual alcohol effects on psychomotor vigilance the morning after intoxication. *Journal of Addiction Research & Therapy, 1,* Article 101. doi:10.4172/2155-6105.1000101

Howland, J., Rohsenow, D. J., Cote, J., Gomez, B., Mangione, T. W., & Laramie, A. K. (2001). Effects of low-dose alcohol exposure on simulated merchant ship piloting by maritime cadets. *Accident Analysis and Prevention, 33,* 257–265. doi:10.1016/S0001-4575(00)00040-3

Howland, J., Rohsenow, D. J., Cote, J., Siegel, M., & Mangione, T. W. (2000). Effects of low-dose alcohol exposure on simulated merchant ship handling power plant operations by maritime cadets. *Addiction, 95,* 719–726. doi:10.1046/j.1360-0443.2000.9557197.x

Huestis, M. A. (2002). Cannabis (marijuana)—Effects on human behavior and performance. *Forensic Science Review, 14,* 16–59.

Hughes, C. E. (2007). Evidence-based policy or policy-based evidence? The role of evidence in the development and implementation of the Illicit Drug Diversion Initiative. *Drug and Alcohol Review, 26,* 363–368. doi:10.1080/09595230701373859

Hunter, J. E., & Schmidt, F. L. (2004). *Methods of meta-analysis: Correcting error and bias in research findings* (2nd ed.). Thousand Oaks, CA: Sage.

Independent Inquiry Into Drug Testing at Work. (2004). *Drug testing in the workplace: The report of the Independent Inquiry Into Drug Testing at Work.* Layerthorpe, York, England: Joseph Rowntree Foundation.

International Center for Alcohol Policies. (1998). *What is a "standard drink"?* (ICAP Reports 5). Washington, DC: Author.

Jackson, K. M., & Sher, K. J. (2003). Alcohol use disorders and psychological distress: A prospective state–trait analysis. *Journal of Abnormal Psychology, 112,* 599–613. doi:10.1037/0021-843X.112.4.599

Jackson, S. E., & Schuler, R. S. (1995). Understanding human resources management in the context of organizations and their environments. *Annual Review of Psychology, 46,* 237–264. doi:10.1146/annurev.ps.46.020195.001321

Jackson, S. E., Schuler, R. S., & Rivero, J. C. (1989). Organizational characteristics as predictors of personnel practices. *Personnel Psychology, 42,* 727–786. doi:10.1111/j.1744-6570.1989.tb00674.x

Jacobson, J. M., Jones, A. L., & Bowers, N. (2011). Using existing employee assistance program case files to demonstrate outcomes. *Journal of Workplace Behavioral Health, 26,* 44–58. doi:10.1080/15555240.2011.540983

Jaffee, W. B., Trucco, E., Teter, C., Levy, S., & Weiss, R. D. (2008). Focus on alcohol and drug abuse: Ensuring validity in urine drug testing. *Psychiatric Services, 59,* 140–142. doi:10.1176/appi.ps.59.2.140

Jager, G., de Win, M. M., Vervaeke, H. K., Schilt, T., Kahn, R. S., van den Brink, W., . . . Ramsey, N. F. (2007). Incidental use of ecstasy: No evidence for harmful effects on cognitive brain function in a prospective fMRI study. *Psychopharmacology, 193,* 403–414. doi:10.1007/s00213-007-0792-1

Jansen, K. L. (2000). A review of the nonmedical use of ketamine: Use, users, and consequences. *Journal of Psychoactive Drugs, 32,* 419–433. doi:10.1080/02791072.2000.10400244

Jansen, K. L., & Darracot-Cankovic, R. (2001). The nonmedical use of ketamine, part two: A review of problem use and dependence. *Journal of Psychoactive Drugs, 33,* 151–158. doi:10.1080/02791072.2001.10400480

Jenkins, A. J. (2007). Pharmacokinetics: Drug absorption, distribution, and elimination. In S. B. Karch (Ed.), *Drug abuse handbook* (2nd ed., pp. 147–205). New York, NY: CRC Press.

Jex, S. M., Beehr, T. A., & Roberts, C. K. (1992). The meaning of occupational stress items to survey respondents. *Journal of Applied Psychology, 77,* 623–628. doi:10.1037/0021-9010.77.5.623

John, O. P., & Srivastava, S. (1999). The Big Five trait taxonomy: History, measurement, and theoretical perspectives. In L. A. Pervin & O. P. John (Eds.), *Handbook of personality: Theory and research* (2nd ed., pp. 102–138). New York, NY: Guilford Press.

Jones, A. W. (2006). Urine as a biological specimen for forensic analysis of alcohol and variability in the urine-to-blood ratio. *Toxicological Reviews, 25,* 15–35. doi:10.2165/00139709-200625010-00002

Jones, S., Casswell, S., & Zhang, J.-F. (1995). The economic costs of alcohol-related absenteeism and reduced productivity among the working population of New Zealand. *Addiction, 60,* 1455–1461. doi:10.1111/j.1360-0443.1995.tb02807.x

Jung, J. (2001). *Psychology of alcohol and other drugs.* Thousand Oaks, CA: Sage.

Kadehjian, L. (2005). Legal issues in oral fluid testing. *Forensic Science International, 150*, 151–160. doi:10.1016/j.forsciint.2004.11.024

Kagel, J. H., Battalio, R. C., & Miles, C. G. (1980). Marihuana and work performance: Results from an experiment. *Journal of Human Resources, 15*, 373–395. doi:10.2307/145289

Kalant, H. (1997). Opium revisited: A brief review of its nature, composition, non-medical use and relative risks. *Addiction, 92*, 267–277.

Kalant, H. (2010). Drug classification: Science, politics, neither, or both? *Addiction, 105*, 1146–1149. doi:10.1111/j.1360-0443.2009.02830.x

Kalechstein, A. D., De La Garza, R., II, Mahoney, J. J., III, Fantegrossi, W. E., & Newton, T. F. (2007). MDMA use and neurocognition: A meta-analytic review. *Psychopharmacology, 189*, 531–537. doi:10.1007/s00213-006-0601-2

Kaner, E. F. S., Dickinson, H. O., Beyer, F., Pienaar, E., Schlesinger, C., Campbell, F., . . . Heather, N. (2009). The effectiveness of brief alcohol interventions in primary care settings: A systematic review. *Drug and Alcohol Review, 28*, 301–323. doi:10.1111/j.1465-3362.2009.00071.x

Kapur, B. M. (1993). Drug-testing methods and clinical interpretations of test results. *Bulletin on Narcotics, 45*, 115–154.

Kashdan, T. B., Vetter, C. J., & Collins, R. L. (2005). Substance use in young adults: Associations with personality and gender. *Addictive Behaviors, 30*, 259–269. doi:10.1016/j.addbeh.2004.05.014

Kawakami, N., Araki, S., Haratani, T., & Hemmi, T. (1993). Relations of work stress to alcohol use and drinking problems in male and female employees of a computer factory. *Environmental Research, 62*, 314–324. doi:10.1006/enrs.1993.1116

Kazanga, I., Tameni, S., Piccinotti, A., Floris, I., Zanchetti, G., & Polettini, A. (2012). Prevalence of drug abuse among workers: Strengths and pitfalls of the recent Italian workplace drug testing (WDT) legislation. *Forensic Science International, 215*, 46–50. doi:10.1016/j.forsciint.2011.03.009

Keay, E., Macdonald, S., Durand, P., Csiernik, R., & Wild, T. C. (2010). Reasons for adopting and not adopting: Employee assistance and drug testing programs in Canada. *Journal of Workplace Behavioral Health, 25*, 65–71. doi:10.1080/15555240903358702

Kendler, K. S., & Baker, J. H. (2007). Genetic influences on measures of the environment: A systematic review. *Psychological Medicine, 37*, 615–626. doi:10.1017/S0033291706009524

Kendler, K. S., Gardner, C., Jacobson, K. C., Neale, M. C., & Prescott, C. A. (2005). Genetic and environmental influences on illicit drug use and tobacco use across birth cohorts. *Psychological Medicine, 35*, 1349–1356. doi:10.1017/S0033291705004964

Kendler, K. S., Karkowski, L. M., Neale, M. C., & Prescott, C. A. (2000). Illicit psychoactive substance use, heavy use, abuse, and dependence in a U.S. population-based sample of male twins. *Archives of General Psychiatry, 57*, 261–269. doi:10.1001/archpsyc.57.3.261

Kendler, K. S., Myers, J., & Prescott, C. A. (2007). Specificity of genetic and environmental risk factors for symptoms of cannabis, cocaine, alcohol, caffeine, and nicotine dependence. *Archives of General Psychiatry, 64,* 1313–1320.

Kenna, G. A., Baldwin, J. N., Trinkoff, A. M., & Lewis, D. C. (2011). Substance use disorders among healthcare professionals. In B. A. Johnson (Ed.), *Addiction medicine* (pp. 1375–1398). New York, NY: Springer.

Kerr, J. S., & Hindmarch, I. (1998). Effects of alcohol alone or in combination with other drugs on information processing, task performance, and subjective responses. *Human Psychopharmacology: Clinical and Experimental, 13,* 1–9. doi:10.1002/(SICI)1099-1077(199801)13:1<1::AID-HUP939>3.0.CO;2-0

Kessler, R. C., & Walters, E. E. (2002). The National Comorbidity Survey. In M. T. Tsuang, M. Tohen, & G. E. P. Zahner (Eds.), *Textbook in psychiatric epidemiology* (2nd ed., pp. 343–361). New York, NY: Wiley. doi:10.1002/0471234311.ch14

Kim, D.-J., Yoon, S.-J., Lee, H.-P., Choi, B.-M., & Go, H. J. (2003). The effects of alcohol hangover on cognitive functions in healthy subjects. *International Journal of Neuroscience, 113,* 581–594. doi:10.1080/00207450390162308

King, K. M., & Chassin, L. (2004). Mediating and moderating effects of adolescent behavioral undercontrol and parenting in the prediction of drug use disorders in emerging adulthood. *Psychology of Addictive Behaviors, 18,* 239–249. doi:10.1037/0893-164X.18.3.239

Kirby, G., Kapoor, K., Das-Purkayastha, P., & Harries, M. (2012). The effect of alcohol on surgical skills. *Annals of the Royal College of Surgeons of England, 94,* 90–93. doi:10.1308/003588412X13171221501627

Kirk, A. K. (2006). Employee assistance program adoption in Australia: Strategic human resource management or "knee-jerk" solutions? *Journal of Workplace Behavioral Health, 21,* 79–95. doi:10.1300/J490v21n01_07

Kirk, A. K., & Brown, D. F. (2003). Employee assistance programs: A review of the management of stress and wellbeing through workplace counselling and consulting. *Australian Psychologist, 38,* 138–143. doi:10.1080/00050060310001707137

Kirsch, I. (1999). Response expectancy: An introduction. In I. Kirsch (Ed.), *How expectancies shape experience* (pp. 3–13). Washington, DC: American Psychological Association.

Kitterlin, M., & Moreo, P. J. (2012). Pre-employment drug testing in the full-service restaurant industry and its relationship to employee work performance factors. *Journal of Human Resources in Hospitality & Tourism, 11,* 36–51. doi:10.1080/15332845.2012.621053

Kleiman, M. A. R. (1999). "Economic cost" measurements, damage minimization and drug abuse control policy. *Addiction, 94,* 638–641.

Knudsen, H. K., Roman, P. M., & Johnson, J. A. (2003). Organizational compatibility and workplace testing: Modeling the adoption of innovative social control processes. *Sociological Forum, 18,* 621–640. doi:10.1023/B:SOFO.0000003006.65704.f1

Knudsen, H. K., Roman, P. M., & Johnson, J. A. (2004). The management of work-place deviance: Organizational responses to employee drug use. *Journal of Drug Issues, 34,* 121–143. doi:10.1177/002204260403400106

Kocher, H. M., Warwick, J., Al-Ghnaniem, R., & Patel, A. G. (2006). Surgical dexterity after a "night out on the town." *ANZ Journal of Surgery, 76,* 110–112. doi:10.1111/j.1445-2197.2006.03664.x

Koelega, H. S. (1989). Benzodiazepines and vigilance performance: A review. *Psychopharmacology, 98,* 145–156. doi:10.1007/BF00444684

Koelega, H. S. (1993). Stimulant drugs and vigilance performance: A review. *Psychopharmacology, 111,* 1–16. doi:10.1007/BF02257400

Kopp, P. (1999). Economic costs calculations and drug policy evaluation. *Addiction, 94,* 641–644.

Kotov, R., Gamez, W., Schmidt, F., & Watson, D. (2010). Linking "big" personality traits to anxiety, depression, and substance use disorders: A meta-analysis. *Psychological Bulletin, 136,* 768–821. doi:10.1037/a0020327

Kouvonen, A., Kivimäki, M., Cox, S. J., Poikolainen, K., Cox, T., & Vahtera, J. (2005). Job strain, effort–reward imbalance, and heavy drinking: A study in 40,851 employees. *Journal of Occupational and Environmental Medicine, 47,* 503–513. doi:10.1097/01.jom.0000161734.81375.25

Kovner, A. R., Elton, J. J., & Billings, J. (2000). Evidence-based management. *Frontiers of Health Services Management, 16,* 3–24.

Kraemer, H. C., Stice, E., Kazdin, A., Offord, D., & Kupfer, D. (2001). How do risk factors work together? Mediators, moderators, and independent, overlapping, and proxy risk factors. *American Journal of Psychiatry, 158,* 848–856.

Kraus, J. F. (2001). The effects of certain drug-testing programs on injury reduction in the workplace: An evidence-based review. *International Journal of Occupational and Environmental Health, 7,* 103–108.

Kunsman, G. W., Manno, J. E., Manno, B. R., Kunsman, C. M., & Przekop, M. A. (1992). The use of microcomputer-based psychomotor tests for the evaluation of benzodiazepine effects on human performance: A review with emphasis on temazepam. *British Journal of Clinical Pharmacology, 34,* 289–301.

Kuoppala, J., Lamminpää, A., & Husman, P. (2008). Work health promotion, job well-being, and sickness absences: A systematic review and meta-analysis. *Journal of Occupational and Environmental Medicine, 50,* 1216–1227. doi:10.1097/JOM.0b013e31818dbf92

Kurtz, N. R., Googins, B., & Howard, W. C. (1984). Measuring success of occupational alcohol programs. *Journal of Studies on Alcohol, 45,* 33–45.

Kurtzman, T. L., Otsuka, K. N., & Wahl, R. A. (2001). Inhalant abuse by adolescents. *Journal of Adolescent Health, 28,* 170–180. doi:10.1016/S1054-139X(00)00159-2

Laaksonen, M., Piha, K., Martikainen, P., Rahkonen, O., & Lahelma, E. (2009). Health-related behaviours and sickness absence from work. *Occupational and Environmental Medicine, 66,* 840–847. doi:10.1136/oem.2008.039248

Labbe, A. K., & Maisto, S. A. (2010). Development of the Stimulant Medication Outcome Expectancies Questionnaire for college students. *Addictive Behaviors, 35*, 726–729. doi:10.1016/j.addbeh.2010.03.010

Lachman, H. M. (2006). An overview of the genetics of substance use disorders. *Current Psychiatry Reports, 8*, 133–143. doi:10.1007/s11920-006-0013-3

Lacy, B. W., & Ditzler, T. F. (2007). Inhalant abuse in the military: An unrecognized threat. *Military Medicine, 172*, 388–392.

Lahtinen, E., Koskinen-Ollonqvist, P., Rouvinen-Wilenius, P., Tuominen, P., & Mittelmark, M. B. (2005). The development of quality criteria for research: A Finnish approach. *Health Promotion International, 20*, 306–315. doi:10.1093/heapro/dai008

Lange, W. R., Cabanilla, B. R., Moler, G., Bernacki, E. J., Frankenfield, D. L., & Fudala, P. J. (1994). Preemployment drug screening at the Johns Hopkins Hospital, 1989 and 1991. *American Journal of Drug and Alcohol Abuse, 20*, 35–46. doi:10.3109/00952999409084055

Lapham, S. C., Gregory, C., & McMillan, G. (2003). Impact of an alcohol misuse intervention for health care workers—1: Frequency of binge drinking and desire to reduce alcohol use. *Alcohol and Alcoholism, 38*, 176–182. doi:10.1093/alcalc/agg047

Larg, A., & Moss, J. R. (2011). Cost-of-illness studies: A guide to critical evaluation. *PharmacoEconomics, 29*, 653–671. doi:10.2165/11588380-000000000-00000

Larson, S. L., Eyerman, J., Foster, M. S., & Gfroerer, J. C. (2007). *Worker substance use and workplace policies and programs* (DHHS Publication No. SMA 07-4273, Analytic Series A-29). Rockville, MD: Substance Abuse and Mental Health Services Administration, Office of Applied Studies.

Lazarus, R. S. (1985). Stress: Appraisal and coping capacities. In A. Eicher, M. M. Silverman, & D. M. Pratt (Eds.), *How to define and research stress* (pp. 5–16). Washington, DC: U.S. Department of Health and Human Services.

Lazarus, R. S., & Folkman, S. (1985). Stress as rubric. In A. Eicher, M. M. Silverman, & D. M. Pratt (Eds.), *How to define and research stress* (pp. 33–38). Washington, DC: U.S. Department of Health and Human Services.

Lee, D., Milman, G., Barnes, A. J., Goodwin, R. S., Hirvonen, J., & Huestis, M. A. (2011). Oral fluid cannabinoids in chronic, daily cannabis smokers during sustained, monitored abstinence. *Clinical Chemistry, 57*, 1127–1136. doi:10.1373/clinchem.2011.164822

Lehman, W. E. K., & Simpson, D. D. (1992). Employee substance use and on-the-job behaviors. *Journal of Applied Psychology, 77*, 309–321. doi:10.1037/0021-9010.77.3.309

Leigh, B. C., & Stacy, A. W. (2004). Alcohol expectancies and drinking in different age groups. *Addiction, 99*, 215–227. doi:10.1111/j.1360-0443.2003.00641.x

Leigh, J. P., & Jiang, W. Y. (1993). Liver cirrhosis deaths within occupations and industries in the California Occupational Mortality Study. *Addiction, 88*, 767–779. doi:10.1111/j.1360-0443.1993.tb02091.x

Lemon, J., Chesher, G., Fox, A., Greeley, J., & Nabke, C. (1993). Investigation of the "hangover" effects of an acute dose of alcohol on psychomotor performance. *Alcoholism: Clinical and Experimental Research, 17*, 665–668. doi:10.1111/j.1530-0277.1993.tb00816.x

Lessem, J. M., Hopfer, C. J., Haberstick, B. C., Timberlake, D., Ehringer, M. A., Smolen, A., & Hewitt, J. K. (2006). Relationship between adolescent marijuana use and young adult illicit drug use. *Behavior Genetics, 36*, 498–506. doi:10.1007/s10519-006-9064-9

Leukefeld, C. G., & Bukowski, W. J. (Eds.). (1991). *Drug abuse prevention: Methodological issues* (DHHS Publication No. ADM91-1761). Washington, DC: Government Printing Office.

Lewin, K. (1936). *Principles of topological psychology*. New York, NY: McGraw-Hill. doi:10.1037/10019-000

Li, G., Baker, S. P., Zhao, Q., Brady, J. E., Lang, B. H., Rebok, G. W., & DiMaggio, C. (2011). Drug violations and aviation accidents: Findings from the U.S. mandatory drug testing programs. *Addiction, 106*, 1287–1292. doi:10.1111/j.1360-0443.2011.03388.x

Lim, D., Sanderson, K., & Andrews, G. (2000). Lost productivity among full-time workers with mental disorders. *Journal of Mental Health Policy and Economics, 3*, 139–146. doi:10.1002/mhp.93

Linnan, L., Bowling, M., Childress, J., Lindsay, G., Blakey, C., Pronk, S., . . . Royall, P. (2008). Results of the 2004 National Worksite Health Promotion Survey. *American Journal of Public Health, 98*, 1503–1509. doi:10.2105/AJPH.2006.100313

Liu, S., Wang, M., Zhan, Y., & Shi, J. (2009). Daily work stress and alcohol use: Testing the cross-level moderation effects of neuroticism and job involvement. *Personnel Psychology, 62*, 575–597. doi:10.1111/j.1744-6570.2009.01149.x

Lockwood, F. S., Klaas, B. S., Logan, J. E., & Sandberg, W. R. (2000). Drug-testing programs and their impact on workplace accidents: A time-series analysis. *Journal of Individual Employment Rights, 8*, 295–306.

Logan, B. K. (2002). Methamphetamine: Effects on human performance and behavior. *Forensic Science Review, 14*, 134–151.

Looby, A., & Earleywine, M. (2007). Negative consequences associated with dependence in daily cannabis users. *Substance Abuse Treatment, Prevention, and Policy, 2*, Article 3. doi:10.1186/1747-597X-2-3

Lowmaster, S. E., & Morey, L. C. (2012). Predicting law enforcement officer job performance with the Personality Assessment Inventory. *Journal of Personality Assessment, 94*, 254–261. doi:10.1080/00223891.2011.648295

Lubman, D. I., Yucel, M., & Lawrence, A. J. (2008). Inhalant abuse among adolescents: Neurobiological considerations. *British Journal of Pharmacology, 154*, 316–326. doi:10.1038/bjp.2008.76

Lundahl, B., & Burke, B. L. (2009). The effectiveness of motivational interviewing: A practice-friendly review of four meta-analyses. *Journal of Clinical Psychology, 65*, 1232–1245. doi:10.1002/jclp.20638

Lyvers, M., Czerczyk, C., Follent, A., & Lodge, P. (2009). Disinhibition and reward sensitivity in relation to alcohol consumption by university undergraduates. *Addiction Research and Theory, 17,* 668–677. doi:10.3109/16066350802404158

Macdonald, S. (1997). Work-place alcohol and drug testing: A review of the scientific evidence. *Drug and Alcohol Review, 16,* 251–259. doi:10.1080/09595239800187431

Macdonald, S., Csiernik, R., Durand, P., Rylett, M., & Wild, T. C. (2006). Prevalence and factors related to Canadian workplace health programs. *Canadian Journal of Public Health, 97,* 121–125.

Macdonald, S., Csiernik, R., Durand, P., Wild, T. C., Dooley, S., Rylett, M., . . . Sturge, J. (2006). Changes in the prevalence and characteristics of Ontario workplace health programs: 1989 to 2003. *Journal of Workplace Behavioral Health, 22,* 53–64. doi:10.1300/J490v22n01_04

Macdonald, S., Hall, W., Roman, P., Stockwell, T., Coghlan, M., & Nesvaag, S. (2010). Testing for cannabis in the work-place: A review of the evidence. *Addiction, 105,* 408–416. doi:10.1111/j.1360-0443.2009.02808.x

Macdonald, S., Lothian, S., & Wells, S. (1997). Evaluation of an employee assistance program at a transportation company. *Evaluation and Program Planning, 20,* 495–505. doi:10.1016/S0149-7189(97)00028-1

Macdonald, S., Wells, S., & Fry, R. (1993). The limitations of drug screening in the workplace. *International Labour Review, 132,* 95–113.

Macdonald, S., Wells, S., & Wild, T. C. (1999). Occupational risk factors associated with alcohol and drug problems. *American Journal of Drug and Alcohol Abuse, 25,* 351–369. doi:10.1081/ADA-100101865

Madsen, I. E. H., Burr, H., Diderichsen, F., Pejtersen, J. H., Borritz, M., Bjnorner, J. B., & Rugulies, R. (2011). Work-related violence and incident use of psychotropics. *American Journal of Epidemiology, 174,* 1354–1362. doi:10.1093/aje/kwr259

Maisto, S. A., Galizio, M., & Connors, G. J. (2008). *Drug use and abuse* (5th ed.). Belmont, CA: Wadsworth.

Mandell, W., Eaton, W. W., Anthony, J. C., & Garrison, R. (1992). Alcoholism and occupations: A review of and analysis of 104 occupations. *Alcoholism: Clinical and Experimental Research, 16,* 734–746. doi:10.1111/j.1530-0277.1992.tb00670.x

Mangione, T. W., Howland, J., Amick, B., Cote, J., Lee, M., Bell, N., & Levine, S. (1999). Employee drinking practices and work performance. *Journal of Studies on Alcohol, 60,* 261–270.

Manheimer, A. (Ed.). (2007). *Alcohol.* New York, NY: Greenhaven Press.

Marchand, A. (2008). Alcohol use and misuse: What are the contributions of occupation and work organization condition? *BMC Public Health, 8,* Article 333. doi:10.1186/1471-2458-8-333

Markon, K. E., Krueger, R. F., & Watson, D. (2005). Delineating the structure of normal and abnormal personality: An integrative hierarchical approach. *Journal of Personality and Social Psychology, 88,* 139–157. doi:10.1037/0022-3514.88.1.139

Marlatt, G. A., & Witkiewitz, K. (2010). Update on harm-reduction policy and intervention research. *Annual Review of Clinical Psychology, 6,* 591–606. doi:10.1146/annurev.clinpsy.121208.131438

Marmot, M. G., North, F., Feeney, A., & Head, J. (1993). Alcohol consumption and sickness absence: From the Whitehall II study. *Addiction, 88,* 369–382. doi:10.1111/j.1360-0443.1993.tb00824.x

Martin, C. S. (2007). Measuring acute alcohol impairment. In S. B. Karch (Ed.), *Drug abuse handbook* (2nd ed., pp. 316–333). New York, NY: CRC Press.

Martin, J. K., Kraft, J. M., & Roman, P. M. (1994). Extent and impact of alcohol and drug use problems in the workplace: A review of empirical evidence. In S. Macdonald & P. M. Roman (Eds.), *Research advances in alcohol and drug problems: Vol. 2. Drug testing in the workplace* (pp. 3–31). New York, NY: Plenum Press.

Masi, D., Altman, L., Benyon, C., Kennish, R., McCann, B., & Williams, C. (2004). Employee assistance programs in the year 2002. In R. W. Manderscheid & M. J. Henderson (Eds.), *Mental health, United States, 2002* (DHHS Publication No. SMA 3938; pp. 209–223). Rockville, MD: Substance Abuse and Mental Health Services Administration.

Matano, R. A., Koopman, C., Wanat, S. F., Winzelberg, A. J., Whitsell, S. D., Westrup, D., . . . Taylor, C. B. (2007). A pilot study of an interactive web site in the workplace for reducing alcohol consumption. *Journal of Substance Abuse Treatment, 32,* 71–80. doi:10.1016/j.jsat.2006.05.020

Mayhew, D. R., Simpson, H. M., Wood, K. M., Lonero, L., Clinton, K. M., & Johnson, A. G. (2011). On-road and simulated driving: Concurrent and discriminant validation. *Journal of Safety Research, 42,* 267–275. doi:10.1016/j.jsr.2011.06.004

Mazas, C. A., Cofta-Woerpel, L., Daza, P., Fouladi, R. T., Vidrine, J. I., Cinciripini, P. M., . . . Wetter, D. W. (2006). At-risk drinking among employed men and women. *Annals of Behavioral Medicine, 31,* 279–287. doi:10.1207/s15324796abm3103_10

McCrae, R. R., & Costa, P. T., Jr. (1997). Personality trait structure as a human universal. *American Psychologist, 52,* 509–516. doi:10.1037/0003-066X.52.5.509

McFarlin, S. K., & Fals-Stewart, W. (2002). Workplace absenteeism and alcohol use: A sequential analysis. *Psychology of Addictive Behaviors, 16,* 17–21. doi:10.1037/0893-164X.16.1.17

McFarlin, S. K., Fals-Stewart, W., Major, D. A., & Justice, E. M. (2001). Alcohol use and workplace aggression: An examination of perpetration and victimization. *Journal of Substance Abuse, 13,* 303–321. doi:10.1016/S0899-3289(01)00080-3

McKinney, A., & Coyle, K. (2004). Next day effects of a normal night's drinking on memory and psychomotor performance. *Alcohol and Alcoholism, 39,* 509–513. doi:10.1093/alcalc/agh099

McLeod, R., Stockwell, T., Stevens, M., & Phillips, M. (1999). The relationship between alcohol consumption patterns and injury. *Addiction, 94,* 1719–1734. doi:10.1046/j.1360-0443.1999.941117199.x

McMullen, J. (Ed.). (2005). *Marijuana*. New York, NY: Greenhaven Press.

Merikangas, K. R. (1990). The genetic epidemiology of alcoholism. *Psychological Medicine, 20*, 11–22. doi:10.1017/S0033291700013192

Merikangas, K. R., Stolar, M., Stevens, D. E., Goulet, J., Preisig, M. A., Fenton, B., . . . Rounsaville, B. J. (1998). Familial transmission of substance use disorders. *Archives of General Psychiatry, 55*, 973–979. doi:10.1001/archpsyc.55.11.973

Meyer, J. S., & Quenzer, L. F. (2005). *Psychopharmacology: Drugs, the brain, and behavior*. Sunderland, MA: Sinauer Associates.

Miller, N. S., Gold, M. S., & Smith, D. E. (Eds.). (1997). *Manual of therapeutics for addictions*. New York, NY: Wiley.

Ministry of Health. (2007). *Alcohol use in New Zealand: Analysis of the 2004 New Zealand Health Behaviours Survey*. Wellington, New Zealand: Author.

Ministry of Health. (2009). *Alcohol use in New Zealand: Key results of the 2007/08 New Zealand Alcohol and Drug Use Survey*. Wellington, New Zealand: Author.

Mintzer, M. Z. (2007). Effects of opioid pharmacotherapy on psychomotor and cognitive performance: A review of human laboratory studies of methadone and buprenorphine. *Heroin Addiction and Related Clinical Problems, 9*, 5–24.

Moffitt, T. E., Caspi, A., & Rutter, M. (2006). Measured gene–environment interactions in psychopathology: Concepts, research strategies, and implications for research, intervention, and public understanding of genetics. *Perspectives on Psychological Science, 1*, 5–27. doi:10.1111/j.1745-6916.2006.00002.x

Monroe, S. M., & Simons, A. D. (1991). Diathesis–stress theories in the context of life stress: Implications for depressive disorders. *Psychological Bulletin, 110*, 406–425. doi:10.1037/0033-2909.110.3.406

Montoya, A. G., Sorrentino, R., Lukas, S. E., & Price, B. H. (2002). Long-term neuropsychiatric consequences of "ecstasy" (MDMA): A review. *Harvard Review of Psychiatry, 10*, 212–220.

Moore, R. S. (1998). The hangover: An ambiguous concept in workplace alcohol policy. *Contemporary Drug Problems, 25*, 49–63.

Moore, R. S., Ames, G. M., Duke, M. R., & Cunradi, C. B. (2012). Food service employee alcohol use, hangovers and norms during and after work hours. *Journal of Substance Use, 17*, 269–276. doi:10.3109/14659891.2011.580414

Moore, R. S., Cunradi, C. B., Duke, M. R., & Ames, G. M. (2009). Dimensions of problem drinking among young adult restaurant workers. *American Journal of Drug and Alcohol Abuse, 35*, 329–333. doi:10.1080/00952990903075042

Moore, S., Grunberg, L., & Greenberg, E. (2000). The relationships between alcohol problems and well-being, work attitudes, and performance: Are they monotonic? *Journal of Substance Abuse, 11*, 183–204. doi:10.1016/S0899-3289(00)00020-1

Morantz, A. (2008). Does post-accident drug testing reduce injuries? Evidence from a large retail chain. *American Law and Economics Review, 10*, 246–302. doi:10.1093/aler/ahn012

Morgan, C. J., & Curran, H. V. (2012). Ketamine use: A review. *Addiction, 107*, 27–38. doi:10.1111/j.1360-0443.2011.03576.x

Morgan, C. J. A., Muetzelfeldt, L., & Curran, H. V. (2010). Consequences of chronic ketamine self-administration upon neurocognitive function and psychological wellbeing: A 1-year longitudinal study. *Addiction, 105,* 121–133. doi:10.1111/j.1360-0443.2009.02761.x

Morgan, M. J. (2000). Ecstasy (MDMA): A review of its possible persistent psychological effects. *Psychopharmacology, 152,* 230–248. doi:10.1007/s002130000545

Mosher, C. J., & Akins, S. (2007). *Drugs and drug policy: The control of consciousness alteration.* Thousand Oaks, CA: Sage.

Moyer, A., Finney, J. W., Swearingen, E., & Vergun, P. (2002). Brief interventions for alcohol problems: A meta-analytic review of controlled investigations in treatment-seeking and non-treatment-seeking populations. *Addiction, 97,* 279–292. doi:10.1046/j.1360-0443.2002.00018.x

Murphy, K. R., & Thornton, G. C., III. (1992). Characteristics of employee drug testing policies. *Journal of Business and Psychology, 6,* 295–309. doi:10.1007/BF01126767

Musshoff, F., & Madea, B. (2007). New trends in hair analysis and scientific demands on validation and technical notes. *Forensic Science International, 165,* 204–215. doi:10.1016/j.forsciint.2006.05.024

Mustanski, B. S., Viken, R. J., Kaprio, J., & Rose, R. J. (2003). Genetic influences on the association between personality risk factors and alcohol use and abuse. *Journal of Abnormal Psychology, 112,* 282–289. doi:10.1037/0021-843X.112.2.282

National Federation of Independent Business. (2004). *Alcohol, drugs, violence and obesity in the workplace.* Nashville, TN: Author.

Neale, M. C., Harvey, E., Maes, H. H. M., Sullivan, P. F., & Kendler, K. S. (2006). Extensions to the modeling of initiation and progression: Applications to substance use and abuse. *Behavior Genetics, 36,* 507–524. doi:10.1007/s10519-006-9063-x

Newcomb, M. (1994). Prevalence of alcohol and other drug use on the job: Cause for concern or irrational hysteria? *Journal of Drug Issues, 24,* 403–416.

Nichols, D. E. (2004). Hallucinogens. *Pharmacology & Therapeutics, 101,* 131–181. doi:10.1016/j.pharmthera.2003.11.002

Nielsen, K., Randall, R., Holten, A.-L., & Gonzalez, E. R. (2010). Conducting organizational-level occupational health interventions: What works? *Work & Stress, 24,* 234–259. doi:10.1080/02678373.2010.515393

Nochajski, T. H. (1993). Instructional set and visual-motor performance. In H.-D. Utzelmann, G. Berghaus, & G. Kroj (Eds.), *Alcohol, drugs, and traffic safety: Proceedings of the 12th International Conference on Alcohol, Drugs, and Traffic Safety* (pp. 625–630). Cologne, Germany: Verlag TUV Rheinland.

Nolan, S. (2008). Drug-free workplace programmes: New Zealand perspective. *Forensic Science International, 174,* 125–132. doi:10.1016/j.forsciint.2007.03.012

Normand, J., Lempert, R. O., & O'Brien, C. P. (1994). *Under the influence? Drugs and the American work force.* Washington, DC: National Academy Press.

Normand, J., Salyards, S. D., & Mahoney, J. J. (1990). An evaluation of pre-employment drug testing. *Journal of Applied Psychology, 75*, 629–639. doi:10.1037/0021-9010.75.6.629

Norström, T. (2006). Per capita alcohol consumption and sickness absence. *Addiction, 101*, 1421–1427. doi:10.1111/j.1360-0443.2006.01446.x

Nutt, D., King, L. A., Saulsbury, W., & Blakemore, C. (2007). Development of a rational scale to assess the harms of drugs of potential misuse. *Lancet, 369*, 1047–1053. doi:10.1016/S0140-6736(07)60464-4

Office of National Drug Control Policy. (2004). *The economic costs of drug abuse in the United States, 1992–2002* (Publication No. 207303). Washington, DC: Executive Office of the President.

O'Malley, P. M., Johnston, L. D., & Bachman, J. G. (1999). Epidemiology of substance abuse in adolescence. In P. J. Ott, R. E. Tarter, & R. T. Ammerman (Eds.), *Sourcebook on substance abuse: Etiology, epidemiology, assessment, and treatment* (pp. 14–31). Boston, MA: Allyn & Bacon.

Oscar-Berman, M., & Marinkovic, K. (2007). Alcohol: Effects on neurobehavioral functions and the brain. *Neuropsychology Review, 17*, 239–257. doi:10.1007/s11065-007-9038-6

Osilla, K. C., dela Cruz, E., Miles, J. N. V., Zellmer, S., Watkins, K., Larimer, M. E., & Marlatt, G. A. (2010). Exploring productivity outcomes from a brief intervention for at-risk drinking in an employee assistance program. *Addictive Behaviors, 35*, 194–200. doi:10.1016/j.addbeh.2009.10.001

Osilla, K. C., Zellmer, S., Larimer, M. E., Neighbors, C., & Marlatt, G. A. (2008). A brief intervention for at-risk drinking in an employee assistance program. *Journal of Studies on Alcohol and Drugs, 69*, 14–20.

Ozminkowski, R. J., & Goetzel, R. Z. (2001). Getting closer to the truth: Overcoming research challenges when estimating the financial impact of worksite health promotion programs. *American Journal of Health Promotion, 15*, 289–295. doi:10.4278/0890-1171-15.5.289

Ozminkowski, R. J., Mark, T. L., Goetzel, R. Z., Blank, D., Walsh, J. M., & Cangianelli, L. (2003). Relationship between urinalysis testing for substance use, medical expenditures, and the occurrence of injuries at a large manufacturing firm. *American Journal of Drug and Alcohol Abuse, 29*, 151–167. doi:10.1081/ADA-120018844

Pagan, J. L., Rose, R. J., Viken, R. J., Pulkkinen, L., Kaprio, J., & Dick, D. M. (2006). Genetic and environmental influences on stages of alcohol use across adolescence and into young adulthood. *Behavior Genetics, 36*, 483–497. doi:10.1007/s10519-006-9062-y

Pardo, Y., Aguilar, R., Molinuevo, B., & Torrubia, R. (2007). Alcohol use as a behavioral sign of disinhibition: Evidence from J. A. Gray's model of personality. *Addictive Behaviors, 32*, 2398–2403. doi:10.1016/j.addbeh.2007.02.010

Parker, D. A., & Farmer, G. C. (1988). The epidemiology of alcohol abuse among employed men and women. In M. Galanter (Ed.), *Recent developments in alcoholism* (pp. 113–130). New York, NY: Plenum Press. doi:10.1007/978-1-4615-7718-8_6

Parker, D. A., & Harford, T. C. (1992). Gender-role attitudes, job competition and alcohol consumption among women and men. *Alcoholism: Clinical and Experimental Research, 16,* 159–165. doi:10.1111/j.1530-0277.1992.tb01359.x

Parks, K. M., & Steelman, L. A. (2008). Organizational wellness programs: A meta-analysis. *Journal of Occupational Health Psychology, 13,* 58–68. doi:10.1037/1076-8998.13.1.58

Parrott, A. C. (1991a). Performance tests in human psychopharmacology (1): Test reliability and standardization. *Human Psychopharmacology: Clinical and Experimental, 6,* 1–9. doi:10.1002/hup.470060102

Parrott, A. C. (1991b). Performance tests in human psychopharmacology (3): Construct validity and test interpretation. *Human Psychopharmacology: Clinical and Experimental, 6,* 197–207. doi:10.1002/hup.470060303

Parrott, A. C. (2001). Human psychopharmacology of ecstasy (MDMA): A review of 15 years of empirical research. *Human Psychopharmacology: Clinical and Experimental, 16,* 557–577. doi:10.1002/hup.351

Parsons, O. A., & Nixon, S. J. (1998). Cognitive functioning in sober social drinkers: A review of the research since 1986. *Journal of Studies on Alcohol, 59,* 180–190.

Patat, A. (2000). Clinical pharmacology of psychotropic drugs. *Human Psychopharmacology: Clinical and Experimental, 15,* 361–387. doi:10.1002/1099-1077(200007)15:5<361::AID-HUP205>3.0.CO;2-1

Patel, A. B., & Fromme, K. (2010). Explicit outcome expectancies and substance use: Current research and future directions. In L. M. Scheier (Ed.), *Handbook of drug use etiology: Theory, methods, and empirical findings* (pp. 147–164). Washington, DC: American Psychological Association.

Patrick, M. E., Wray-Lake, L., Finlay, A. K., & Maggs, J. L. (2010). The long arm of expectancies: Adolescent alcohol expectancies predict adult alcohol use. *Alcohol and Alcoholism, 45,* 17–24. doi:10.1093/alcalc/agp066

Patterson, C. R., Bennett, J. B., & Wiitala, W. L. (2005). Healthy and unhealthy unwinding: Promoting health in small business. *Journal of Business and Psychology, 20,* 221–247. doi:10.1007/s10869-005-8261-5

Pearlin, L. I., Menaghan, E. G., Lieberman, M. A., & Mullan, J. T. (1981). The stress process. *Journal of Health and Social Behavior, 22,* 337–356. doi:10.2307/2136676

Pearson, T. A., & Manolio, T. A. (2008). How to interpret a genome-wide association study. *JAMA, 299,* 1335–1344. doi:10.1001/jama.299.11.1335

Peirce, R. S., Frone, M. R., Russell, M., Cooper, M. L., & Mudar, P. (2000). A longitudinal model of social contact, social support, depression, and alcohol use. *Health Psychology, 19,* 28–38. doi:10.1037/0278-6133.19.1.28

Pelfrene, E., Vlerick, P., Moreau, M., Mak, R. P., Kornitzer, M., & De Backer, G. (2004). Use of benzodiazepine drugs and perceived job stress in a cohort of working men and women in Belgium: Results from the BELSTRESS study. *Social Science & Medicine, 59,* 433–442. doi:10.1016/j.socscimed.2003.11.002

Perez, A. Y., Kirkpatrick, M. G., Gunderson, E. W., Marrone, G., Silver, R., Foltin, R. W., & Hart, C. L. (2008). Residual effects of intranasal methamphetamine on sleep, mood, and performance. *Drug and Alcohol Dependence, 94,* 258–262. doi:10.1016/j.drugalcdep.2007.10.011

Peter, R., & Siegrist, J. (1997). Chronic work stress, sickness absence, and hypertension in middle managers: General or specific sociological explanations? *Social Science & Medicine, 45,* 1111–1120. doi:10.1016/S0277-9536(97)00039-7

Pfeffer, J., & Sutton, R. I. (2006). *Hard facts, dangerous half-truths, and total nonsense: Profiting from evidence-based management.* Boston, MA: Harvard Business School Press.

Pickering, A. D., & Gray, J. A. (1999). The neuroscience of personality. In L. A. Pervin & O. P. John (Eds.), *Handbook of personality: Theory and research* (2nd ed., pp. 277–299). New York, NY: Guilford Press.

Pidd, K., Berry, J. G., Harrison, J. E., Roche, A. M., Driscoll, T. R., & Newson, R. S. (2006). *Alcohol and work: Patterns of use, workplace culture and safety* (Injury Research and Statistics Series No. 28). Adelaide, Australia: Australian Institute of Health and Welfare.

Pierce, A. (2007). Workplace drug testing outside the U.S. In S. B. Karch (Ed.), *Drug abuse handbook* (pp. 765–775). New York, NY: CRC Press.

Pil, K., & Verstraete, A. (2008). Current developments in drug testing in oral fluid. *Therapeutic Drug Monitoring, 30,* 196–202. doi:10.1097/FTD.0b013e318167d563

Plant, M. A. (1978). Occupation and alcoholism: Cause or effect? A controlled study of recruits to the drink trade. *International Journal of the Addictions, 13,* 605–626.

Plomin, R., & Caspi, A. (1999). Behavioral genetics and personality. In L. A. Pervin & O. P. John (Eds.), *Handbook of personality: Theory and research* (2nd ed., pp. 251–276). New York, NY: Guilford Press.

Plomin, R., DeFries, J. C., McClearn, G. E., & McGuffin, P. (2008). *Behavioral genetics* (5th ed.). New York, NY: Worth.

Posthuma, D., Beem, A. L., de Geus, E. J. C., Van Baal, G. C. M., von Hjelmborg, J. B., Iachine, I., & Boomsma, D. I. (2003). Theory and practice in quantitative genetics. *Twin Research, 6,* 361–376. doi:10.1375/136905203770326367

Pragst, F., & Balivova, M. A. (2006). State of the art in hair analysis for detection of drug and alcohol abuse. *Clinica Chimica Acta, 370,* 17–49. doi:10.1016/j.cca.2006.02.019

Prat, G., Adan, A., Perez-Pamies, M., & Sanchez-Turet, M. (2008). Neurocognitive effects of alcohol hangover. *Addictive Behaviors, 33,* 15–23. doi:10.1016/j.addbeh.2007.05.002

Prat, G., Adan, A., & Sanchez-Turet, M. (2009). Alcohol hangover: A critical review. *Human Psychopharmacology: Clinical and Experimental, 24,* 259–267. doi:10.1002/hup.1023

Prescott, C. A. (2002). Sex differences in the genetic risk for alcoholism. *Alcohol Research & Health, 26,* 264–273.

Prescott, C. A., Madden, P. A. F., & Stallings, M. C. (2006). Challenges in genetic studies of the etiology of substance use and substance use disorders: Introduction to the special section. *Behavior Genetics, 36,* 473–482.

Price, D. L., & Flax, R. A. (1982). Alcohol, task difficulty, and incentives in drill press operation. *Human Factors, 24,* 573–579.

Price, D. L., & Hicks, T. G. (1979). The effects of alcohol on performance of a production assembly task. *Ergonomics, 22*, 37–41. doi:10.1080/00140137908924587

Price, D. L., & Liddle, R. J. (1982). The effect of alcohol on a manual arc welding task. *Welding Journal, 61*, 15–19.

Price, D. L., Radwan, M. A. E., & Tergou, D. D. (1986). Gender, alcohol, pacing, and incentive effects on an electronics assembly task. *Ergonomics, 29*, 393–406. doi:10.1080/00140138608968273

Prottas, D. J., Diamante, T., & Sandys, J. (2011). The U.S. domestic workforce use of employee assistance support services: An analysis of ten years of data. *Journal of Workplace Behavioral Health, 26*, 296–312. doi:10.1080/155552 40.2011.618431

Quest Diagnostics Incorporated. (2004). *Increased use of amphetamines linked to rising workplace drug use, according to Quest Diagnostics' 2003 Drug Testing Index* [Press release]. Lyndhurst, NJ: Author.

Quest Diagnostics Incorporated. (2010). *The Drug Testing Index.* Lyndhurst, NJ: Author.

Quest Diagnostics Incorporated. (2011). *The Drug Testing Index.* Lyndhurst, NJ: Author.

Ragland, D. R., Greiner, B. A., Krause, N., Holman, B. L., & Fisher, J. M. (1995). Occupational and nonoccupational correlates of alcohol consumption in urban transit drivers. *Preventive Medicine, 24*, 634–645. doi:10.1006/pmed.1995.1099

Ramaekers, J. G., Kauert, G., Theunissen, E. L., Toennes, S. W., & Moeller, M. R. (2009). Neurocognitive performance during acute THC intoxication in heavy and occasional cannabis users. *Journal of Psychopharmacology, 23*, 266–277. doi:10.1177/0269881108092393

Ramchand, R., Pomeroy, A., & Arkes, J. (2009). *The effects of substance use on workplace injuries.* Santa Monica, CA: Rand Corporation.

Ranganathan, M., & D'Souza, D. C. (2006). The acute effect of cannabinoids on memory in humans: A review. *Psychopharmacology, 188*, 425–444. doi:10.1007/s00213-006-0508-y

Rees, K., Allen, D., & Lader, M. (1999). The influences of age and caffeine on psychomotor and cognitive function. *Psychopharmacology, 145*, 181–188. doi:10.1007/s002130051047

Rehm, J., Baliunas, D., Brochu, S., Fischer, B., Gnam, W., Patra, J., . . . Taylor, B. (2006). *The costs of substance use in Canada 2002.* Ottawa, Ontario, Canada: Canadian Centre on Substance Abuse.

Reuter, P. (1993). Prevalence estimation and policy formulation. *Journal of Drug Issues, 23*, 167–184.

Reuter, P. (1999). Are calculations of the economic costs of drug abuse either possible or useful? *Addiction, 94*, 635–638.

Rice, D. P. (1999). Economic costs of substance abuse, 1995. *Proceedings of the Association of American Physicians, 111*, 119–125. doi:10.1046/j.1525-1381.1999.09254.x

Rice, D. P., Kelman, S., Miller, L. S., & Dunmeyer, S. (1990). *The economic costs of alcohol and drug abuse and mental illness: 1985.* Washington, DC: U.S. Department of Health and Human Services.

Richman, J. A., Rospenda, K. M., Nawyn, S. J., Flaherty, J. A., Fendrich, M., Drum, M. L., & Johnson, T. P. (1999). Sexual harassment and generalized workplace abuse among university employees: Prevalence and mental health correlates. *American Journal of Public Health, 89*, 358–363. doi:10.2105/AJPH.89.3.358

Rinaldi, R. C., Steindler, E. M., Wilford, B. B., & Goodwin, D. (1988). Clarification and standardization of substance abuse terminology. *JAMA, 259*, 555–557. doi:10.1001/jama.1988.03720040047025

Roche, A., & Pidd, K. (2006). *Workers' alcohol use and absenteeism*. Adelaide, Australia: Flinders University, National Centre for Education and Training on Addiction.

Roche, A. M., Pidd, K., Berry, J. G., & Harrison, J. E. (2008). Workers' drinking patterns: The impact on absenteeism in the Australian work-place. *Addiction, 103*, 738–748. doi:10.1111/j.1360-0443.2008.02154.x

Roche, A. M., Pidd, K., Bywood, P., & Freeman, T. (2008). Methamphetamine use among Australian workers and its implications for prevention. *Drug and Alcohol Review, 27*, 334–341. doi:10.1080/09595230801919478

Roese, N. J., & Sherman, J. W. (2007). Expectancy. In A. W. Kruglanski & E. Tory Higgins (Eds.), *Social psychology: Handbook of basic principles* (2nd ed., pp. 91–115). New York, NY: Guilford Press.

Rohsenow, D. J., Howland, J., Arnedt, J. T., Almeida, A. B., Greece, J., Minsky, S., . . . Sales, S. (2010). Intoxication with bourbon versus vodka: Effects on hangover, sleep, and next-day neurocognitive performance in young adults. *Alcoholism: Clinical and Experimental Research, 34*, 509–518. doi:10.1111/j.1530-0277.2009.01116.x

Rohsenow, D. J., Howland, J., Minsky, S. J., & Arnedt, J. T. (2006). Effects of heavy drinking by maritime academy cadets on hangover, perceived sleep, and next-day ship power plant operation. *Journal of Studies on Alcohol, 67*, 406–415.

Roman, P. M. (1980). Medicalization and social control in the workplace: Prospects for the 1980s. *Journal of Applied Behavioral Science, 16*, 407–422. doi:10.1177/002188638001600309

Roman, P. M. (2002). Missing work: The decline in infrastructure and support for workplace alcohol intervention in the United States, with implications for developments in other nations. In W. Miller & C. Weisner (Eds.), *Changing substance abuse through health and social systems* (pp. 197–210). New York, NY: Kluwer/Plenum. doi:10.1007/978-1-4615-0669-0_15

Roman, P. M., & Baker, S. C. (2002). Alcohol and drug problem management in the workplace. In J. C. Thomas & M. Hersen (Eds.), *Handbook of mental health in the workplace* (pp. 371–380). Thousand Oaks, CA: Sage.

Roman, P. M., & Blum, T. C. (1995). *Employers*. In R. H. Coombs & D. M. Ziedonis (Eds.), *Handbook on drug abuse prevention* (pp. 129–158). Englewood Cliffs, NJ: Prentice Hall.

Roman, P. M., & Blum, T. C. (1999). Externalization and internalization as frames for understanding workplace deviance: The management of alcohol and drug abuse. *Research in the Sociology of Work, 8,* 139–164.

Roman, P. M., & Blum, T. C. (2002). The workplace and alcohol problem prevention. *Alcohol Research & Health, 26,* 49–57.

Roman, P. M., & Knudsen, H. K. (2009). Drug testing, the workplace, and other applications. In L. M. Cohen, A. Young, D. E. McChargue, T. R. Leffingwell, & K. L. Cook (Eds.), *Pharmacology and treatment of substance abuse: Evidence- and outcome-based perspectives* (pp. 465–476). New York, NY: Routledge.

Romero, R., Kuivaniemi, H., Tromp, G., & Olson, J. M. (2002). The design, execution, and interpretation of genetic association studies to decipher complex diseases. *American Journal of Obstetrics and Gynecology, 187,* 1299–1312. doi:10.1067/mob.2002.128319

Roos, E., Lahelma, E., & Rahkonen, O. (2006). Work–family conflicts and drinking behaviours among employed men and women. *Drug and Alcohol Dependence, 83,* 49–56. doi:10.1016/j.drugalcdep.2005.10.009

Rospenda, K. M. (2002). Workplace harassment, services utilization, and drinking outcomes. *Journal of Occupational Health Psychology, 7,* 141–155. doi:10.1037/1076-8998.7.2.141

Rospenda, K. M., Fujishiro, K., Shannon, C. A., & Richman, J. A. (2008). Workplace harassment, stress, and drinking behavior over time: Gender differences in a national sample. *Addictive Behaviors, 33,* 964–967. doi:10.1016/j.addbeh.2008.02.009

Rospenda, K. M., Richman, J. A., & Shannon, C. A. (2009). Prevalence and mental health correlates of harassment in the workplace: Results from a national study. *Journal of Interpersonal Violence, 24,* 819–843. doi:10.1177/0886260508317182

Rospenda, K. M., Richman, J. A., Wislar, J. S., & Flaherty, J. A. (2000). Chronicity of sexual harassment and generalized workplace abuse: Effects on drinking outcomes. *Addiction, 95,* 1805–1820. doi:10.1046/j.1360-0443.2000.9512180510.x

Rosta, J. (2008). Hazardous alcohol use among hospital doctors in Germany. *Alcohol and Alcoholism, 43,* 198–203. doi:10.1093/alcalc/agm180

Rousseau, D. M., & McCarthy, S. (2007). Educating managers from an evidence-based perspective. *Academy of Management Learning & Education, 6,* 84–101. doi:10.5465/AMLE.2007.24401705

Roxburgh, S. (1998). Gender differences in the effect of job stressors on alcohol consumption. *Addictive Behaviors, 23,* 101–107. doi:10.1016/S0306-4603(97)00025-7

Roy-Byrne, P. P., & Cowley, D. S. (1990). The use of benzodiazepines in the workplace. *Journal of Psychoactive Drugs, 22,* 461–465. doi:10.1080/02791072.1990.10472220

Rutter, M., Moffitt, T. E., & Caspi, A. (2006). Gene–environment interplay and psychopathology: Multiple varieties but real effects. *Journal of Child Psychology and Psychiatry, 47,* 226–261. doi:10.1111/j.1469-7610.2005.01557.x

Saitz, R. (1998). Introduction to alcohol withdrawal. *Alcohol Health & Research World, 22,* 5–12.

Salonsalmi, A., Laaksonen, M., Lahelma, E., & Rahkonen, O. (2009). Drinking habits and sickness absence: The contribution of working conditions. *Scandinavian Journal of Public Health, 37,* 846–854. doi:10.1177/1403494809350519

Sayette, M. A. (1999). Does drinking reduce stress? *Alcohol Research & Health, 23,* 250–255.

Schafer, J., & Brown, S. A. (1991). Marijuana and cocaine effect expectancies and drug use patterns. *Journal of Consulting and Clinical Psychology, 59,* 558–565. doi:10.1037/0022-006X.59.4.558

Schat, A. C. H., Frone, M. R., & Kelloway, E. K. (2006). Prevalence of workplace aggression in the U.S. workforce: Findings from a national study. In E. K. Kelloway, J. Barling, & J. Hurrell (Eds.), *Handbook of workplace violence* (pp. 47–89). Thousand Oaks, CA: Sage.

Schreier, J. W. (1987). *Substance abuse in organizations 1971–1986: Realities, trends, reactions.* Milwaukee, WI: Far Cliffs Consulting.

Schults, T. F. (2007). Current legal issues in workplace drug testing. In S. B. Karch (Ed.), *Drug abuse handbook* (pp. 878–893). New York, NY: CRC Press.

Schwenk, C. R. (1998). Marijuana and job performance: Comparing the major streams of research. *Journal of Drug Issues, 28,* 941–970.

Science of Genetics Review Group. (2010). *Science of genetics review.* Bethesda, MD: National Institute on Drug Abuse.

Scott, J. C., Woods, S. P., Matt, G. E., Meyer, R. A., Heaton, R. K., Atkinson, J. H., & Grant, I. (2007). Neurocognitive effects of methamphetamine: A critical review and meta-analysis. *Neuropsychology Review, 17,* 275–297. doi:10.1007/s11065-007-9031-0

Segel, J. E. (2006). *Cost-of-illness studies: A primer.* Triangle Park, NC: RTI International.

Shain, M. (1990). Health promotion programs and the prevention of alcohol abuse: Forging a link. In P. M. Roman (Ed.), *Alcohol problem intervention in the workplace: Employee assistance programs and strategic alternatives* (pp. 163–179). New York, NY: Quorum.

Shain, M., & Groeneveld, J. (1980). *Employee-assistance programs.* Lexington, MA: Lexington Books.

Sher, K. J., Bartholow, B. D., & Wood, M. D. (2000). Personality and substance use disorders: A prospective study. *Journal of Consulting and Clinical Psychology, 68,* 818–829. doi:10.1037/0022-006X.68.5.818

Sher, K. J., Trull, T. J., Bartholow, B. D., & Vieth, A. (1999). Personality and alcoholism: Issues, methods, and etiological processes. In K. E. Leonard & H. T. Blane (Eds.), *Psychological theories of drinking and alcoholism* (2nd ed., pp. 54–105). New York, NY: Guilford Press.

Sher, K. J., Wood, M. D., Wood, P. K., & Raskin, G. (1996). Alcohol outcome expectancies and alcohol use: A latent variable cross-lagged panel study. *Journal of Abnormal Psychology, 105,* 561–574. doi:10.1037/0021-843X.105.4.561

Sieck, C. J., & Heirich, M. (2010). Focusing attention on substance abuse in the workplace: A comparison of the workplace interventions. *Journal of Workplace Behavioral Health, 25,* 72–87. doi:10.1080/15555240903358744

Silber, B. Y., Croft, R. J., Papafotiou, K., & Stough, C. (2006). The acute effects of *d*-amphetamine and methamphetamine on attention and psychomotor performance. *Psychopharmacology, 187,* 154–169. doi:10.1007/s00213-006-0410-7

Single, E. W. (1988). The availability theory of alcohol related problems. In C. D. Chaudron & D. A. Wilkinson (Eds.), *Theories of alcoholism* (pp. 325–351). Toronto, Ontario, Canada: Addiction Research Foundation.

Single, E. (2009). Why we should still estimate the costs of substance abuse even if we needn't pay undue attention to the bottom line. *Drug and Alcohol Review, 28,* 117–121. doi:10.1111/j.1465-3362.2008.00040.x

Single, E., Collins, D., Easton, B., Harwood, H., Lapsley, H., Kopp, P., & Wilson, E. (2001). *International guidelines for estimating the costs of substance abuse: 2001 edition.* Geneva, Switzerland: World Health Organization.

Smith, A. M., Longo, C. A., Fried, P. A., Hogan, M. J., & Cameron, I. (2010). Effects of marijuana on visuospatial working memory: An fMRI study in young adults. *Psychopharmacology, 210,* 429–438. doi:10.1007/s00213-010-1841-8

Smith, A., Wadsworth, E., Moss, S., & Simpson, S. (2004). *The scale and impact of illegal drug use by workers* (Research Report No. 93). London, England: Health and Safety Executive.

Snow, D. L., Swan, S. C., & Wilton, L. (2003). A workplace coping-skills intervention to prevent alcohol abuse. In J. B. Bennett & W. E. K. Lehman (Eds.), *Preventing workplace substance abuse: Beyond drug testing to wellness* (pp. 57–96). Washington, DC: American Psychological Association. doi:10.1037/10476-002

Snowden, C. B., Miller, T. R., Waehrer, G. M., & Spicer, R. S. (2007). Random alcohol testing reduced alcohol-involved fatal crashes of drivers of large trucks. *Journal of Studies on Alcohol and Drugs, 68,* 634–640.

Solowij, N., & Battisti, R. (2008). The chronic effect of cannabis on memory: A review. *Current Drug Abuse Reviews, 1,* 81–98. doi:10.2174/1874473710801010081

Spada, M. M., Moneta, G. B., & Wells, A. (2007). The relative contribution of metacognitive beliefs and expectancies on drinking behavior. *Alcohol and Alcoholism, 42,* 567–574. doi:10.1093/alcalc/agm055

Spector, P. E., Zapf, D., Chen, P. Y., & Frese, M. (2000). Why negative affectivity should not be controlled in job stress research: Don't throw out the baby with the bath water. *Journal of Organizational Behavior, 21,* 79–95. doi:10.1002/(SICI)1099-1379(200002)21:1<79::AID-JOB964>3.0.CO;2-G

Spell, C. S., & Blum, T. C. (2001). Organizational adoption of preemployment drug testing. *Journal of Occupational Health Psychology, 6,* 114–126. doi:10.1037/1076-8998.6.2.114

Spell, C. S., & Blum, T. C. (2005). Adoption of workplace substance abuse prevention programs: Strategic choice and institutional perspectives. *Academy of Management Journal, 48,* 1125–1142. doi:10.5465/AMJ.2005.19573113

Spetch, A., Howland, A., & Lowman, R. L. (2011). EAP utilization patterns and employee absenteeism: Results of an empirical, 3-year longitudinal study in a national Canadian retail corporation. *Consulting Psychology Journal: Practice and Research, 63*, 110–128. doi:10.1037/a0024690

Spicer, R. S., & Miller, T. R. (2005). Impact of a workplace peer-focused substance abuse prevention and early intervention program. *Alcoholism: Clinical and Experimental Research, 29*, 609–611. doi:10.1097/01.ALC.0000158831.43241.B4

Stallones, L., & Kraus, J. E. (1993). The occurrence and epidemiologic features of alcohol-related occupational injuries. *Addiction, 88*, 945–951. doi:10.1111/j.1360-0443.1993.tb02112.x

Steele, P. D. (1989). A history of job-based alcoholism programs: 1955–1972. *Journal of Drug Issues, 19*, 511–532.

Steele, P. D. (1995). A history of job-based alcoholism programs: 1972–1980. *Journal of Drug Issues, 25*, 397–422.

Steele, P. D. (1998, September). *Employee assistance programs: Then, now, and in the future.* Paper presented at the Center for Substance Abuse Prevention's Knowledge Exchange Workshop, Tacoma, WA.

Stein, R. A., & Strickland, T. L. (1998). A review of the neuropsychological effects of commonly used prescription medications. *Archives of Clinical Neuropsychology, 13*, 259–284.

Stephens, R., Ling, J., Heffernan, T. M., Heather, N., & Jones, K. (2008). A review of the literature on the cognitive effects of alcohol hangover. *Alcohol and Alcoholism, 43*, 163–170. doi:10.1093/alcalc/agm160

Steptoe, A., Wardle, J., Lipsey, Z., Mills, R., Oliver, G., Jarvis, M., & Kirschbaum, C. A. (1998). Longitudinal study of workload and variations in psychological well-being, cortisol, smoking, and alcohol consumption. *Annals of Behavioral Medicine, 20*, 84–91. doi:10.1007/BF02884453

Sterud, T., Hem, E., Ekeberg, O., & Lau, B. (2007). Occupational stress and alcohol use: A study of two nationwide samples of operational police and ambulance personnel in Norway. *Journal of Studies on Alcohol and Drugs, 68*, 896–904.

Stewart, W. F., Ricci, J. A., Chee, E., & Morganstein, D. (2003). Lost productive work time costs from health conditions in the United States: Results from the American Productivity Audit. *Journal of Occupational and Environmental Medicine, 45*, 1234–1246. doi:10.1097/01.jom.0000099999.27348.78

Stone, A. A., Turkkan, J. S., Bachrach, C. A., Jobe, J. B., Kurtzman, H. S., & Cain, V. S. (Eds.). (2000). *The science of self-report: Implications for research and practice.* Mahwah, NJ: Erlbaum.

Storr, C. L., Trinkoff, A. M., & Anthony, J. C. (1999). Job strain and non-medical drug use. *Drug and Alcohol Dependence, 55*, 45–51. doi:10.1016/S0376-8716(98)00181-1

Stough, C., King, R., Papafotiou, K., Swann, P., Ogden, E., Wesnes, K., & Downey, L. A. (2012). The acute effects of 3,4-methylenedioxymethamphetamine and d-methamphetamine on human cognitive functioning. *Psychopharmacology, 220*, 799–807. doi:10.1007/s00213-011-2532-9

Strauss, E., Sherman, E. M. S., & Spreen, O. (2006). *A compendium of neuropsychological tests: Administration, norms, and commentary.* New York, NY: Oxford University Press.

Streufert, S., Pogash, R., Braig, D., Gingrich, D., Kantner, A., Landis, R., . . . Severs, W. (1995). Alcohol hangover and managerial effectiveness. *Alcoholism: Clinical and Experimental Research, 19,* 1141–1146. doi:10.1111/j.1530-0277.1995. tb01592.x

Streufert, S., Pogash, R., Roache, J., Severs, W., Gingrich, D., Landis, R., . . . Kantner, A. (1994). Alcohol and managerial performance. *Journal of Studies on Alcohol, 55,* 230–238.

Streufert, S., Satish, U., Pogash, R., Gingrich, D., Landis, J. R., Lonardi, L., . . . Roache, J. D. (1996). Effects of alprazolam on complex human functioning. *Journal of Applied Social Psychology, 26,* 1912–1930. doi:10.1111/j.1559-1816.1996.tb00105.x

Stuck, M., English, A. J., & Chandler, W. S. (1998). Comparison of positive screening and confirmatory results. *Professional Safety, 43,* 34–36.

Sullivan, W. C. (1905). Industrial alcoholism. *Economic Review, 15,* 150–163.

Swan, G. E., Carmelli, D., & Cardon, L. R. (1996). The consumption of tobacco, alcohol, and coffee in Caucasian male twins: A multivariate genetic analysis. *Journal of Substance Abuse, 8,* 19–31. doi:10.1016/S0899-3289(96)90055-3

Swena, D. D., & Gaines, W., Jr. (1999). Effect of random drug screening on fatal commercial truck accident rates. *International Journal of Drug Testing, 2,* 1–13.

Swendsen, J., Conway, K. P., Degenhardt, L., Glantz, M., Jin, R., Merikangas, K. R., . . . Kessler, R. C. (2010). Mental disorders as risk factors for substance use, abuse and dependence: Results from the 10-year follow-up of the National Comorbidity Survey. *Addiction, 105,* 1117–1128. doi:10.1111/j.1360-0443.2010.02902.x

Swift, R., & Davidson, D. (1998). Alcohol hangover: Mechanisms and mediators. *Alcohol Health & Research World, 22,* 54–60.

Tait, R. J., MacKinnin, A., & Christensen, H. (2011). Cannabis use and cognitive function: 8-year trajectory in a young adult cohort. *Addiction, 106,* 2195–2203. doi:10.1111/j.1360-0443.2011.03574.x

Taylor, B., Irving, H. M., Kanteres, F., Room, R., Borges, G., Cherpitel, C., . . . Rehm, J. (2010). The more you drink, the harder you fall: A systematic review and meta-analysis of how acute alcohol consumption and injury or collision risk increase together. *Drug and Alcohol Dependence, 110,* 108–116. doi:10.1016/j.drugalcdep.2010.02.011

Taylor, F. W. (1915). *Principles of scientific management.* New York, NY: Harper.

Temple, E. C., Brown, R. E., & Hine, D. W. (2011). The "grass ceiling": Limitations in the literature hinder our understanding of cannabis use and its consequences. *Addiction, 106,* 238–244. doi:10.1111/j.1360-0443.2010.03139.x

Terracciano, A., Löckenhoff, C. E., Crum, R. M., Bienvenu, J., & Costa, P. T. (2008). Five-factor model personality profiles of drug users. *BMC Psychiatry, 8,* Article 22. Retrieved from http://www.biomedcentral.com/1471-244x/8/22

Teter, C. J., & Guthrie, S. K. (2001). A comprehensive review of MDMA and GHB: Two common club drugs. *Pharmacotherapy, 21,* 1486–1513. doi:10.1592/phco.21.20.1486.34472

Thavorncharoensap, M., Teerawattananon, Y., Yothasamut, J., Lertpitakpong, C., & Chaikledkaew, U. (2009). The economic impact of alcohol consumption: A systematic review. *Substance Abuse Treatment, Prevention, and Policy, 4,* Article 20. doi:10.1186/1747-597X-4-20

Thomas, C. (1997). Drug testing in the workplace. *New Zealand Journal of Industrial Relations, 22,* 159–169.

Torrealday, O., Stein, L. A. R., Barnett, N., Golembeske, C., Lebau, R., Colby, S. M., & Monti, P. M. (2008). Validation of the Marijuana Effect Expectancy Questionnaire—Brief. *Journal of Child & Adolescent Substance Abuse, 17,* 1–17. doi:10.1080/15470650802231861

Tourangeau, R., Rips, L. J., & Rasinski, K. (2000). *The psychology of survey response.* New York, NY: Cambridge University Press.

Trice, H. M., Beyer, J. M., & Hunt, R. E. (1978). Evaluating implementation of a job-based alcoholism policy. *Journal of Studies on Alcohol, 39,* 448–465.

Trice, H. M., & Schonbrunn, M. (1981). A history of job-based alcoholism programs: 1900–1955. *Journal of Drug Issues, 11,* 171–198.

Trice, H. M., & Sonnenstuhl, W. J. (1990). On the construction of drinking norms in work organizations. *Journal of Studies on Alcohol, 51,* 201–220.

Trinkoff, A. M., Storr, C. L., & Wall, M. P. (1999). Prescription-type drug misuse and workplace access among nurses. *Journal of Addictive Diseases, 18,* 9–17. doi:10.1300/J069v18n01_02

Trinkoff, A. M., Zhou, Q., Storr, C. L., & Soeken, K. L. (2000). Workplace access, negative proscriptions, job strain, and substance use in registered nurses. *Nursing Research, 49,* 83–90. doi:10.1097/00006199-200003000-00004

Tsanaclis, L., & Wicks, J. F. C. (2007). Patterns of drug use in the United Kingdom as revealed through analysis of hair in a large population sample. *Forensic Science International, 170,* 121–128. doi:10.1016/j.forsciint.2007.03.033

Turkkan, J. S. (2000). General issues in self-report. In A. A. Stone, J. S. Turkkan, C. A. Bachrach, J. B. Jobe, H. S. Kurtzman, & V. S. Cain (Eds.), *The science of self-report: Implications for research and practice* (pp. 1–2). Mahwah, NJ: Erlbaum.

Uhl, G. R. (2004). Molecular genetic underpinnings of human substance abuse vulnerability: Likely contributions to understanding addiction as a mnemonic process. *Neuropharmacology, 47*(Suppl. 1), 140–147. doi:10.1016/j.neuropharm.2004.07.029

Upmark, M., Moller, J., & Romelsjo, A. (1999). Longitudinal, population-based study of self reported alcohol habits, high levels of sickness absence, and disability pensions. *Journal of Epidemiology and Community Health, 53,* 223–229. doi:10.1136/jech.53.4.223

U.S. Department of Health and Human Services. (1998). *Preliminary results from the 1997 National Household Survey on Drug Abuse.* Washington, DC: Government Printing Office.

U.S. Department of Health and Human Services. (1999). *Substance use and mental health characteristics by employment status* (DHHS Publication No. SMA 99-3311). Washington, DC: U.S. Government Printing Office.

U.S. Department of Health and Human Services. (2000). *Healthy People 2010* (2nd ed., Vol. 2). Washington, DC: U.S. Government Printing Office.

U.S. Department of Health and Human Services. (2009). *Results from the 2008 National Survey of Drug Use and Health: Detailed tables*. Rockville, MD: Author.

U.S. Department of Labor. (1990). *An employer's guide to dealing with substance abuse*. Washington, DC: Author.

U.S. Office of Management and Budget. (2000). *Standard occupational classification manual*. Lanham, MD: Bernan Press.

Vahtera, J., Poikolainen, K., Kivimäki, M., Ala-Mursula, L., & Pentti, J. (2002). Alcohol intake and sickness absence: A curvilinear relation. *American Journal of Epidemiology, 156*, 969–976. doi:10.1093/aje/kwf138

Vasse, R. M., Nijhuis, F. J. N., & Kok, G. (1998). Associations between work stress, alcohol consumption, and sickness absence. *Addiction, 93*, 231–241. doi:10.1046/j.1360-0443.1998.9322317.x

Veazie, M. A., & Smith, G. S. (2000). Heavy drinking, alcohol dependence, and injuries at work among young workers in the United States labor force. *Alcoholism: Clinical and Experimental, 24*, 1811–1819. doi:10.1111/j.1530-0277.2000.tb01985.x

Verkes, R. J., Gijsman, H. J., Pieters, M. S. M., Schoemaker, R. C., de Visser, S., Kuijpers, M., . . . Cohen, A. F. (2001). Cognitive performance and serotonergic function in users of ecstasy. *Psychopharmacology, 153*, 196–202. doi:10.1007/s002130000563

Vermeeren, A., & Coenen, A. M. L. (2011). Effects of the use of hypnotics on cognition. *Progress in Brain Research, 190*, 89–103. doi:10.1016/B978-0-444-53817-8.00005-0

Verster, J. C. (2008). The alcohol hangover—A puzzling phenomenon. *Alcohol and Alcoholism, 43*, 124–126. doi:10.1093/alcalc/agm163

Verster, J. C., van Duin, D., Volkerts, E. R., Schreuder, A. H. C. L., & Verbaten, M. N. (2003). Alcohol hangover effects on memory functioning and vigilance performance after an evening of binge drinking. *Neuropsychopharmacology, 28*, 740–746. doi:10.1038/sj.npp.1300090

Verster, J. C., & Volkerts, E. R. (2004). Clinical pharmacology, clinical efficacy, and behavioral toxicity of alprazolam: A review of the literature. *CNS Drug Reviews, 10*, 45–76. doi:10.1111/j.1527-3458.2004.tb00003.x

Verstraete, A. G. (2004). Detection times of drugs of abuse in blood, urine, and oral fluid. *Therapeutic Drug Monitoring, 26*, 200–205. doi:10.1097/00007691-200404000-00020

Verstraete, A. G., & Pierce, A. (2001). Workplace drug testing in Europe. *Forensic Science International, 121*, 2–6. doi:10.1016/S0379-0738(01)00445-5

Verstraete, A. G., & Walsh, J. M. (2007). Point of collection testing of alternative specimens (other than urine). In S. B. Karch (Ed.), *Drug abuse handbook* (pp. 898–908). New York, NY: CRC Press.

Vogel-Sprott, M. (1992). *Alcohol tolerance and social drinking*. New York, NY: Guilford Press.

Wadsworth, E. J. K., Moss, S. C., Simpson, S. A., & Smith, A. P. (2006). Cannabis use, cognitive performance and mood in a sample of workers. *Journal of Psychopharmacology (Oxford, England), 20*, 14–23. doi:10.1177/0269881105056644

Wadsworth, E. J. K., Simpson, S. A., Moss, S. C., & Smith, A. P. (2004). Recreational drug use: Patterns from a South Wales self-report survey. *Journal of Psychopharmacology (Oxford, England), 18*, 228–237. doi:10.1177/0269881104042627

Walsh, D. C. (1982). Employee assistance programs. *The Milbank Memorial Fund Quarterly. Health and Society, 60*, 492–517. doi:10.2307/3349803

Walsh, D. C., Elinson, L., & Gostin, L. (1992). Worksite drug testing. *Annual Review of Public Health, 13*, 197–221. doi:10.1146/annurev.pu.13.050192.001213

Walsh, J. M. (2008). New technology and new initiatives in U.S. workplace testing. *Forensic Science International, 174*, 120–124. doi:10.1016/j.forsciint.2007.03.011

Walsh, J. M., & Trumble, J. G. (1991). The politics of drug testing. In R. H. Coombs & L. J. West (Eds.), *Drug testing: Issues and options* (pp. 22–49). New York: Oxford University Press.

Wang, M., Liu, S., Zhan, Y., & Shi, J. (2010). Daily work–family conflict and alcohol use: Testing the cross-level moderation effects of peer drinking norms and social support. *Journal of Applied Psychology, 95*, 377–386. doi:10.1037/a0018138

Warner, J. (1995). Good help is hard to find: A few comments about alcohol and work in preindustrial England. *Addiction Research, 2*, 259–269. doi:10.3109/16066359509005211

Washton, A. M., & Gold, M. S. (1987). Recent trends in cocaine abuse as seen from the "800-cocaine" hotline. In A. M. Washton & M. S. Gold (Eds.), *Cocaine: A clinician's handbook* (pp. 10–22). New York, NY: Guilford Press.

Watt, K., Purdie, D. M., Roche, A. M., & McClure, R. J. (2004). Risk of injury from acute alcohol consumption and the influence of confounders. *Addiction, 99*, 1262–1273. doi:10.1111/j.1360-0443.2004.00823.x

Webb, G. R., Redman, S., Hennrikus, D. J., Kelman, G. R., Gibberd, R. W., & Sanson-Fisher, R. W. (1994). The relationships between high-risk and problem drinking and the occurrence of work injuries and related absences. *Journal of Studies on Alcohol, 55*, 434–446.

Webb, G., Shakeshaft, A., Sanson-Fisher, R., & Havard, A. (2009). A systematic review of work-place interventions for alcohol-related problems. *Addiction, 104*, 365–377. doi:10.1111/j.1360-0443.2008.02472.x

Weiss, P. A., Hitchcock, J. H., Weiss, W. U., Rostow, C., & Davis, R. (2008). The Personality Assessment Inventory borderline, drug, and alcohol scales as predictors of overall performance in police officers: A series of exploratory analyses. *Policing and Society, 18*, 301–310. doi:10.1080/10439460802091708

Weiss, R. M. (2005). Overcoming resistance to surveillance: A genealogy of the EAP discourse. *Organization Studies, 26*, 973–997. doi:10.1177/0170840605054600

Wennig, R. (2000). Threshold values in toxicology—Useful or not? *Forensic Science International, 113*, 323–330. doi:10.1016/S0379-0738(00)00254-1

Westermeyer, J. (1988). The pursuit of intoxication: Our 100-century-old romance with psychoactive substances. *American Journal of Drug and Alcohol Abuse, 14*, 175–187. doi:10.3109/00952999809001545

Wetherell, A. (1996). Performance tests. *Environmental Health Perspectives, 104*(Suppl. 2), 247–273.

Widiger, T. A., Verheul, R., & van den Brink, W. (1999). Personality and psychopathology. In L. A. Pervin & O. P. John (Eds.), *Handbook of personality: Theory and research* (2nd ed., pp. 347–366). New York, NY: Guilford Press.

Wiese, J. G., Shlipak, M. G., & Browner, W. S. (2000). The alcohol hangover. *Annals of Internal Medicine, 132*, 897–902.

Wiesner, M., Windle, M., & Freeman, A. (2005). Work stress, substance use, and depression among young adult workers: An examination of main and moderator effect models. *Journal of Occupational Health Psychology, 10*, 83–96. doi:10.1037/1076-8998.10.2.83

Williams, J. F., & Storck, M. (2007). Inhalant abuse. *Pediatrics, 119*, 1009–1017. doi:10.1542/peds.2007-0470

Williams, M., Mohsin, M., Weber, D., Jalaludin, B., & Crozier, J. (2011). Alcohol consumption and injury risk: A case-crossover study in Sydney, Australia. *Drug and Alcohol Review, 30*, 344–354. doi:10.1111/j.1465-3362.2010.00226.x

Williams, M. E. (Ed.). (2007). *Hallucinogens*. New York, NY: Greenhaven Press.

Wittenborn, J. R. (1979). Effects of benzodiazepines on psychomotor performance. *British Journal of Clinical Pharmacology, 7*(Suppl. 1), 61S–67S.

Wolff, K., Farrell, M., Marsden, J., Monteiro, M. G., Ali, R., Welch, S., & Strang, J. (1999). A review of biological indicators of illicit drug use, practical considerations and clinical usefulness. *Addiction, 94*, 1279–1298. doi:10.1046/j.1360-0443.1999.94912792.x

Wolkenberg, R. C., Gold, C., & Tichauer, E. R. (1975). Delayed effects of acute alcoholic intoxication on performance with reference to work safety. *Journal of Safety Research, 7*, 104 118.

World Health Organization. (2004). *Neuroscience of psychoactive substance use and dependence*. Geneva, Switzerland: Author.

Wu, L.-T., & Ringwalt, C. L. (2006). Inhalant use and disorders among adults in the United States. *Drug and Alcohol Dependence, 85*, 1–11. doi:10.1016/j.drugalcdep.2006.01.017

Young, S. E., Rhee, S. H., Stallings, M. C., Corley, R. P., & Hewitt, J. K. (2006). Genetic and environmental vulnerabilities underlying adolescent substance use and problem use: General or specific? *Behavior Genetics, 36*, 603–615. doi:10.1007/s10519-006-9066-7

Zacny, J. P. (1995). A review of the effects of opioids on psychomotor and cognitive performance in humans. *Experimental and Clinical Psychopharmacology, 3*, 432–466. doi:10.1037/1064-1297.3.4.432

Zacny, J. P. (1996). Should people taking opioids for medical reasons be allowed to work and drive? *Addiction, 91*, 1581–1584. doi:10.1111/j.1360-0443.1996.tb02263.x

Zacny, J. P., & Gutierrez, S. (2011). Subjective, psychomotor, and physiological effects of oxycodone alone and in combination with ethanol in healthy volunteers. *Psychopharmacology, 218*, 471–481. doi:10.1007/s00213-011-2349-6.

Zhang, A., Huang, L. X., & Brittingham, A. M. (1999). *Worker drug use and workplace policies and programs: Results from the 1994 and 1997 National Household Survey on Drug Abuse* (DHHS Publication No. SMA 99-3352). Washington, DC: U.S. Government Printing Office.

Zhang, Z., & Snizek, W. E. (2003). Occupation, job characteristics, and the use of alcohol and other drugs. *Social Behavior and Personality, 31*, 395–412. doi:10.2224/sbp.2003.31.4.395

Zhu, J., Tews, M. J., Stafford, K., & George, R. T. (2011). Alcohol and illicit substance use in the food service industry: Assessing self-selection and job-related risk factors. *Journal of Hospitality & Tourism Research, 35*, 45–63. doi:10.1177/1096348010388640

Zwerling, C. (1993). Current practice and experience in drug and alcohol testing. *Bulletin on Narcotics, 45*, 155–196.

Zwerling, C., Ryan, J., & Orav, E. J. (1990). The efficacy of preemployment drug screening for marijuana and cocaine in predicting employment outcome. *JAMA, 264*, 2639–2643. doi:10.1001/jama.1990.03450200047029

INDEX

Health status, 150. *See also* Workplace
    health promotion
Heather, N., 87
Heavy substance use. *See also* Binge
    drinking
    with educational programs,
        196–197
    genetic and environmental factors
        in, 60–61
    single occasion of, 125
    in temporal order, 7–8
    WWP interventions for, 191–192
Heffernan, T. M., 87
Heishman, S. J., 105
Helander, A., 200–201
Hem, E., 35
Heritability, 59–61, 65
Hermansson, U., 200–201
Hertz, R. P., 129–130
HHS (Health and Human Services), 145
Hicks, T. G., 88
Highley-Marchington, J. C., 184
High-risk occupations, 46
Historical background
    of employee assistance programs,
        178–181
    of psychoactive drugs, 3–5
    of workplace drug testing, 144–146
    of workplace wellness programs,
        187–188
Hodgins, D. C., 72
Hoffmann, J. P., 46, 169
Holder, H. D., 179
Howland, A., 184
Howland, J., 90
Human capital approach, 128–129

IIDTW (Independent Inquiry into Drug
    Testing at Work), 150–151, 166
Illicit drug use/impairment. *See also*
    specific headings
    and absenteeism, 118–119
    after work, 40–42
    with age, 49–50
    and alcohol, 208
    with chronic marijuana use, 101
    defining, 16–19
    and dependence rates, 32–34
    detection of, 156, 161
    with gender, 49–50

    with occupation, 49–50
    prevalence rates for, 30–32
    speculation about, 7
    testing for, 155–156, 207
    in workplace, 40–42
Illness, cost of, 127–131
Immunoassary screening tests,
    162–163
Impairment. *See specific headings*
Inaccurate reporting, 8–9
Inadequate measurement, 10
Inconsistencies, 131
Independent Inquiry into Drug Testing at
    Work (IIDTW), 150–151, 166
Individual differences, 80
Industrial alcoholism programs, 178
Information dissemination, 5–10
Inhalants
    classification and effects of, 15–16
    psychopharmacology of, 108–109
    testing for, 156
    as unscheduled drugs, 18–19
Injunctive norms, 71
Injury. *See* Job injuries
Internal organizational environment,
    164–165
International Center for Alcohol
    Policies, 202
International workforce/workplace
    drug testing in, 149–153
    prevalence rates in, 34–35, 42–44
The Internet
    drug-free workplace advisor on, 206n1
    interventions on, 197–201
    misinformation on, 6
Interplay, gene–environment, 62–63
Interventions. *See also specific headings*
    brief, 198–201
    educational, 190–198
    preventive, 187–188
    screening, 198–201
    web-based, 197–198
    workplace, 178
Intoxication
    defined, 20–21
    in preindustrial workplace, 4
    and substance use, 137–140
Ipsos MORI Social Research Institute
    (MORI), 150–151
Isolation, 7–8

ABOUT THE AUTHOR

Michael R. Frone PhD, is a social–organizational psychologist and a senior research scientist at the Research Institute on Addictions, University at Buffalo, State University of New York. His research has focused on employee mental health, physical health, and substance use. He also has conducted research on stressful life events and alcohol use, the measurement and outcomes of alcohol and marijuana expectancies, and motivational models of alcohol use and alcohol-related problems. Dr. Frone has conducted or collaborated on several national surveys. He has published numerous book chapters and journal articles, and coedited the volumes *The Psychology of Workplace Safety* and the *Handbook of Work Stress*. He was an associate editor for the *Journal of Occupational Health Psychology* and has served on the editorial boards of the *Journal of Applied Psychology*, the *Journal of Occupational Health Psychology*, the *Journal of Organizational Behavior*, *Organizational Behavior and Human Decision Processes*, and *Organizational Research Methods*. Dr. Frone also has served as an ad hoc reviewer for 25 scientific journals covering a number of substantive areas, such as organizational behavior and management, psychology and sociology of health, and alcohol and drug use.